Nanomedicine for Cancer Diagnosis and Therapy

Arshi Malik • Sarah Afaq •
Mohammed Tarique
Editors

Nanomedicine for Cancer Diagnosis and Therapy

Springer

Editors
Arshi Malik
Department of Clinical Biochemistry, College of Medicine
King Khalid University
Abha, Saudi Arabia

Sarah Afaq
Department of Clinical Biochemistry, College of Medicine
King Khalid University
Abha, Saudi Arabia

Mohammed Tarique
Center for Interdisciplinary Research in Basic Sciences
Jamia Millia Islamia
New Delhi, India

ISBN 978-981-15-7563-1 ISBN 978-981-15-7564-8 (eBook)
https://doi.org/10.1007/978-981-15-7564-8

This Springer imprint is published by the registered company Springer Nature Singapore Pte Ltd.
The registered company address is: 152 Beach Road, #21-01/04 Gateway East, Singapore 189721, Singapore

Contents

About the Editors

Arshi Malik is an Assistant Professor at the Department of Biochemistry, College of Medicine, King Khalid University. Previously, he worked as a Research Associate at the Wellman Laboratories of Photo medicine and Photobiology, Massachusetts General Hospital, Harvard Medical School, and as an Assistant Researcher at the University of Wisconsin. His main research interest is in chemoprevention and chemotherapy using various natural agents. He has extensive experience with human tissue cultures, orthotopic/ecotopic implantations of tumors in rodents, tail vein injections, and surgery on small animals. He is a member of various scientific societies, including the American Association of Cancer Research, USA, and Society of Investigative Dermatology, USA. To date, he has published 30 research articles in peer-reviewed international journals and has contributed one book chapter.

Sarah Afaq is an Assistant Professor at the Department of Biochemistry, College of Medicine, King Khalid University. Previously, she was an honorary associate at the Department of Surgery, University of Wisconsin, Madison, USA, and an Assistant Professor at the Department of Biochemistry, Roorkee College of Pharmacy, Roorkee, India. She has extensive experience in human cancer and embryonic stem cell lines as well as blood screening for anti-DNA antibodies in Systemic Lupus Erythematosus patients, as well as nanotechnology-based techniques for the design and delivery of drug molecules. She is a member of numerous scientific societies, including the Clinical Immunology Society, USA and International Society for Stem Cell Research, USA. To date, she has published more than 20 research articles in peer-reviewed international journals.

Mohammed Tarique is a Dr. D.S. Kothari Postdoctoral Fellow at the Center for Interdisciplinary Research in Basic Sciences (CIRBSc), Jamia Millia Islamia, India. Holding a Ph.D. in Plasmodium Biology from the International Centre for Genetic Engineering and Biotechnology, New Delhi, India. His research focuses on understanding the biology of Plasmodium towards the development of novel drugs. He has published more than 20 research articles in peer-reviewed international journals. Currently serves on the editorial boards of numerous journals, including the International Research Journal of Engineering and Technology, American Journal of BioScience, and Cell & Cellular Life Sciences Journal.

Nanoparticles for Cancer Therapy

1

Megala Jayaraman, Parijat Dutta, Jayesh Telang, and Sabari Krishnan B. B.

Abstract

Oncology and nanotechnology can be considered as the synergic driving force of biomedical science, one being the cause for the other to flourish. With improving technical advances and prognostic strategies, cancer nanomedicine has shed light on novel therapeutic, imaging, and diagnostic techniques by minimizing the side effects which are otherwise caused by free drugs. In this book chapter, we reviewed different types of nanoparticles and their application in major cancer types such as that of the blood, lungs, breast, prostate, etc., with special emphasis on their pharmacokinetic properties and the novel findings and discoveries in the budding stages of nanotechnology. The chapter briefly discusses the "golden age" of cancer nanotechnology, where experiments and researches have grown factorially due to the seemingly boundless combinations of nanoparticles and drug conjugates. We have also reviewed the novel nanobioinformatic researches which have advanced in this decade, with more importance given to molecular dynamics and biological simulations. The chapter ends by discussing the available cancer nanomedicine approved by various drug regulatory boards and that are in clinical trials, focussing on the ongoing research in this field such as *mi*RNA-based nanomedicine, and nanobots, which may be the future of targeted personalized medicine.

Megala Jayaraman, Parijat Dutta, Jayesh Telang, and Sabari Krishnan B. B. contributed equally with all other contributors.

M. Jayaraman (✉) · P. Dutta · J. Telang · S. Krishnan B. B.
Department of Genetic Engineering, Faculty of Engineering and Technology, SRM Institute of Science and Technology, Chennai, Tamil Nadu, India
e-mail: megalaj@srmist.edu.in; pn9553@srmist.edu.in; jp3744@srmist.edu.in; sb6909@srmist.edu.in

A. Malik et al. (eds.), *Nanomedicine for Cancer Diagnosis and Therapy*,
https://doi.org/10.1007/978-981-15-7564-8_1

Keywords

Cancer · Nanomedicine · Nanoparticles · Pharmacokinetics · Nanobioinformatics

1.1 Introduction

1.1.1 Cancer and its Types

Cancer is a generic term used to represent a large group of diseases involving abnormal cell growth that can affect any site in the body and, on a later stage, spread to a different location by a process called metastasis. It is the second-largest cause of death worldwide (World Health Organization 2018). As of 2018, more than 18 million cases were reported globally, and it is estimated that by 2040, the numbers can go as high as 29.5 million people (Global Cancer Observatory 2018). A tumor is a term used to refer to a mass of rapidly dividing undifferentiated cells, and this cell mass forms the basis of all cancers. Not all tumors are cancerous, but if left untreated or provided suitable conditions, they can thrive and metastasize to other organs causing both specific and non-specific signs and symptoms like fever, cachexia, bleeding, etc. (Grange et al. 2002). In theory, metastatic cancer can occur in any part of the body. Still, it is more dependent on the "seed-and-soil theory" by Dr. Stephen Paget (1855–1926), which means that like the favorable conditions that a seed needs to germinate and thrive, metastatic cancerous cells need a favorable microenvironment to support their growth. These cells somehow "know" to select such a site, invade, and proliferate (Langley and Fidler 2011).

1.1.2 Nanomedicine

Nanomedicine is simply the medical application of nanotechnology. According to the National Nanotechnology Initiative, nanotechnology was defined as "the manipulation of matter with at least one dimension sized from 1–100 nm" (Austin Birmingham Court n.d.). Similarly, nanomedicine, according to the European Science Foundation, is defined as: "it is a technique [nanomedicine] that uses nano-sized tools for the diagnosis, prevention, and treatment of disease and to gain an increased understanding of the complex underlying pathophysiology of the disease. The ultimate goal is to improve quality of life" (European Science Foundation 2005). The nanomedical field not only includes the key to the potential cure for many disorders but also gives us a new understanding of the biological impact of these molecules at a nanoscale level. Though nanomedicine is a new field of research, its foundation stone was laid in the seventeenth century using colloidal gold and solutions containing gold salt by Dr. Francis Anthony and Nicholas Culpepper, in 1618 and 1656, respectively (Contributors n.d.-a). The modern medical applications of this field flourished after a deep understanding of the biological mechanisms of drug uptake, immunology, and cell signaling and communication, such as the Nobel prize-winning works of Sir Élie Metchnikoff and Dr. Paul Ehrlich in 1908 on phagocytosis and cell-specific diagnosis and therapy (Astruc 2015). With progressing computational, electronic, and molecular advancements, nanotechnology is being successfully incorporated into biomolecular machine simulations and nanoelectronic devices as well as inert drug carrier systems and nanobots. Here, we will be looking more into the nanomaterials and their properties which can act as drug carriers for difficult-to-target disorders, like cancer, and specific in vivo imaging applications. Though nanomaterials and nanoparticles can be considered synonymous terms, we need to understand that nanomaterials are aggregate molecules that embody nanoparticles at least in one of their dimensions for enhancing their functional properties (Buzea et al. 2007) but for convenience, here we may use these terms interchangeably.

Though nanomedicine is a new scientific discipline, there is a significant surge of research, especially in targeted therapy, and manpower within a short time. This may be due to its enormous advantage over conventional drug therapies due to the following main reasons (Ventola 2012; Wang et al. 2013):

- Similar molecular sizes biomolecules and nanoparticles make them more tunable, designable, and target-specific, thus reducing the chance for side-effects such as immune response against the drug;
- Engineered nanomaterials overcome several rheological, thermodynamic, and metabolic limitations of conventional drugs, such as solubility, permeability, and bioavailability;
- Reliable optical and electronic properties of nanostructures make them good candidates for less radiotoxic in vivo imaging applications;
- The encapsulated structure of nanodrug carriers and their nanosize (increased surface area) gives them the advantage to carry concentrated amounts of therapeutic drugs to the target, causing a significantly high impact on the target cell;
- Nanomaterials that are responsive to stresses like temperature or pH alteration, which in turn cause nanostructural modifications, form the basis of a controlled drug delivery strategy.

1.2 Evolution of Cancer Therapy

The historical evidence of cancer dates back to 1600 BC in the Egyptian Edwin Smith Papyrus, which had likely indications of breast cancer. Aulus Cornelius Celsus (25 BC–50 AD) translated "*karkinos*", the Greek term proposed by Hippocrates for the crab-like appearance of the blood vessels in a cancerous tumor of the breast, into "cancer", the Latin term meaning "crab". In the 1870s, Dr. Campbell de Morgan defined the metastatic property of cancer, which defined this disorder as more contagious (Grange et al. 2002).

1.2.1 Surgery and Adjuvant Therapies

Celsus had recommended surgery as the treatment strategy for curing cancer, but Galen of Pergamon disagreed with Celsus and recommended the use of laxatives. This non-invasive treatment strategy had been largely accepted and practiced for thousands of years (Grange et al. 2002). Though there was a successful uplift of medicine in the consecutive years, cancer treatment progressed very slowly, mostly due to poor knowledge about its pathophysiology, genetics, and treatment options. The most important treatment strategy now and then was *surgery*, and it is to be noted that there were swift surgical procedures even before the introduction of anesthetic medication. But when anesthesia was introduced in the 1840s, time-consuming and successful surgical operations, such as radical mastectomy for breast cancer, were performed by pioneers like Dr. Christian Albert Theodore Billroth, Dr. William Sampson Handley, and Dr. William Stewart Halsted. With advanced technology and modern surgical instruments, by the twentieth century, surgeons were able to minimize the amount of tissue removed during the procedure. Followed by this, instead of mastectomy, lumpectomy (or the primary tumor removal) was done for breast cancer patients, osteoma, and soft tissue tumor removal without the need for amputation, etc. (Medical and Editorial Content Team and American Cancer Society 2014). Coupled with these surgical procedures, chemotherapy and radiotherapy were also performed to destroy any cancerous cells left in place or the system.

Chemotherapy is an effective anti-cancer treatment using a drug cocktail that targets the fast-growing cells of the body, but they show high non-specificity and adverse side-effects such as immunosuppression, anemia, hair loss, etc., in the patient. Some of the main chemotherapeutic drugs are 5-fluorouracil (5FU), cyclophosphamide, vincristine, vinblastine, cisplatin, and methotrexate. Due to its immunosuppressive effect, there is a chance of getting pathogenic disorders that can prove fatal. However, the non-specificity and thus the side-effects of chemotherapeutics were found to have reduced with the development of adjuvant therapeutic strategies (Contributors n.d.-b). *Radiotherapy*, on the other hand, is less non-specific and targets the tumor with high doses of ionizing radiation, besides its side-effects such as nausea and vomiting, radiation-induced hypopituitarism, secondary neoplasms, etc. The dosage depends on the type of cancer and typically ranges from 20–60 Gy (Contributors n.d.-c).

More advanced and targeted therapies were devised in the following years such as *cryotherapy*, which uses a spray stream of liquid nitrogen to freeze and kill the cancerous cells, *laser therapy* to cut through or "vaporize" the abnormal cells, and *rhizotomy* (also called radiofrequency ablation, or fulguration) which uses medium frequency alternating current (350–500 Hz) to heat and kill the cancerous cells, especially in less commonly affected organs (Contributors n.d.-d).

1.2.2 Hormone Therapy

Hormone therapy is another effective treatment strategy for cancers of the organs influenced highly by developmental hormones, such as breast and prostate cancers. The work by Colonel Sir George Thomas Beatson in the 1890s on establishing the relationship between ovaries and breast development and the indication of an "unknown" control (now known as estrogen) of metastatic breast cancer progression by the ovaries led to the development of many hormone-based therapeutics like tamoxifen and aromatase inhibitors like anastrozole and letrozole, which predominantly have anti-estrogenic activity. Similarly, the work by Dr. Charles Brenton Huggins in 1941 on metastatic prostate cancer and its relation with testicular hormones helped design drugs such as finasteride and dutasteride, which have anti-androgenic effects (Medical and Editorial Content Team and American Cancer Society 2014). Generally, these hormones act as growth and survival factors to tumor cells and by using hormone therapy, these hormones or their precursors are inhibited or suppressed from binding to their specific receptor in the tumor cell (as shown by aromatase inhibitors) or are increased in the bloodstream to initiate a negative feedback mechanism by the pituitary gland (as shown by gonadotropin-releasing hormone analogs). Octreotide, a somatostatin analog, is used as an inhibitory hormone therapy administered in combination with other medications, mainly for cancers associated with the gastrointestinal tract and accessory organs (DeVita et al. 2008).

1.2.3 Immunotherapy

Immunotherapy is a treatment strategy that recruits antibodies or other specific biomolecules to target and destroy cancerous cells. This technique came into being when mass productions of monoclonal antibodies were made possible by George Jean Franz Köhler and César Milstein in the 1970s (MG et al. 2015), but it took nearly four decades for optimizing and studying its side-effects. Immunotherapy is classified into two: *activation immunotherapy* and *suppressive immunotherapy*. Activation immunotherapy is used to stimulate the immune system of patients to fight against cancerous cells, whereas the latter reduces the immune response, mainly for autoimmune disorders and allergies (Contributors n.d.-e). The first therapeutic monoclonal antibodies for treating lymphoma and breast cancer were rituximab and trastuzumab, respectively and were approved in the late 1990s (Medical and Editorial Content Team and American Cancer Society 2014). With advanced technology, more immunotherapeutic drugs were developed. Some of the immunostimulant drugs, mainly monoclonal antibodies, used for cancer therapy are ipilimumab, which targets the cytotoxic T-lymphocyte-associated protein 4 (CTLA4 or CD152), nivolumab, and pembrolizumab, which target the programmed cell death protein-1 (PD1 or CD279). On April 29, 2010, the United States Food and Drug Administration (USFDA) approved the use of an immunostimulant vaccine called Sipuleucel-T, which introduces protein subunits into the patient's system to help the immune cells target hormone-refractory prostate cancer cells, specifically (Contributors n.d.-f).

1.2.4 Cancer Therapy with Nanomedicine

Though there are plenty of therapeutic options for treating cancer, most of the strategies have non-specificity as a common drawback, at least to some extent, leading to adverse effects. After the development of the first-generation targeted drug therapy by Dr. Ehrlich and Alfred Bertheim in the 1910s, a new gateway of medical and therapeutic applications was wide open. Arsphenamine (also known as Compound 606, or SALVARSAN), the first targeted drug, was thus found and proved to be a comparatively "less toxic" targeted drug against *Treponema pallidum pallidum* and *Trypanosoma brucei* ssp. which causes syphilis and sleeping sickness, respectively, in humans (MG et al. 2015; Contributors n.d.-g). This also marked the beginning of more targeted drug therapy strategies, such as chemotherapy, which arguably targets only fast-dividing cells. Also, Dr. Ehrlich proposed the foundational idea of *Zauberkugeln* or "magic bullets", which is the fancy term for a drug that can be targeted to a particular pathogen or infected cell, causing very little or no side-effects to the patient at all. This thought was novel due to the added advantages of targeted drug therapy over the conventional modes, such as specificity in drug target and delivery even in difficult-to-reach areas of the body, improved safety and biocompatibility triggering experiments with potent drugs once consider fatal due to interference from host metabolic pathways, improved pharmacokinetics, pharmacodynamics, etc. (Onoue et al. 2014). However, Dr. Ehrlich's idea of magic bullets was made a complete reality by Peter Paul Speiser and Patrick Couvrer in 1977 when they formulated the fundamental principles of nanomedicines, which greatly account for the advantages of this novel field (European Inventor Award-European Patent Office 2017).

Tumor-targeting nanodrugs, which are the main focus of this text, were developed and gained clinical recognition in the 1990s (Tran et al. 2017). Over the years, nanodrugs have evolved dramatically, especially in their specificity and drug-release qualities. The milestone discoveries of nanoparticles, especially nanodrugs, are listed in Table 1.1 (Wang et al. 2013; Tran et al. 2017; Nano.gov-US National Nanotechnology Initiative n.d.; Cunha et al. 2018; Shi et al. 2010; Jiang et al. 2020; Nanotechnology panel-American Chemistry Council n.d.; Pisanic Ii et al. 2014; Akakuru et al. 2018; Ainslie Lab n.d.; He et al. 2019).

1.3 Nanoparticles in Cancer Therapy

In this section, we have reviewed and compiled the important basic information about protein-based, magnetic, inorganic, lipid-based, targeted, polymeric, and multifunctional nanoparticles and modern co-therapeutic nanoparticles such as QDs and DNA nanoparticles. Like any other extracellular material, nanomaterials

Table 1.1 The major milestones of nanoparticle and cancer nanomedical research

Year	Event
400–1800s	Lycurgus cup, the vibrant colors of stained glass in cathedrals, and lustrous ceramic glazes in mosques Use of nanowires and nanotubes in Damascus steel
1847	Michael Faraday reported the optical properties of colloidal "ruby" gold nanoparticles, leading to the birth of nanoscience
1950	Hydrogels were developed
1952	The first sustained molecule-release formulation
1959	Dr. Richard P. Feynman delivered his famous lecture, *There's Plenty of Room at the Bottom: An Invitation to Enter the New Field of Physics*, at the annual American Physical Society meeting at Caltech
1964	Sustained delivery of low-molecular-weight compounds using silicone polymers was demonstrated
1965	Liposomes were used as drug-delivery vehicles
1971	Dr. Judah Folkman proposed the idea of anti-angiogenesis therapy for cancer treatment
1974	Dr. Norio Taniguchi of Tokyo Science University coined the term "nanotechnology"
1976	The first controlled-release polymer system for ionic molecules and macromolecules was developed
1978	Details about the first dendrimer (also known as arborols and cascade molecules) were published Cisplatin was approved as a chemotherapeutic agent against testicular and ovarian cancer by the USFDA
1979	Polymeric nanoparticles were used for cancer therapy
1980	The first targeted polyethylene glycol (PEG)ylated liposome was developed Dr. Alexei Ekimov and Dr. Louis E. Brus discovered quantum dots (QDs) in solid matrices and colloidal solutions
1982	Dr. Nadrian C. Seeman developed DNA nanotechnology
1986	Dr. Hiroshi Maeda and (Dr.) Yasuhiro Matsumura discovered the enhanced permeability and retention (EPR) effect of macromolecular drugs
1987	Dr. Dennis J. Slamon et al. found human epidermal growth factor receptor 2 (*HER2*)/*Neu* oncogene, also known as *ERBB2*, as a potential contributor to tumor cell proliferation
1990	The first polymer-drug conjugate was approved by the USFDA ADAGEN®, a PEG-adenosine deaminase conjugate drug was approved by the USFDA Colloidal iron oxide nanoparticles (colloidal IONs) were developed
1993	Paclitaxel was approved by the USFDA for medical use
1994	Long circulating poly(lactic-co-glycolic acid) (PLGA)-PEG nanoparticles were developed
1995	CAELYX® and DOXIL®, PEGylated liposomal formulations of doxorubicin (DXR), were approved for treating AIDS-related Kaposi's sarcoma, and breast and ovarian cancers
1996	Ferumoxide, a magnetic resonance imaging (MRI) agent, was developed DAUNOXOME®, a liposomal formulation of daunorubicin (DNR) citrate, was approved by the USFDA for treating Kaposi's sarcoma
1998	Goserelin acetate implant was approved by the USFDA for treating breast and prostate cancer by suppressing gonadocorticoids Trastuzumab was approved by the USFDA

(continued)

Table 1.1 (continued)

Year	Event
	Drug delivery using microneedles was first implemented First oligonucleotide treatment for cytomegalovirus retinitis Dr. Andrew Z. Fire and Dr. Craig C. Mello published their work on RNA interference (RNA*i*) in *Caenorhabditis elegans* Dr. Paul Alivisatos and Dr. S. M. Nie developed water-soluble bioconjugated QDs
1999	Controlled-release microchips were developed Polymersome was developed
2000	MYOCET®, a non-PEGylated liposomal formulation of DXR, was approved by the USFDA for treating metastatic breast cancer
2001	The first liposome-based small interfering RNA (*si*RNA) delivery system was developed QD-to-fluorophore FRET bioassays and QD-mediated photoelectric detection of DNA were developed
2002	The first clinical study of the targeted polymer-drug conjugate was conducted Silicone hydrogel was developed QD-mediated in vivo detection of redox-active proteins was performed
2003	Multiphoton QD imaging was developed LIPUSU®, a liposomal formulation of paclitaxel (PTX), was approved in China for treating metastatic gastric cancer
2004	Bevacizumab was approved by the USFDA for treating metastatic colon cancer
2005	ABRAXANE®, protein-bound or liposomal formulations of PTX, was approved by the USFDA for treating non-small cell lung cancer, pancreatic adenocarcinoma, and breast cancer Particle replication in non-wetting template (PRINT) platform was used for designing encapsulated bioactive agents The single QD homogenous nanosensor was developed
2006	Dr. Paul W. H. Rothemund developed the technique of DNA *origami* ONCASPAR® (Pegaspargase) was approved by the USFDA for treating acute lymphoblastic leukemia (ALL) Fumiaki Koizumi et al. developed NK012, an SN-38–releasing nanodevice
2007	GENEXOL®PM, a specialized nanoformulation of PTX, was approved in Korea for treating *HER2*$^{-}$ breast cancer DEPOCYT®, a long-lasting liposomal formulation of cytarabine, was approved by the USFDA for treating lymphoma, leukemia, and solid tumors Simultaneous imaging, therapy, and drug-delivery sensing by QD aptamers were developed
2008	First targeted delivery of *si*RNA in humans using nanoparticles entered clinical trials Co-delivery of drugs and *si*RNA to treat multidrug resistance
2009	MEPACT®, a liposomal formulation of mifamurtide, was approved by the European Medical Agency (EMA) for treating osteogenic sarcoma Non-blinking QDs were developed
2010	Methoxy-PEG (mPEG)-poly(D,L-lactide)taxol was developed as a PTX carrier Polyamidoamine (PAMAM) dendrimers were synthesized Dendrimersomes were first described Real-time fluorescence correlation spectroscopy monitoring of intracellular protein interactions was possible
2011	Cell membrane-coated nanoparticles were developed to evade the immune system

(continued)

Table 1.1 (continued)

Year	Event
2012	MARQIBO®, a liposomal formulation of vincristine, was approved by the USFDA for treating ALL NANOTHERM® was developed for thermotherapy Docetaxel (DTX)-derived formulations were used to treat a large number of cancers QD-mediated FRET relay system was developed
2013	KADCYLA® (trastuzumab emtansine, a drug-antibody conjugate) was approved by the USFDA for treating *HER2*$^+$ breast cancer Biosynthesis of QDs was possible
2014	PTX injection concentrate for nanodispersion was approved in India for treating metastatic breast cancer Protein biomarkers were found for predicting the EPR effect
2015	Targeted upconverting nanoparticles were developed for photodynamic therapy Ferumoxytol-based imaging agent was developed to predict EPR and therapeutic response ONIVYDE®, a liposomal formulation of irinotecan, was approved by the USFDA for treating metastatic pancreatic cancer
2016	DHP107, a lipid-based PTX formulation, was approved in Korea for treating advanced gastric cancer after failure in first-line chemotherapy
2017	VYXEOS®, a liposomal formulation of DNR and cytarabine, was approved by the USFDA for treating acute myelogenous leukemia Curcumin nanoparticles were used for ovarian cancer
2018	APEALEA®, a water-soluble PTX-micelle formulation, was approved by the EMA for treating ovarian, peritoneal, and fallopian tube cancer

make use of endocytosis for cellular entry. Generally, nanomaterials rely on any of the five main mechanisms of endocytosis for cellular entry. They are (Sahay et al. 2010; Zhao and Stenzel 2018):

- *Phagocytosis*: the process of recognizing, binding, and engulfing nanoparticles by the target cells with the help of opsonins. Since opsonization plays an important role in phagocytosis, nanoparticles that have a higher affinity for opsonins undergo phagocytosis.
- *Clathrin-mediated endocytosis*: the process involves the binding of nanoparticles on cell surface receptors, followed by engulfing the nanoparticle–receptor complex into a clathrin-1-coated pit. Polymeric and DNA nanoparticles generally use this pathway for cellular entry.
- *Caveolae-mediated endocytosis*: the process of binding of nanoparticles onto the lipid-raft domain, which is coupled caveolins and cavins, and engulfing the complex into an iconic flask-shaped structure called caveola, which means "little caves" in Latin, and delivering them to lysosomes or other organelles. A sub-type of this mode of endocytosis is called *potocytosis*, by which the cargo is delivered directly to the cytoplasm (Mineo and Anderson 2001). Most lipid-based nanoparticles, QDs, and some protein-based and inorganic nanoparticles make use of these pathways to enter the target cell.

- *Clathrin- and caveolae-independent endocytosis*: the process involves the binding of nanoparticles to certain receptors that activate pathways that include proteins such as CDC42, RhoA, Arf6, flotillin, etc., triggering vesicle formation. This pathway of cell entry is mainly used by folate-linked nanoparticles.
- *Macropinocytosis*: a special case of clathrin- and caveolae-mediated endocytosis, which involves transient activation of tyrosine kinase receptors by growth factors or pathogenic entities that cause membrane ruffles leading to the formation of macropinosomes. Mainly, polymeric and lipid-based nanoparticles and nanoparticles with surface antigens use this mode of cellular entry.

1.3.1 Protein Nanoparticles

The beneficial effects of nanoparticles in drug-delivery systems lie in the fact that we can control various physicochemical parameters of the nanoparticles such as size, surface area, and surface characteristics so that the drugs can exhibit their optimum effect (Hong et al. 2020). Many studies that have been going on regarding this particular topic have shown the efficiency of protein nanoparticles as a drug-delivery system because of their biodegradability and low toxicity. Due to their small size, they are transmitted through the cells by endocytosis (Jacob et al. 2018), and their non-antigenic property becomes one of the added advantages (Verma and Garg 2001). The half-life, activity, and stability of these nanoparticles can be ameliorated by shielding them from renal clearance and enzymatic degradation (Hong et al. 2020). Thus protein nanoparticles have become a new tool in different kinds of targeted therapies (including lung therapy (Mottaghitalab et al. 2017), tumor therapy (Lohcharoenkal et al. 2014)), especially for cancer therapy (Verma and Garg 2001).

Protein nanoparticles can be prepared by the following three techniques:

- Chemical methods (including emulsion (Hong et al. 2020; Yang et al. 2007; Sturesson and Carlfors 2000; Wang and Uludag 2008) and complex coacervation (Nisha et al. 2004)),
- Physical methods (including nanospray drying (Oliveira et al. 2013) and electrospray techniques (Wu et al. 2009)), and
- Self-assembly (Batrakova et al. 2006) and desolvation (Zhao et al. 2015a).

Albumin-bound nanocarrier system (~130 nm) is one of the most current impactful approaches in cancer therapy (Lohcharoenkal et al. 2014). Several kinds of research have proven the potentiality of albumin to accumulate in solid tumors (Takakura et al. 1990), thus using it in targeted delivery of anti-tumor drugs. One such example is the USFDA-approved albumin-bound PTX used for the treatment of metastatic breast cancer (Gradishar 2006). While the standard PTX formulation allows a dosage of 175 $mg.m^{-2}$ of body surface area, this nanoformulation allows a dosage of up to 260 $mg.m^{-2}$ (Nyman et al. 2005). Another successful approach towards cancer therapy was the administration of *si*RNA. It was found that *si*RNA delivery systems using cationic bovine serum albumin (CBSA) protected *si*RNA from degrading, making CBSA an excellent choice for *si*RNA delivery and in the treatment of metastatic lung cancer (Han et al. 2014). Gliadin- (a type of prolamin which is a component of gluten) based nanoparticles has been proven to be very useful in the treatment of colon cancer (Lohcharoenkal et al. 2014). Gliadin nanoparticles carrying cyclophosphamide, an anti-cancer drug, successfully persuade apoptosis in breast cancer cells (Gulfam et al. 2012). Multiple studies have successfully exhibited the use of milk-protein nanoparticles. Cisplatin and flutamide, anti-cancer drugs used primarily against testicular and ovarian cancer and prostate cancer, respectively, have shown remarkable results in cancer-curing with side-effects such as toxicity and birth defects. Nanoparticle researches such as cisplatin-loaded casein nanoparticles have been shown to inhibit tumor growth in mice models bearing hepatic tumors in a more specific and less toxic manner (Zhen et al. 2013). Similarly, flutamide-loaded casein nanoparticles were proved to be successful in prostate cancer-bearing rats (Elzoghby et al. 2013). DXR-carrying lactoferrin (derived from cow milk) nanoparticles were used as an oral delivery system for the treatment of hepatocellular carcinoma (Schneider et al. 1984). The field of protein nanoparticles in cancer research is still in its nascent state. The number of data exhibiting the treatment efficiency of these nanoparticles is very few; therefore, more research works need to be carried out in this field for establishing conclusory statements.

1.3.2 Magnetic Nanoparticles

It was in the late 1970s, the concept of using magnetic nanoparticles as a drug-delivery system got recognized (Senyei et al. 1978; Mosbach and Schröder 1979). The drug–carrier complex injected into the subject accumulates at the tumor location by the external high-gradient magnetic field generated through natural magnetic forces. The ability to identify and target a specific tumor in vivo makes magnetic nanoparticles beneficial. It reduces the systemic distribution of cytotoxic compounds and increases the uptake of drugs at particular sites, thereby enabling a comparatively lower dose to work efficiently (Dobson 2006). Magnetic nanoparticles are mostly used in cancer research as carriers of chemotherapeutic drugs, occasionally herbal and traditional medicines (Chen et al. 2014; Unsoy et al. 2014; Chen et al. 2010a; Ramazanov et al. 2020). They are also used in some recent techniques in cancer therapy like photodynamic therapy (Agostinis et al. 2011; Janko et al. 2019), magnetic hyperthermia (Yin et al. 2014; Jose et al. 2020), and photothermal therapy (Estelrich and Busquets 2018). As mentioned earlier, the property of *si*RNA protection is used in the case of *si*RNA-functionalized IONs. In a recent study, it was shown that this complex knocks down the anti-apoptotic gene *birc5* (baculoviral inhibitor of apoptosis repeat-containing 5) that encodes for survivin. Survivin is a member of the inhibitor-of-apoptosis family and it is overexpressed in most cancer types. A significant uplift was observed in the rate of apoptosis in subjected tumor cells and it was concluded that the downregulation of *birc5* expression was successful (Wang et al. 2016; Yigit et al. 2012). A separate study was conducted by encapsulating IONs (MAGNEVIST® or FERIDEX®) with *COX-2*-specific *si*RNA into PEGylated liposomes and delivering into breast cancer xenografts in female SCID mice. The downregulation of COX-2 (cyclooxygenase-2) was observed in the target subjects (Mikhaylova et al. 2009). Another interesting study was done to detect prostate cancer by MRI and deliver the drugs to the tumor tissue simultaneously with the help of superparamagnetic IONs (SPIONs). The magnetic nanoparticle was cross-linked with RNA aptamer which was distinct for prostate-specific membrane antigen (PSMA). DXR molecules, intercalated in the RNA strands, are released when the nanoparticles are taken up by the cancer cells. The cancer cells are killed eventually exhibiting a slower tumor growth rate (Yu et al. 2011). The field of using nanoparticles in cancer therapy is progressing gradually. However, there are several concerns to be dealt with when it comes to using them in human systems. The first challenge is to get proper control over the size and magnetization of the particles. Second, being the bioavailability, which makes drug-conjugated nanoparticles a step ahead of free drugs, is also very important. There are some toxic side-effects reported to be associated with magnetic nanoparticles such as the production of reactive oxygen species, chromosomal damage, and leakage of lactate dehydrogenase (Singh et al. 2010). We need to optimize their target-specific interaction and elimination from the body, thus helping reduce these side-effects to a great extent (Yigit et al. 2012).

1.3.3 Inorganic Nanoparticles

Inorganic nanoparticles are widely recognized due to their ability to form specific compounds with unique physicochemical properties (Sun et al. 2014). Among all of them, gold (Au) has been used the most as it exhibits low toxicity. The strong affinity of Au to thiol and amine functional groups makes the surface modification of Au nanoparticles easier (Patra et al. 2008). In 1978, the approval of cisplatin as an anti-tumor agent by the USFDA encouraged researchers to find other metals that can contribute to cancer therapy. It has been proven that the addition of Au in anti-tumor compounds increases the anti-tumor property of that compound (Berners-Price et al. 1987; Haiduc and Silvestru 1989). The radioisotope of Au, ^{198}Au, has been extensively used in the treatment of different cancers such as nasopharyngeal carcinoma, head and neck cancer, and prostate cancer (Bhattacharya and Mukherjee 2008). A strategy of combining platinum nanoparticles with radiation by fast ions was also applied for performing hadron therapy. These approaches are expected to ameliorate cancer therapy protocols (Porcel et al. 2010). The use of transition metals for therapeutic purposes is a growing field in inorganic nanoparticle-based cancer therapy research. Inorganic photoactivated chemotherapy (PACT) offers great potential in cancer therapy. After photoexcitation, the metal complex follows different pathways for their decay resulting in the release of radiative energy, thus losing the ligands or transferring the energy to a nearby species. Some d-block metals such as titanium (Ti), vanadium (V), chromium (Cr), manganese (Mn), iron (Fe), cobalt (Co), copper (Cu), ruthenium (Ru), rhodium (Rh), rhenium (Re), osmium (Os), iridium (Ir), platinum (Pt), and Au are extensively researched for their potential in PACT (Farrer et al. 2009). However, titanium dioxide (TiO_2), though possessing anti-tumor properties (Thevenot et al. 2008), is not allowed to use in human subjects due to the logistic limitations of introducing UV light in vitro (Bhattacharyya et al. 2011). Studies have shown that treating B16F10 melanoma cells, JHU prostate cancer cells, 3T3 fibroblasts, and lung carcinoma cells with alcohol-, amine-, and carboxylic acid-functionalized TiO_2 were able to kill the cells (Thevenot et al. 2008). The treatment of cancer becomes challenging because of the heterogeneous nature of cancer cells. The use of inorganic nanoparticles could be an approach towards this heterogeneity. Understanding and targeting interactions between stromal cells and tumor cells and the leaky vasculature around tumor cells are possible areas yet to be completely addressed (Patra et al. 2008; Jain 1999).

1.3.4 Lipid Nanoparticles

Being biocompatible, lipid nanoparticles have less chance of showing toxic effects. Drug entrapment is also better here as it provides a hydrophobic environment for the solubilization of drugs (Chaudhari et al. 2020). In the 1960s, after liposomes were discovered (Düzgüneş and Gregoriadis 2005) as a novel drug-delivery system, it has been proved to be extremely useful because of the different advantages that they exhibit over conventional drug therapies and contemporary nanoparticle formulations. These spherical structures consist of a phospholipid bilayer with an aqueous center (Cho et al. 2008). Liposomal chemotherapeutics are also being evaluated relentlessly for cancer therapy researches (Hofheinz et al. 2005). The USFDA had approved liposomal DXR (MYOCET® and DOXIL®) (Markman 2006) and liposomal DNR (DAUNOXOME®) as medications against metastatic breast cancer and AIDS-related Kaposi's sarcoma, respectively (Rivera 2003; Rosenthal et al. 2002). While liposomes play an important role in the vesicular delivery system, solid lipid nanoparticles (SLNs) are used mainly for particulate delivery. As the name suggests, solid lipids are composed of lipids that are solid at body temperature and room temperature (Das and Chaudhury 2011; Wissing et al. 2004). Glyceryl tristearate, COMPRITOL® 888 ATO (a mixture of glyceryl behenate esters), glycerol monostearate, and PRECIROL® ATO 5 (a mixture of glycerol palmitostearate esters) are some of the solid lipids that are extensively used (Khosa et al. 2018). Though these SLNs show efficacy, biodegradability, and biocompatibility (Krishna Sailaja et al. 2011; Shidhaye et al. 2008), their structural stability remains a major problem (Chaudhari et al. 2020). Besides the use of synthetic chemotherapeutics, researchers demonstrated the success of naturally occurring phytochemicals and mycochemicals over cancer clinically. The use of curcumin (abundant in *Curcuma longa*), ursolic acid (a component of the epicuticular wax on apples), epigallocatechin-3-gallate (abundant in *Camellia sinensis*), piperine (found in *Piper* sp.), cassic acid (found in *Cassia reticulata* and some species of the *Rheum*), resveratrol (abundant in the skins of grapes and peanuts), linalool (present in almost all aromatic plants), capsaicin (abundant in chili peppers), wogonin (found in *Scutellaria baicalensis*), orcinol glucoside (derived from lichens), pomegranate (*Punica granatum*) extract, lemonal (found in the essential oils of almost all "lemony" plants), gambogic acid (derived from *Garcinia hanburyi*), soursop (*Annona muricata*) fruit extract, quercetin, β-carotene, and α-tocopherol are some of the many natural chemical options used by researchers to conquer cancer. With changing active-molecule chemistry, the composition of lipid nanoenvelopes can also change. The lipid derivatives used for these studies were oleic acid, phosphatidylcholines, behenic acid, stearic acid, lecithins, palmitic acid, cholesterol, myristyl esters, and even *murumuru* (*Astrocaryum murumuru*) butter (Chaudhari et al. 2020).

1.3.5 Targeted Nanoparticles

The active targeting of nanoparticle drug delivery involves the addition of specific ligands to the nanoenvelope to increase the rate of cellular internalization (Blanco et al. 2012). Several ligands have exhibited promising results in this area including antibodies, aptamers, and some small molecules (Blanco et al. 2012; Kumar et al. 2020). Among these ligands, the most commonly used ones are antibodies due to their better efficacy and targeted cytotoxicity than their non-targeted relatives (Kumar et al. 2020). However, the main challenge of these conjugated systems is to sustain the functionality of both ligands and nanoparticles. Some of the other challenges faced by targeted nanoparticles are:

- Controllability in the number of ligands per nanoparticle and their orientation (Karra et al. 2013),
- Ensuring both in vitro and in vivo stability of the final conjugated nanoparticle (Kumar et al. 2020), and
- Reliability of conjugation procedures for the clinical applications (Karra et al. 2013).

Unlike the proteinaceous nature of antibody-based ligands, aptamers are short (20–80 nucleotides long) nucleic acid-based ligands that have come into the limelight recently. The advantages of using aptamers are their small size, better penetration into biological systems (Veiseh et al. 2010), their ability to selectively target cancerous cells (Tan et al. 2011), etc. The use of A10 aptamers by including cisplatin and PTX in nanoparticles is the current area of exploration in the delivery of several anti-cancer agents, especially in prostate cancer (Farokhzad et al. 2004). The drawback of these aptamers is that they are quite expensive (Blanco et al. 2012). The use of cell surface receptors in targeted drug delivery is another research-dense area in cancer therapy. The tracing of epidermal growth factor (EGF) in aerosol administrations of gelatin nanoparticles revealed that they had accumulated in orthotopic lung adenocarcinomas in SCID mice (Tseng et al. 2008). Also, when a tumor growth factor-beta-1 (TGF-β1) antisense-expressing construct was delivered using nanoparticles, it showed great potential against TGF-β1/TGF-β1 receptor-mediated tumorigenic pathways (Sun et al. 2012). Here, the main goal is to target overexpressed receptors or growth factor ligands in specific cancers and select them for strategic cell killing utilizing monoclonal or polyclonal antibodies (Kumar et al. 2020).

1.3.6 Polymeric Nanoparticles

Polymeric nanoparticles are sub-micron-sized, solid colloidal particles with their drug component encapsulated within a polymeric coat. These nanoparticles, apart from other nanoparticles, can be easily synthesized, are cost-effective, biodegradable, non-immunogenic, and get readily dispersed in aqueous media (Bolhassani et al. 2014). The polymer capsule can have a natural, semi-natural, or synthetic origin. Chitosan, a linear polysaccharide with conjugated monomeric units of β-(1→4)-linked D-glucosamine and N-acetyl-D-glucosamine, commercially obtained by the alkaline deacetylation of chitin, the structural compound of the exoskeletons of crustaceans, is one of the most widely used semi-natural polymers for nanoenvelope development. Besides chitosan, other animal-derived polymers such as glycogen (Gálisová et al. 2020), albumin, and glycosaminoglycans like heparin (Bolhassani et al. 2014) and hyaluronic acid, algae-derived polymers like alginate, galactosans, and carrageenan, plant-derived polymers like starch, cellulose, and resins, and bacterium-derived polymers such as dextran are also used (Patra et al. 2018). Synthetic polymers used for this purpose are mainly poly(lactic-co-glycolic acid) (PLGA), and polymeric derivatives of acrylamide, vinyl alcohol, and ethylene glycol. The choice of the polymer is determined by the chemical nature of the active compound that it carries. Generally, cationic polymers (typically produced by treatment with cationic agents like cetrimonium bromide) are used to encapsulate drugs and therapeutic proteins having a net negative charge or to adsorb nucleic acids onto their surface. The disadvantage observed in most of the polymeric nanoformulations is its instability and disintegration with varying physical parameters such as pH. However, the introduction of charged groups to the envelope has been shown to improve its stability to a considerable level (Lombardo et al. 2019). The main applications of these nanoparticles are in the target-specific delivery of genes, *si*RNAs, therapeutic proteins, small molecule drugs, and nanoimaging probes like fluorescent dyes or semiconductor QDs. Extensive research is being done in various fields of cancer therapy using polymeric nanoparticles, including thermotherapy, and the main cell lines and in vivo models chosen are for hepatocellular carcinoma and breast cancer.

1.3.7 Multifunctional Nanoparticles

Nanoparticle research is truly a fathomless domain with applications in all possible fields. We have seen that the development of specialized target-specific nanoparticles was indeed a revolution, especially in the medical and drug-delivery fields. However, the administration of different cocktails of nanoparticles for different functions, say, for cancer cell targeting as well as fluorescent imaging of the cells, was quite challenging until the development of multifunctional or multimodal nanoparticles. Ideally, a multifunctional nanoparticle can have ligands and cores of all types, ranging from therapeutic molecules to imaging molecules, but due to multiple constraints, it is difficult to develop a multifunctional nanoparticle with all desired qualities. Multifunctional nanoparticles, as mentioned, have multiple functions and can be broadly said to have four functions (Babu et al. 2014):

- To target the cell or molecule of interest,
- To invade the target cell,
- To release the drug in a controlled manner, and
- To give out "signals of success".

Though the basic structure of multifunctional nanoparticles is the same as that of a typical nanoparticle, i.e., having a metallic or drug-based core surrounded by lipids, polymers, or small molecules, they include additional molecules for target cell invasion, such as PEG, and imaging, such as fluorescent dye molecules, mostly on their surface. Quantitative and qualitative analyses of such systems have shown the enormous potential of these nanoparticles in faster and accurate disease prognosis and treatment.

1.3.8 Quantum Dots

QDs are, fundamentally, semiconductor nanocrystals that consist of elements used in conventional photodiodes such as lead sulfide, cadmium selenide, indium phosphide, etc. They are used mainly for in vivo imaging due to their fluorescent properties, exhibited by exciton formation and narrow photoexcitation peak. Theoretically, they are considered to be point dipoles with dimension-dependent optical and thermodynamic properties. The term "quantum dots" was coined by M. A. Reed et al. in 1986, but such structures were discovered by Dr. Alexey I. Ekimov in solid matrices (Contributors n.d.-h) and Dr. Louis E. Brus in colloidal suspension, in 1981 and 1984, respectively (Contributors n.d.-i). In biomedical as well as nanomedical fields, fluorescent dyes, recombinant fluorescent proteins, and bioluminescent substrates such as cyanines, rGFP, and luciferins are used for imaging studies, especially in vitro, but possess limitations. QDs have played an important role in tumor cell imaging in vivo, ex vivo, and in vitro. They are either targeted actively, i.e., by the use of tumor-specific ligands, or passively, thanks to the EPR effect, which is the accumulation of molecules of certain sizes like liposomes and nanoparticles administered intravenously in the cancer cells rather than in normal cells because of leaky tumor vasculature. They are specifically used for cell trafficking and immunohistochemical studies, biomarker determination, sentinel lymph node mapping, neural and vasculature imaging. Actively targeted QDs were used in the detection and analysis of prostate cancer using PSMA, breast cancer using

HER2, ovarian cancer using mucin-16, and pancreatic cancer using transferrin receptor-1, antigen claudin-4, and urokinase plasminogen activator (uPA) receptor as ligands. However, despite their highly specific and accurate imaging properties, they pose the threat of heavy metal poisoning and unwanted immune response (Fang et al. 2012). The study by Amdursky et al. (2010) revealed that diphenylalanine peptide nanotubes in specific conditions show optical properties like that of QDs as well as self-assembling, and this can be a better option for tackling the problem of heavy metal poisoning. Still, more studies on the nanotoxicology of QDs are needed to understand the after-effects of this limitation to devise new QD-development strategies.

1.3.9 DNA Nanoparticles

We have come across different types of therapeutic nanoparticles so far, from micelles to multimodal, and learned their functional versatility. However, considering its structural versatility, we reach a common point of discussion that is either on lipid molecules or polymers such as PEG. It was in 1980s, a new wave of change hit the shores of nanobiotechnology when Dr. Nadrian C. Seeman started designing DNA structures with desired structural characteristics, a less common approach since DNA was always "linked" to genetic information. Since then, a revolutionary take-off of nanoparticle design took place, with the freedom to take over the complementary binding of the DNA bases and with the aid of self-assembling as well as externalized folding strategies, forming almost all possible symmetric three-dimensional structures [such as the famous DNA "smiley face" (Rothemund 2006)], which is the fundamental concept of DNA *origami*, the inspirational creativeness of Dr. Paul W. K. Rothemund in 2006. The molecular understanding of natural, complex DNA structures such as the replication fork, Holliday junction, and cross-over models was the kick start to the development of this field. The novelty of this field converted what we call genetic "defects" into nanostructural "assets". DNA nanomedicine considers three fundamental DNA conformations as the base of any DNA-based drug vectors: *linear*, *branched*, and *cross-linked*. The most widely used topology is linear DNA due to its simplicity and ability to interact with functional proteins. The latter two topologies have more advantageous applications considering their stable structure and crystallographic features. DNA, considered as a nanostructure, has led to the development of molecular sensors, targeted drug vehicles such as DNA dendrimers, controlled drug-release systems, and even nanomachines such as DNA clamp (Campolongo et al. 2010; Seeman 2003; Seeman 2010; University of Montreal 2013). DNA nanotechnology has been successfully used in cancer diagnosis and treatment over the past 40 years. DNA *origami*, DNA hydrogels, DNA structures with signal amplification properties, DNA conjugates of metallic, fluorescent, and magnetic nanoparticles, deoxyribozymes, and two-dimensional nanosheets are some of the therapeutic applications of DNA nanotechnology in medicine (Chen et al. 2018). With improvising techniques in DNA nanotechnology such as nanoinformatics and designing DNA-based nanomotors and nanobots, we can confirm that tomorrow's hope and scope lie in biomedical and nanomedical research.

1.4 Pharmacokinetics of Cancer Nanodrug Carriers

Nanodrug carriers are being extensively learned for their mechanism of action, both extracellular and intracellular. This is very important to determine or design the path by which the target cell decides for processing the drug-carrying nanostructures. Pharmacokinetics is the study of relationship between drug dosage and its concentration in the body over time and is best explained by the ADME scheme, which translates into drug absorption, distribution, metabolism, and excretion. The different pharmacokinetic parameters under each section of this scheme are used to determine the pharmacokinetic properties of any drug. The typical absorption parameters are mainly related to that of drug bioavailability, such as area-under–concentration-time curve (AUC), maximum plasma concentration (C_{max}), and the time taken to reach C_{max} (T_{max}). The distribution parameter is mainly the volume of distribution (V_{d}), whereas the main parameter of metabolism is elimination half-life ($t_{1/2}$). Excretion of the drug is generally quantified as the average drug clearance rate (CL). Table 1.2 shows the fold comparison of some important pharmacokinetic properties of cancer drugs and their nanoparticle formulation.

1.5 Cancer Nanomedical Research

1.5.1 Initial Advancements in Nanoparticle Research

Like other medical researches, extensive research has been done in nanodrug development, especially for treating cancerous conditions. According to PubMed publication statistics, nearly 40,000 papers have been published till now with novel findings on cancer nanoparticle research, starting from 1980, of which approximately 6% are about clinical cancer-nanotechnological and anti-cancer nanomedical research. We can see a significant growth curve in the research density of nanoparticle technology, particularly in cancer therapy, after the beginning of the twenty-first century. The numbers increased from 25 research papers in 1999 to more than 5000 in the year 2019 alone, cumulatively about 36,400 papers over a span of 21 years that is on average about five research papers per day! This indeed was the "golden age" of cancer nanoparticle research. These statistics are the indications of our improving understanding of drug molecules and nanoparticles, creativity, and human nature of the "research by one, results for all" motto.

The main clinical models used for cancer-nanomedicine research are cancerous cell lines, animal models, and human or human xenograft models, as well as in silico-evaluated models. Cancer-nanomedicine research can be classified into four broad categories: (1) nanodrug development, (2) nanodrug modification, (3) comparative studies, and (4) in silico studies. These classes show the advantageous effects

Table 1.2 A comparison of the pharmacokinetic parameters of free drug versus nanoparticle formulation of the same drug (Chou et al. 2013; Abdifetah and Na-Bangchang 2019)

Name of free drug and drug-nanoparticle formulation	Mode(s) of administration (dosage in mg/kg body weight of model) (reference)	The fold difference in parameters compared to the free drug					
		AUC	C_{max}	T_{max}	V_d	$t_{1/2}$	CL
PTX	Intravenous (10) (Feng et al. 2007)	–	–	–	–	–	–
PTX-PLGA/ATPGS		0.77	–	–	–	**20.24**	–
5FU	Intravenous (30) (Li et al. 2008)	–	–	–	–	–	–
5FU-PBLG/PEG		0.92	0.27	–	**1.65**	**378.41**	–
DXR	Intravenous (5) (Agarwal et al. 2009)	–	–	–	–	–	–
DXR-PAD/PPI		**3.16**	–	**4.88**	–	–	0.32
DTX	Intravenous (15) (Senthilkumar et al. 2008)	–	–	–	–	–	–
DTX-PLGA		**1.55**	0.82	–	–	**1.70**	0.64
DTX-PLGA/mPEG/2 kDa		**2.44**	0.89	–	–	**3.58**	0.41
DTX-PLGA/mPEG/5 kDa		**2.74**	0.93	–	–	**3.76**	0.36
DXR	Oral (10) (Kalaria et al. 2009)	–	–	–	–	–	–
DXR-PLGA		**3.64**	**2.38**	**6**	–	–	–
DXR	Intravenous (2) (Yu et al. 2009)	–	–	–	–	–	–
DXR-CHGC		**6.61**	–	–	–	–	0.15
DXR	Intravenous (5) (Jain et al. 2010)	–	–	–	–	–	–
DXR-SLN		**3.04**	0.83	–	–	**3.58**	0.32
DXR-MSLN		**4.95**	0.79	–	–	**9.31**	0.19
PTX	Intravenous (10) (Zabaleta et al. 2012)	–	–	–	–	–	–
PTX-PVM/MA	Oral (10) (Zabaleta et al. 2012)	–	–	–	–	–	–
PTX-PVM/MA/PEG2000		**7.57**	**10.5**	**1.52**	–	0.34	–
PTX-PVM/MA/PEG6000		**4.32**	**9.5**	0.79	–	0.23	–
PTX-PVM/MA/PEG10000		**1.76**	**7**	0.87	–	1.07	–
Sirolimus	Intravenous (10) (Woo et al. 2012)	–	–	–	–	–	–
Sirolimus-PLA/PEG		**3.15**	**3.91**	1	–	–	–
DTX	Intravenous (40) (Ernsting et al. 2012)	–	–	–	–	–	–
DTX-CMC/PEG		**38.64**	**17.12**	–	0.13	**5.22**	0.02
DTX	Intravenous (1.5) (Ho et al. 2012)	–	–	–	–	–	–
DTX-PMCCL/PEG		**2.36**	–	–	0.47	**1.60**	0.29

(continued)

Table 1.2 (continued)

Name of free drug and drug-nanoparticle formulation	Mode(s) of administration (dosage in mg/kg body weight of model) (reference)	The fold difference in parameters compared to the free drug					
		AUC	C_{max}	T_{max}	V_d	$t_{1/2}$	CL
DTX	Intravenous (10) (Yu et al. 2013)	–	–	–	–	–	–
DTX-PLGA		**1.19**	0.64	1	1.14	**2.09**	0.75
DTX-PLA/ATPEGS		**2.13**	0.69	1	**5.57**	**13.29**	0.5
DTX	Oral (10) (Saremi et al. 2013)	–	–	–	–	–	–
DTX-chitosan/GSH/PMMA		**10.60**	0.75	**2.5**	**–**	**8.76**	–
DTX	Intravenous (2.5) (Qiao et al. 2013)	–	–	–	–	–	–
DTX-PALA		**1.51**	**–**	**–**	**–**	**1.53**	0.74
DXR	Oral (10) (Guo et al. 2014)	–	–	–	–	–	–
DXR-chitosan/12 kDa		1.01	0.89	1	–	1.03	0.94
DXR-chitosan/ATPEGS/15 kDa		1.11	0.82	1	–	1.49	0.85
DXR-chitosan/ATPEGS/22 kDa		**2.36**	1.16	1	–	**2.52**	0.42
PTX (in TAXOL®)	Intravenous (6) (Bernabeu et al. 2014)	–	–	–	–	–	–
PTX (in ABRAXANE®)		0.71	–	–	**12.25**	1.18	1.18
PTX-PECL/ATPGS		**2.69**	–	–	**4.17**	**11.87**	0.32
DTX	Intravenous (1) (Lee et al. 2014)	–	–	–	–	–	–
DTX-PS/PDLLA		1.33	–	–	**1.75**	**2.34**	0.43
ESC8	Intravenous (2) (Andey et al. 2015)	–	–	–	–	–	–
ESC8-corn oil	Oral (50) (Andey et al. 2015)	–	–	–	–	–	–
ESC8-liposome	Oral (20) (Andey et al. 2015)	–	–	–	–	–	–
ESC8-SLN		**1.97**	**1.83**	1.08	0.55	1.08	0.5
ESC8-NSLC		**1.78**	**1.63**	1.09	0.61	1.09	0.55
ATZ	Intravenous (1) (Shavi et al. 2015)	–	–	–	–	–	–
ATZ-PLGA		**4.77**	**–**	**–**	**4.49**	**21.59**	0.19
ATZ-PLA		**19.32**	**–**	**–**	**1.84**	**35.49**	0.05
ATZ-PECL		**19.82**	**–**	**–**	**1.62**	**32.29**	0.05
ATPS	Intraperitoneal (100) (Gao et al. 2016)	–	–	–	–	–	–
ATPS-NE		0.56	0.57	**1.8**	–	0.46	**1.8**
NCP	Intravenous (50) (Shalaby et al. 2016)	–	–	–	–	–	–
NCP-mPEG/1.9 kDa		1.28	0.87	–	–	**4.48**	–
NCP-PECL/mPEG/2.0 kDa		0.32	0.56	–	–	**3.12**	–
MPT	Oral (30) (Zhang et al. 2016)	–	–	–	–	–	–
MPT-Ch		**3.15**	**2.19**	1.47	–	1.33	–

(continued)

Table 1.2 (continued)

Name of free drug and drug-nanoparticle formulation	Mode(s) of administration (dosage in mg/kg body weight of model) (reference)	The fold difference in parameters compared to the free drug					
		AUC	C_{max}	T_{max}	V_d	$t_{1/2}$	CL
GTB	Intravenous (2) (Khare et al. 2016)	–	–	–	–	–	–
GTB-PLGA		**2.17**	–	–	–	2	0.46
GTB-PLGA/mPEG		**3.24**	–	–	–	**19**	0.31
DXR	Intravenous (4) (Lee et al. 2016)	–	–	–	–	–	–
DXR-CSA/DCA		1.47	–	–	**16.78**	**2.15**	0.69
DXR-CSA/DCA/PEG		**2.44**	**–**	**–**	**2.85**	**5.46**	0.60
DXR	Intravenous (5) (Chao et al. 2017)	–	–	–	–	–	–
DXR-PECL/mPEG		**5.97**	**2.12**	–	0.67	**4.54**	0.15
DNR	Intravenous (4) (Varghese et al. 2016)	–	–	–	–	–	–
DNR-soya lecithin/PLGA		0.76	–	–	1.42	1.19	1.24
DTX	Intravenous (25) (Vardhan et al. 2017)	–	–	–	–	–	–
DTX-PHBV		**1.62**	0.38	**12**	**14.57**	**8.21**	0.43
DTX trihydrate	Oral (20) (Khurana et al. 2017)	–	–	–	–	–	–
DTX-LCG-SNELS		**10.86**	**4.60**	0.43	–	–	–
DTX-MCG-SNELS		**8.76**	**1.77**	0.84	–	–	–
DTX (serum)	Intravenous (5) (Rafiei and Haddadi 2017)	–	–	–	–	–	–
DTX-PLGA		**3.91**	–	–	0.39	1.41	0.27
DTX-PLGA/PEG		**5.46**	–	–	0.76	**3.69**	0.19
DTX (liver)	Intravenous (5) (Rafiei and Haddadi 2017)	–	–	–	–	–	–
DTX-PLGA		1.48	–	–	–	1.32	0.66
DTX-PLGA/PEG		**2.42**	–	–	–	**3.09**	0.53
DTX (kidney)	Intravenous (5) (Rafiei and Haddadi 2017)	–	–	–	–	–	–
DTX-PLGA		**2.07**	**–**	**–**	**–**	**1.54**	0.51
DTX-PLGA/PEG		0.85	–	–	–	0.65	1.19
DTX (heart)	Intravenous (5) (Rafiei and Haddadi 2017)	–	–	–	–	–	–
DTX-PLGA		0.89	–	–	–	0.52	1.14
DTX-PLGA/PEG		0.56	–	–	–	0.46	**1.91**
DTX (lungs)	Intravenous (5) (Rafiei and Haddadi 2017)	–	–	–	–	–	–
DTX-PLGA		0.52	–	–	–	0.59	**2.11**
DTX-PLGA/PEG		0.31	–	–	–	0.33	**4.32**
MTX	Intravenous (5) (Madhwi et al. 2017)	–	–	–	–	–	–
MTX-GPLGA		**4.21**	–	–	0.8	**1.74**	–
TMZ (plasma)	Intraperitoneal (3) (Sharma et al. 2018)	–	–	–	–	–	–
TMZ-chitosan/PAMAM		0.82	–	–	–	1.48	–

(continued)

Table 1.2 (continued)

Name of free drug and drug-nanoparticle formulation	Mode(s) of administration (dosage in mg/kg body weight of model) (reference)	The fold difference in parameters compared to the free drug					
		AUC	C_{max}	T_{max}	V_d	$t_{1/2}$	CL
TMZ (brain)	Intraperitoneal (3) (Sharma et al. 2018)	–	–	–	–	–	–
TMZ-chitosan/PAMAM		1.11	–	–	1.35	**1.76**	0.77
DNR	Oral (10) (Ahmad et al. 2019)	–	–	–	–	–	–
DNR-PLGA		**6.22**	**7.14**	1	–	**2.19**	–
DNR-chitosan/PLGA		**11.29**	**13.24**	1	–	**2.79**	–

ATPGS α-Tocopheryl polyethylene glycol succinate,*PBLG* Poly(γ-benzyl-L-glutamate), *PAD* Poly (aldehydrodextran), *PPI* Polypropylene imine, *CHGC* Cholesterol-modified glycol chitosan, *MSLN* Mannosylated SLN, *PVM/MA* Poly(vinyl methyl ether-co-maleic anhydride), *CMC* Carboxymethylcellulose, *PMCCL* Poly(2-methyl-2-carboxytrimethylene carbonate-co-D,L-lactide), *PLA* Poly(lactic acid), *GSH* reduced L-glutathione, *PMMA* Poly(methyl methacrylate), *PALA* Semi-polyamidoamine-b-poly(D,L-lactic acid), *PECL* Poly(ε-caprolactone), *PS/PDLL* Poly (styrene)-b-poly(D,L-lactide), *ESC-8* Estrone derivative, *NSLC* Nanostructured lipid carriers, *ATZ* Anastrozole, *ATPS* α-Tocopherol succinate, *NE* nanoemulsion, *NCP* Noscapine, *MPT* Mifepristone, *GTB* Gemcitabine, *CSA* Chondroitin sulfate A, *DCA* Deoxycholic acid, *PHBV* Poly (3-hydroxybutyrate-co-3-hydroxyvalerate), *L/MCG* Long–/Medium-chain fatty acid glyceride, *SNELS* Self-nanoemulsifying lipidic nanomicelles systems, *MTX* Methotrexate, *GPLGA* Glycine-linked PLGA

The values in **bold** are the pharmacokinetic parameters of the drug-nanoparticle formulation which are 50% or more ($\geq$1.5) than that of the free drug

of drug-nanoparticle conjugate over the native drug on treating the particular disorder, with special emphasis on nanoscale drug modulations to existing cancer medications, drug-to-drug conjugations, natural drug design, and nanoimaging. As indicated in the publication statistics above, it is difficult to include the enormous data produced in the "golden age" due to multiple constraints, and there is a scope for those researches alone to be a book chapter. Therefore, here, we present a detailed description of cancer nanoparticle research in the initial stages of cancer nanodrug research (till 2008) and in silico research carried out after 2010, with a brief explanation of the mainstream research on the golden age.

The mainstream researches in the initial stages of cancer nanotechnology were mainly focused on nanodrug development by optimizing the conditions of encapsulation and ligand binding, thus improving its bioavailability and specificity. These studies had background support from clinical validation by in vitro and in vivo cancer studies, mainly in human and murine cancer cell lines, forming the foundation of many kinds of research done in the later stages.

In these initial stages, the approach towards cancer nanoparticle development was quite challenging and time-taking. The researchers would have gone through many procedures such as drug identification, thermodynamic estimation, target identification, ligand identification, nanoparticle design, and its administration in each trial. We honor their hard work and dedication, which bear as resources and experimental protocol for researchers even now. The choice of experimenting with chemotherapeutic drugs was a brilliant idea since the drug was very effective with the only disadvantage of serious side-effects due to non-specificity. Encapsulating these potent drugs in target-specific nanoenvelopes was a possible strategy to overcome this disadvantage of chemotherapeutic drugs. As shown by Jiang et al. in 1995, the effect of lyophilized aclacinomycin-A–poly(isobutyl cyanoacrylate) nanoparticles on human hepatocellular carcinoma cell line QGY-7703 was clinically satisfactory when compared to native aclacinomycin-A treatment. They showed a concentration-dependent cytotoxic effect of the drug-nanoparticle conjugate in vitro and a 20% more tumor inhibition rate than its native drug in nude mice with orthotopic human hepatoma transplantation (Jiang et al. 1995). A promising therapeutic strategy for human gastric carcinoma by Qu et al. (2006) showed that intraperitoneal administration of mitomycin-C–activated carbon nanoparticles in nude mice models resulted in an effective payload with on-target delivery, without showing the typical adverse effects of mitomycin-C poisoning such as leukopenia and thrombocytopenia. Camptothecin, a topoisomerase poison, first derived from *Camptotheca acuminata*, was used in Chinese traditional medicine for cancer treatment. Several derivatives of camptothecin, like 9-nitrocamptothecin (rubitecan), a potent drug against pancreatic cancer, and other solid tumors, were developed and showed great clinical outcomes. However, the major problem with this drug is its low bioavailability and solubility (Contributors n.d.-j). The development of NK012, an SN-38-releasing nanodevice developed by Koizumi et al. (2006), was a milestone in camptothecin-based anti-cancer treatment. SN-38, also known as 7-ethyl-10-hydroxy-camptothecin, was encapsulated in polymeric micelles by self-assembly, which was demonstrated to have anti-cancer activity in lung, colon, and colorectal cancer cell lines and bulky tumors such as SBC-3/*Neo* and SBC-3/*VEGF*. The work by Derakhshandeh et al. (2007) demonstrated the encapsulation of rubitecan in biodegradable poly (DL-lactide-co-glycolide) nanoparticles by nanoprecipitation method. This novel formulation improved the longevity of drug release up to 160 h, thus claiming that such nanoparticle formulations can have clinical importance for anti-cancer drug development (Derakhshandeh et al. 2007). A study by Chen et al. (2007) showed that MTX conjugated AuNPs can effectively suppress tumor growth in lung carcinoma mice model with ascites. The nanoparticle formulation also showed high cytotoxicity in several such cell lines, suggesting the effectiveness of MTX-AuNP conjugate over free MTX (Chen et al. 2007). The synthesis of SPIONs, coated with bifunctional amine-PVA linkers linking anti-cancer drugs such as 5-fluorouridine (5FUD) and DXR, by Hanessian et al. (2008), revealed the success of 5FUD-SPIONs over DXR-SPIONs due to difference in linkage parameters, suggesting the necessity of linker optimization. A more brilliant nanostructural design, the poly-L-lysine/hydroxyapatite/carbon nanotube hybrid nanocomposite, as designed by Ding et al. (2008) to target CA19–9, an important clinical marker for pancreatic cancer, unfolded a new definition to semiconductor-based biosensor designs. Besides these "conventional" nanodrug-delivery methods, magnetic thermotherapy is a novel technique that uses the heat generated by magnetic nanoparticles to destroy a target cancerous cell. The temperature generated in this technique is due to a "tug of war" between rapid flips (called Néel relaxations) in the magnetic domain of the nanoparticle when exposed to an alternating magnetic field and the inherent anisotropy energy of the material (Web Team, Weekly Technology Times 2016). The work by Jordan et al. (2006) in rats with RG-2 cells implanted to their brains was one of the first papers to show that localized interstitial thermotherapy caused necrosis in areas where an accumulation of magnetic nanoparticles took place, thus it could be a good option for anti-malignant brain tumor therapies if optimized.

1.5.2 Nanomedical Research Using Plant-Derived Compounds

Natural (plant-based) traditional drugs have widely gained recognition due to their organic nature and minimum side-effects. Nanoparticle researchers did not leave this stone unturned. These researches can be a symbol of sustainable research, with the underlying message of the ability of particulate enhancement that can elevate the function and recognition of these traditional drugs. A combination of these medications with nanoparticles has also improved their scientific and technical understanding in a target-specific manner. Curcumin, vincristine (*Catharanthus roseus*), resveratrol, kaempferol, PTX (*Taxus brevifolia*), and silymarin (*Silybum marianum*) are some of the main phytochemicals which are proven to have anti-cancer effects (Patra et al. 2018). Heat-killed *Mycobacterium vaccae* had gained the attention of researchers for its immunostimulating effects against tuberculosis and cancer (Zuany-Amorim et al. 2002). Tian and Groves (1999) employed this novel finding by isolating the active compounds of the bacterial lysate and found it to be high molecular weight proteoglycans, some of them being PS4A and PS4α. The team after thorough in vitro and in vivo experimentation in murine sarcoma model S180 with these native molecules found that activated macrophages played an important role in their anti-tumor effect leading them to develop optimized Chs nanoparticles, as potent carriers of PS4A and PS4α (Tian and Groves 1999). Cucurbitacin B, a triterpene found in pumpkins and gourds as their defense against herbivores, was proved for its potent anti-oral squamous cell carcinoma (OSCC) activity. Yang et al. (2001) selected purified cucurbitacin B and encapsulated it in a PLA coat, a biodegradable carrier material, using the solvent evaporation method. By injecting via the peri-cancer submucosa, the nanodrug formulation was able to reach its target site of cervical lymph nodes, from where it enters the lymphatic capillaries feeding the OSCC (Yang et al. 2001). Quercetin, a plant flavonoid, abundant in red onions, kale, and *Ginkgo biloba*, had been shown to have potential chemotherapeutic properties with a disadvantage of hydrophobicity (Vafadar et al. 2020). Yuan et al. (2006) formulated a nanodrug–carrier system for quercetin using PEGylated liposomes, using the rotary evaporation method and tested in hepatocellular carcinoma H22 models of BALB/c mice. They found that the novel nanoliposomes aggregated in the cancerous tissues and more importantly showed the inhibition of malignant ascites, one of the symptoms of hepatocellular cancer (Yuan et al. 2006). Curcumin being a polyphenol is less dispersible in aqueous media, but *nanocurcumin* was able to overcome this allowing greater bioavailability.

Bisht et al. (2007) developed this novel formulation which is curcumin encapsulated in a polymer coating made of N-isopropyl acrylamide with N-vinyl-2-pyrrolidone and PEG-monoacrylate. The formulation was tested in human pancreatic cancer cell lines and was found to have inhibitory effects on cancerous cell growth by induction of apoptosis and inhibition of the NFκB signaling pathway and downregulation of pro-inflammatory cytokines; thus being a novel application in both cancer and inflammation treatment (Bisht et al. 2007).

1.5.3 Nanomedical Research Using Gene Therapeutic Strategies

Other than small therapeutic molecules being delivered using nanodrug carriers, specific therapeutic genes could also be transferred target-specifically. Most of the gene therapy options involve viral vectors for gene transfection, but non-specificity remains a limiting factor to some extent. The work by Ramesh et al. (2004) claims to be one of the first works that demonstrated a non-viral vector-based gene transfer method involving nanoparticles. The team recruited dioleoyl-3-trimethylammonium propane (DOTAP)-cholesterol-based nano-assemblies to transfer human melanoma differentiation-associated gene 7 (*mda7*) into in vivo-lung tumor xenograft models and syngeneic murine models and showed potential growth-inhibitory activity in primary as well as disseminated lung tumor cells and tumor vascularization (Ramesh et al. 2004). The work by Ohtani et al. (2007) on nanoparticle-mediated gene transfer of cytochrome b561 domain-containing protein 2 (*CYB561D2*, also known as *101F6*) along with ascorbate, showed effective inhibition of lung tumorigenesis and proliferation. Besides direct gene transfer for therapeutic protein production, Pirollo et al. (2007) demonstrated the transfer of anti-*HER2 si*RNA in an immunoliposome-based delivery complex with pH-sensitive peptides attached, into a pancreatic cancer model. The nanoformulation showed significant tumor growth inhibition in the model (Pirollo et al. 2007).

1.5.4 Nanomedical Research Using In Vivo Imaging Techniques

Lawaczeck et al. 1997 studied the nanoimaging properties of SPIONs, mostly consisting of γ-Fe_2O_3 (SH U555A) coated with tumor-targeting carboxydextran in rat tumor models. This MRI nanoparticle had a dosage-dependent half-life with improved tumor-to-liver contrast and very few side-effects (Lawaczeck et al. 1997). A similar nanoimaging study done by Turetschek et al. (2001) used NC100150, ultrasmall SPIONs with oxidizing starch coating, and estimated its magnetic resonance angiographic (MRA) properties in rats with mammary tumors. NC100150 was found to have greater microvascular permeability and density which elevates its scope as a potential MRA agent of tumor microvasculature (Turetschek et al. 2001). A comparative study done by Varallyay et al. (2002) suggested that ferumoxtran, an ultrasmall SPION, can be an effective MR contrast agent in most malignant intracranial tumors. Another comparative study done by de Lussanet et al. (2003) in mice model with human colon carcinoma showed that ultrasmall SPIONs had equivalent results in contrast-enhanced MRI as well as for most of the pharmacokinetic parameters of the nanoparticle when compared with gadopentetate dimeglumine, a gadolinium-based contrast agent. Gadolinium-based contrast agents, especially gadodiamide, are used extensively for MRI of intracranial and spinal disorders but pose adverse side-effects such as nephrogenic systemic fibrosis and kidney failure (Ibrahim et al. 2020). A method for deep magnetic resonance lymphangiography, as proposed by Kobayashi et al. (2003), used dendrimer-based MRI contrasting agents for tracking pathophysiological changes in the lymphatic vessels tested in inflammatory mice models. A report on a multicenter phase II trial by Daldrup-Link et al. (2003) for nanoimaging techniques in human volunteers (63 women with primary breast lesion, 26 cases had benign, whereas the rest had malignant tumor) using NC100150 (*Clariscan*™ Feruglose) emphasized the significant difference in the endothelial transfer coefficient (K^{PS}) of these carbohydrate-PEG-coated, ultrasmall SPIONs between benign and malignant tumor and proposed a criterion for differentiating benign and malignant tumor concerning their microvascular properties, which is $K^{PS} > 0$ for carcinomas (73%) and $K^{PS} < 0$ for benign tumors (73%). With developing technology, more nanoscale molecules with high functionality and specificity were developed for deep and precise cancer cell imaging, like radiolabeled monoclonal antibodies (Mitra et al. 2006) and semiconductor QDs and fluorescent probes coupled with target-recognition properties (Xing et al. 2006). A commendable work was done by Estrada et al. (2006) on human urothelial carcinoma tested in rats and ex vivo showing a distinct behavioral profile leading them to develop an assay system, called *EViTAS*, the acronym for ex vivo tumor assay system, which can be considered a base for oncobehavioral profiling studies, beneficial mostly to cancers of histological indifferences. Advanced in vivo imaging techniques take multiple parameters into account at a time, thus reducing non-specificity and enhancing precise deep imaging using nanoparticles. This is done using multimodal nanostructures, having more than one determinant molecule or probe, exclusively for nanoimaging experiments, with predominant applications in tumor margin visualization. The work by Tréhin et al. (2006) suggests the use of multimodal nanoparticles in tumor boundary determination in murine models of gliosarcoma and colon carcinoma using cross-linked SPIONs and Cy5.5 fluorescent dye. Experimented in NOD/SCID mouse models implanted with under-glycosylated mucin-1-positive ($uMUC1^+$) human pancreatic adenocarcinoma cells, Capan-2, Medarova et al. (2006) used dual-modality probes, which are again cross-linked SPIONs with peptides targeting uMUC1, the tumor-specific antigen, with conjugated Cy5.5 fluorescent dye.

1.5.5 Mainstream Research in the "Golden Age" of Nanotechnology

Here, we consider the research conducted from the early 2000s until 2019 as the "golden age"-research due to the coinciding advancements of both nanotechnology and biotechnology. The mainstream cancer researches were done in cell lines as well as animal models of liver, brain, lung, pancreas, colon, head and neck, breast, and prostate cancers. As a continuation of the research done in the late twentieth century, "golden age" research mainly focused on target-specific nanodrug development, particularly with nanoliposome, multifunctional nano-coats, immunoliposomes, and semiconductor QDs. With an improved understanding of the science behind these materials, specialized nanoparticles did not find any reason to turn back, leading to an outburst in nanoparticle development. Also, the discovery of novel oncotherapeutics and chemotherapeutics during this period increased its possibilities factorially. These outcomes were further optimized with improved nanotoxicological studies, particularly in brilliant non-cancer models such as chick embryos. A complete array of comparative studies, most of them claiming the advantages of nanoencapsulated or nano-conjugated drugs over the free drugs, was widely published in this period. The timescale of this "golden age" may shift in the upcoming years as novel technological advancements are made. Who knows that an era of drug-free treatment is waiting!

1.5.6 Nanomedical Research Using Computational and Nanobioinformatic Tools

The impelling charisma of nanoparticles and nanodrug formulations has a significant contribution from the bioinformatic validatory algorithms and computer simulation modeling techniques, which enable research in an easier, faster, and targeted manner. The field of "nanobioinformatics" is indeed a feed to the ever-growing demands for novel therapeutics and targeted drug therapy, mostly at the nanoscale level. From 2011, there has been an increase in the number of in silico works on cancer nanomedicine, with insight into its pharmacodynamic properties. The work by Patra and Dasgupta (2012) was one such research in which the determining parameters of nanoparticles such as size, electric properties, surface functionalization, and cell-matrix adhesion properties, were experimentally trailed and optimized. The team showed the classification of AuNPs according to their hydrodynamic diameter and *zeta* potential using the *k*-clustering technique. The work claims that though there is a complex interplay between size, zeta potential, surface, and adhesion properties of nanoparticles in its cell-targeted activities, the ratio of zeta potential to surface area plays an important indicator for determining optimal cellular response (Patra and Dasgupta 2012). The work by Chou et al. (2013), however, studied the spatiotemporal responses of anti-cancer nanoparticles and found valuable data which led them to suggest that long half-life in plasma and high interstitial diffusivity of nanoparticles are the key features to produce a significant uniform spatial distribution of nanoparticles in the interstitium. Another important aspect of cancer drug-research is to overcome the major challenge of cancer cell drug resistance. The work by Zhao et al. (2015b) shows a promising nanocoassembling strategy of 10-hydroxycamptothecin and DXR, against drug-resistant invasive breast ductal carcinoma cells (MCF-7R), even without a carrier envelope.

In silico molecular dynamic studies showed that DXR molecules tend to assemble around 10-hydroxycamptothecin through intermolecular forces. This nanosize clustering improved the intracellular drug retention of DXR up to two folds and proved to be more cytotoxic to those cells synergistically (Zhao et al. 2015b). In 2016, Han et al. showed that by modifying vorinostat, a USFDA-approved histone deacetylase inhibitor that was used extensively as a treatment molecule against cutaneous T-cell lymphoma, by adding a disulfide linkage could produce a prodrug with improved efficacy. The new drug was SAHA-S-S-VE, i.e., suberanilohydroxamic acid linked to vitamin E hemisuccinate by a disulfide bond, and it exhibits low critical aggregation concentration, excellent payload capacity, and permeability and bioavailability capacities in nanodrug-delivery systems, exceeding that of the free form of the drug (Han et al. 2016). In 2018, Wang et al. showed the possibility of combining molecules of opposing natures. The study showed the self-assembly of two antimetabolites clofarabine, a hydrophobic purine-2′-deoxyribonucleoside analog used to cure certain types of ALL, and raltitrexed, a hydrophilic folate analog, a thymidylate synthase inhibitor and thus a chemotherapeutic agent, into stable nanostructures by molecular recognition. This novel drug synergy showed positive results in both in vitro and in vivo studies by suppressing the G1 phase of the cell cycle and quenching the deoxynucleotide reservoirs of the cells with improved therapeutic properties (Wang et al. 2018). Besides these in silico molecular dynamic studies, this novel drug showed improved performance in both in vitro and in vivo studies (Han et al. 2016). The extent of nanodrug modeling has also started to search for encapsulating natural products as mentioned in Kunjiappan et al.'s (2018) work. *Dunaliella bardawil*, a unicellular photosynthetic green alga, is widely studied for its biopharmaceutical applications. In this paper, *D. bardawil* biomass was encapsulated in N-succinyl chitosan nanoparticles and was used to target *HRas* proto-oncogene in silico, and HepG2, a hepatocellular carcinoma cell line, for cytotoxic studies. The nanoparticles showed significant affinity to the binding pockets of the proto-oncogene, and the increased active-molecule content in *D. bardawil* biomass, such as β-carotenoids, showed anti-cancer properties when coupled with nanodrug carriers (Kunjiappan et al. 2018). Variation in the inherent properties of cell adhesion molecules is one of the hallmarks of metastasis and Nardelli et al. (2018) focused on $\alpha_v\beta_3$ integrin, one of the most overexpressed receptor proteins in tumor vasculature. $\alpha_v\beta_3$ integrin is a receptor of vitronectin, an important glycoprotein that promotes cell adhesion and spreading, and like most of the integrin ligands, vitronectin too possesses an Arg-Gly-Asp (RGD) peptide sequence as the main binding motif (Contributors n.d.-k). The team claims that the succinimide ring of the conjugated product of c(CGisoDGRG) and 4-(N-maleimidomethyl)cyclohexane-1-carboxamide, which is responsible for $\alpha_v\beta_3$ integrin stabilization, can be a key motif in many future drugs which are intended to target tumors which occur by integrin modulation, with increasing efficacy if delivered using a nanodrug carrier (Nardelli et al. 2018). Like integrin, modulations to CD44, a cell surface glycoprotein, are also observed in cell-to-cell miscommunications and noise. Hyaluronic acid, the only non-sulfated mucopolysaccharide, is a potential ligand for three receptor groups, viz. CD44, intercellular adhesion molecule-1 (ICAM1), and the receptor of hyaluronan-mediated motility (RHAMM) (Contributors n.d.-l). The work by Sargazi et al. (2018) showed that conjugation of hyaluronic acid with PEGylated magnetic nanoparticles carrying mitoxantrone was very effective and target-specific against $CD44^+$ cancer cells. Molecular docking with in vitro and in vivo validation studies revealed that this nanodrug formulation has a higher binding affinity to CD44 than free hyaluronate (Sargazi et al. 2018). A more advanced approach in nanodrug delivery was made by Xu and Kleinstreuer (2018) using a novel computer simulation model of the human hepatic artery system in which the hydrodynamic interactions of multifunctional nanoparticles with red blood cells were studied. They showed that shear-induced diffusion, which is a major migration mechanism for microparticles as well as nanoparticles, played an important role in the transport of nanoparticles even in large arteries, thus developing a scope for direct nanodrug delivery to arteries aiding tumor growth (Xu and Kleinstreuer 2018). Follow-up work by the team proposed that besides shear-induced diffusion, the creation of a cell-free layer due to RBC migration away from the endothelial lining caused a dip in the lateral transport of nanoparticles to its cancerous target, which can be modulated for precise targeting of nanodrugs (Xu and Kleinstreuer 2019).

1.6 Nanomedicine in Cancer Diagnosis and Treatment

As we have seen, nanoparticles can be utilized for the efficient delivery of anti-cancer drugs, diagnosis of cancer in its early stages, and in vivo imaging in a targeted or non-targeted manner without triggering side-effects. The high scope of nanoparticles for cancer research and treatment is due to the EPR effect of nanoparticles which allows their greater accumulation in tumor cells rather than in normal cells. Nanoparticles modified with aptamers or any other targeting molecules enhance the drug delivery to desired tumor sites. Nanoparticles with theranostic properties can be used for integrated cancer diagnosis, disease progression monitoring, and therapeutic efficacy determination. They can also be utilized for designing immunoassays involving nanomaterial-embedded microchips for cancer diagnosis and contrast agents for in vivo imaging studies.

1.6.1 Immunoassays Using Nanomaterial-Embedded Microchips

Tumor cells from the primary tumor site can shed and enter the bloodstream (through the process of intravasation). These tumor cells are called circulating tumor cells (CTCs). University of California, Los Angeles, has developed a unique concept of cell affinity substrates called NanoVelcro. It involves the use of nanostructured substrates that are coated with CTC-capture agents like antibodies or aptamers for immobilization of CTCs (Lin et al. 2014). NanoVelcro CTC assay is highly efficient due to the strong affinity between CTCs and CTC-capture agent-embedded nanostructure substrate complex. This assay can be used for the enumeration,

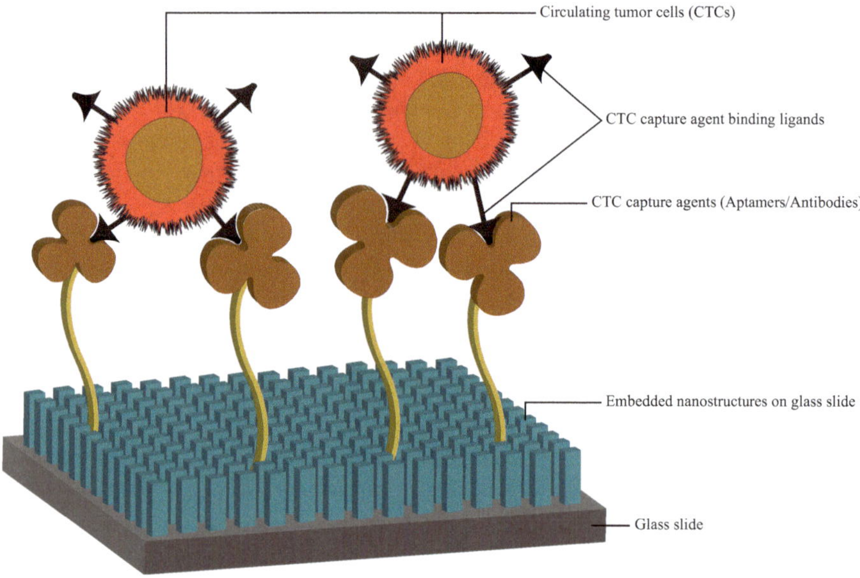

Fig. 1.1 An illustration of the binding of CTCs to the CTC-capture agents which are embedded on a NanoVelcro surface

detection, and isolation of CTCs (Chen et al. 2016). Some microchips, called herringbone chips (HBCs), are made of imprinted poly(dimethylsiloxane) (PDMS) components on a glass slide with a herringbone pattern. The PDMS component was responsible for creating microvortices to enhance the interaction between CTCs and CTC-capture agent-coated surfaces. The enumeration of CTCs can also be performed by first-generation NanoVelcro CTC assay, which involves the use of patterned silicon nanowire substrate conjugated with biotinylated anti-epithelial cell adhesion molecule (EpCAM) to capture CTCs as a result of EpCAM expression on the cancer cells. CTCs can be identified based on CK and CD45 fluorescence signals using fluorescence microscopy. This enumeration assay was performed with more than 100 samples collected from patients with metastatic castration-resistant prostate cancer (mCRPC). Figure 1.1 illustrates the binding of CTCs in a NanoVelcro CTC assay.

QDs can be integrated with nanobiochips for the detection of prominent cancer markers like *ERBB2*, cancer antigen 125 (CA125), and carcinoembryonic antigen (CEA) using saliva and serum. Nanobiochips involve the principle of sandwich immunoassay where antigen-capture is performed by microporous bead array made of agarose, supported within a microfluidics ensemble and antibodies labeled with QDs. The utilization of QD probes allows signal amplification that is 30 times better than that of standard molecular fluorophores (Jokerst et al. 2009).

1.6.2 In Vivo Imaging Using Nanoparticle Contrast Agents

Nanoparticles can be used as delivery vehicles of special probes that help in vivo imaging by overcoming the limitations of conventional imaging techniques such as sensitivity, resolution, penetration, cost-effectiveness, and clinical relevance. A novel nanoliposomal imaging agent, CF800 developed by Zheng et al. can be used for near-infrared (NIR) fluorescence imaging and CT imaging. CF800 has two FDA-approved drugs encapsulated in it, viz. indocyanine green and iohexol. CF800 provided enhanced imaging in CT image analysis of lung tumors. IONs specific to cell surface receptors of cancer cells can be used as MR contrast agents for improved detection of cancer cells, which are claimed to be completely non-harmful and biodegradable (Zheng et al. 2015). Amino-terminal fragment-conjugated IONs (ATF-IONs), which are IONs conjugated to the amino-terminal fragment of uPA protein, can be used to detect human breast cancer. ATF-IONs bind specifically to uPA receptors which are overexpressed on breast cancer cells and are internalized in those cells, causing its accumulation in cancer cells, which in turn generate strong contrast when detected by an MRI scanner at a magnetic field strength of 3 T. This provides enhanced detection of breast cancer cells. These nanoparticles can also be incorporated with drugs for specific drug delivery and response to the therapy can be monitored (Yang et al. 2009). Figure 1.2 illustrates how ATF-IONs act as strong MR contrast agents in imaging breast cancer cells.

Similarly, T-lymphocytes specific to cancer cells can also be labeled with highly derivatized cross-linked iron oxide nanoparticle (CLIONs-HD) for in vivo MRI tracking of injected CLION-HD–labeled lymphocytes and therefore for tracking the state of tumors (Kircher et al. 2003).

1.6.3 Theranostic Nanomedicine

Theranostic nanomedicine is an integrated treatment platform for diagnosis, delivery of targeted therapy, and monitoring the response of the therapy (Sumer and Gao 2008). It offers a promising strategy to track the pharmacokinetics and pharmacodynamic properties of the drug and disease progression or regression. It is simply an application of nanosciences in the diagnosis and therapeutics of a particular disease. Ultrasound-mediated chemotherapy has been established involving the administration of phase-shift drug-loaded nanodroplets (PSDNs), which could vaporize into microbubbles under the influence of ultrasound by acoustic droplet vaporization (ADV). These acoustic PSDNs accumulate in the tumor tissues using targeted delivery and further get converted into microbubbles. Exposure to ultrasonic waves causes these bubbles to expand by ADV inducing mechanical stress, which causes cell corrosion and damage (called sonoporation) and enhances cell permeability and tumor cell ablation through ultrasound and drugs loaded in nanodroplets. According to Chen et al., hydrogen-bonded multilayers of tannic acid and poly (N-vinylpyrrolidone) microcarriers can provide high ultrasound imaging contrast and could deliver encapsulated therapeutics under both low-intensity diagnostic

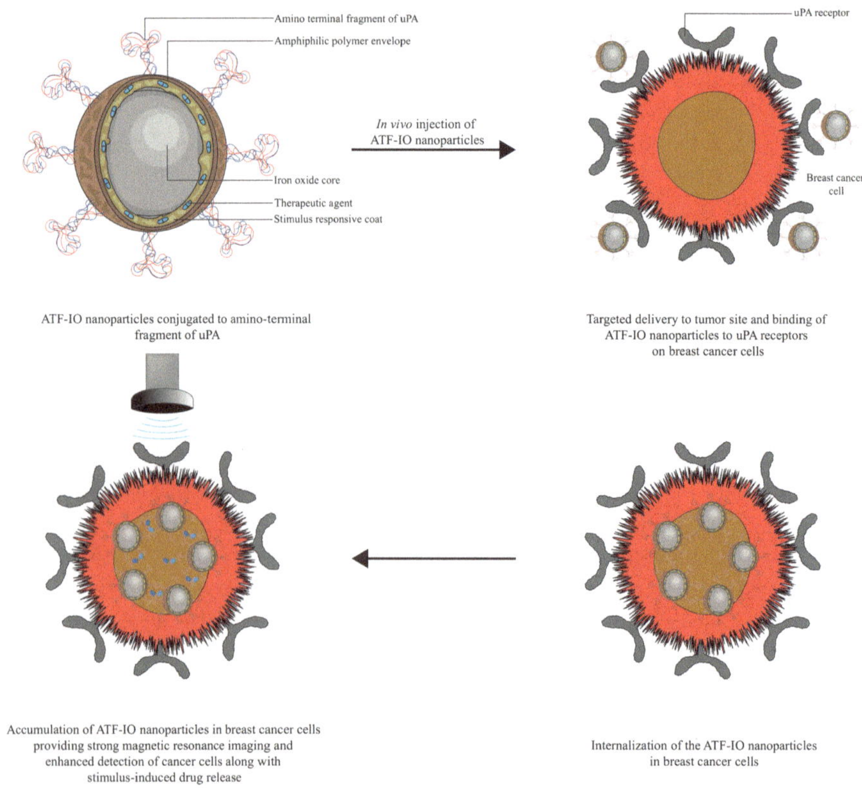

Fig. 1.2 An illustration of the working of ATF-IONs as strong MRI contrast agents

(power intensities of 0.1 W.cm^{-2}) and high-intensity therapeutic (>10 W.cm^{-2}) ultrasonic exposure to tumor tissues. Ultrasound-responsive nanodroplets have a perfluorocarbon (PFC) core and a shell composed of lipids and polymers (Ma et al. 2017). Figure 1.3 illustrates how PFC-core nanodroplets are used for ultrasound-mediated chemotherapy.

As mentioned, the detection of CTCs can help in cancer diagnosis and in predicting whether a patient with metastatic cancer is responding to a certain therapy. Since the concentration of CTCs in the bloodstream is very low, their detection is very challenging. Aptamer-conjugated magnetic or plasmonic nanoparticles can be used for the detection of CTCs. Aptamers specific to CTCs can be conjugated with Au-coated magnetic core nanoparticles and can be incubated with CTC suspension followed by magnetic separation. This approach was used for the detection and separation of *HER2*$^{+}$ SK-BR-3 breast cancer cells from a suspension at a very low concentration (~0.001%). Cy3-modified S6 aptamer was used for targeting SK-BR-3 breast cancer cells via *HER2*, thus combining target-specific therapeutic effect as well as imaging qualities (Fan et al. 2014).

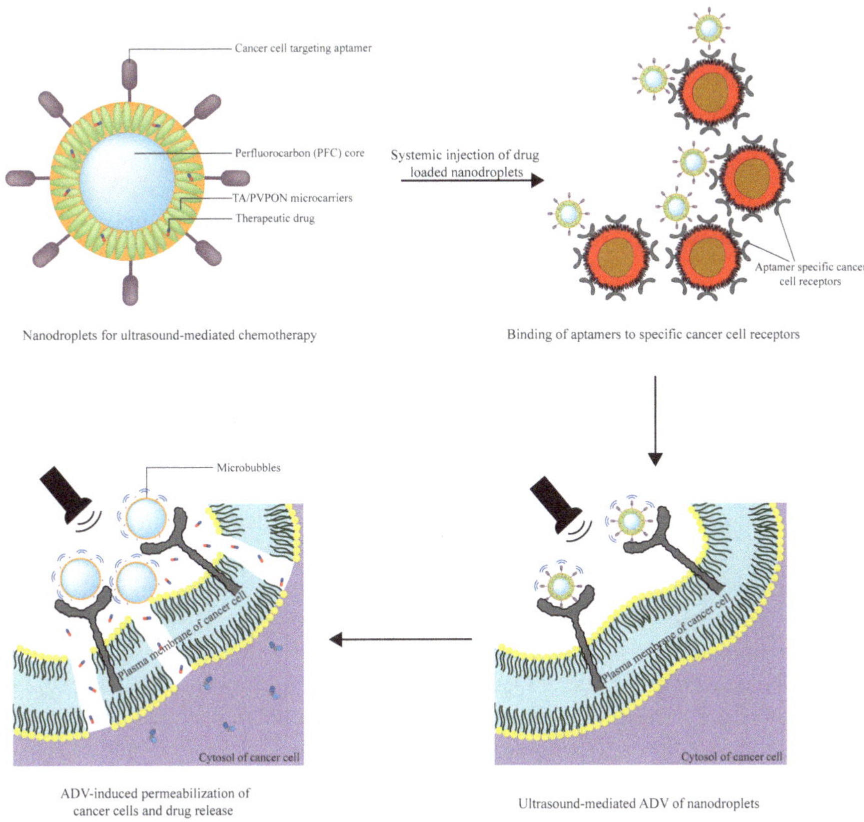

Fig. 1.3 An illustration of the working of PFC-core nanoparticles in ultrasound-mediated chemotherapy

1.6.4 Cancer Nanodrug Release Systems and Personalized Cancer Nanomedicine

The idea of using nanoparticles as personalized cancer nanomedicine gained a crucial role after the discovery of the EPR effect, which has allowed the use of nanoparticles for drug delivery, molecular imaging, and diagnosis of cancer. Applications of nanotechnology in cancer research and treatment have made tremendous progress over the past decades. Liposomal nanoformulations (for example, DOXIL® and MYOCET®) were the first class of therapeutic nanoparticles to receive clinical approval for cancer treatment. Encapsulating drugs in liposomes has shown improvement in pharmacokinetics and biodistribution. Also, they allow the co-delivery of multiple active pharmaceutical ingredients to provide a synergistic effect for better results (Shi et al. 2017). Nanoparticles provide a safe and effective way of drug delivery to target cells.

1.7 Current Research and Prospects

1.7.1 Smart Nanocarrier-Based Drug-Delivery Systems for Cancer Therapy

A smart nanocarrier system in cancer therapy consists of (Hossen et al. 2019):

- A smart nanocarrier that carries anti-cancer drug(s) to the target site,
- A proper targeting mechanism for locating the site, and
- A specific technique to release the payload in the site.

When nanoparticles are used for transporting modules for other substances, they are known as nanocarriers. A typical nanocarrier cannot carry and release drugs in the right concentration at the right target site under the right stimulus, but smart nanocarriers possess all those qualities besides evading the immune responses of the host system (Peer et al. 2007; Lee et al. 2015; Liu et al. 2016). Some nanocarriers and their smart properties are discussed here:

1. *Functionalized liposomes* overcome the shortcomings of conventional liposomes. They can differentiate between healthy and cancerous cells (Hossen et al. 2019). Smart liposomes can respond to the changes in pH, light, ultrasound, redox reaction potentials, and radiations (Noble et al. 2014; Sapra and Allen 2003; Sawant and Torchilin 2012; Ruoslahti 2012). The recent advancement of cancer drug therapy employs chemotherapy with liposomal co-delivery (Zununi Vahed et al. 2017), a type of adjuvant therapy.
2. *Smart micelles* can actively target cancer cells after being ligated with different ligands like therapeutic peptides, folic acids, aptamers, etc. (Sutton et al. 2007). An experiment carried out by Seo et al. has shown that micelle-based co-delivery systems can carry genes with anti-cancer drugs (Seo et al. 2015).
3. *Smart dendrimers* can be synthesized by modifying the dendritic surface by adding carbohydrates, aptamers, and proteins, etc. The modification is mainly performed for actively targeting the cancer site. The dendritic contrast agent for the imaging of tumors has shown to have great potential (Ye et al. 2013).

Several other smart nanocarriers are also being researched and have evolved to be a great alternative for conventional cancer therapy. However, the toxicity of nanocarriers in the human system remains a concern (Ferrari 2005; Sanhai et al. 2008). Studies are being conducted either to subtilize the toxicity or to come up with new nanocarrier systems with low toxicity (Hossen et al. 2019).

1.7.2 RNA Delivery Using Nanoparticles

RNA molecules such as micro-RNAs (*mi*RNAs) and *si*RNAs have the capability of silencing genes and regulating expressions of certain genes in tumor cells that promote malignancy or contribute to cancer in any way. These RNAs can be delivered through liposome-polycation-hyaluronan (LPH) nanoparticles. Successful studies have been made for the systemic delivery of *mi*RNAs and *si*RNAs using LPH nanoparticles into experimental murine lung metastasis models. These nanoparticles were modified with GC4 single-chain antibody fragments (scFv), specifically targeting B16F10 melanoma cells. The *si*RNAs delivered successfully downregulated c-Myc, mouse double -2 homolog (MDM2), and vascular endothelial growth factor (VEGF) protein expressions, and *mi*RNA (miR-34a) induced apoptosis, inhibited survivin expression and downregulated MAPK pathway in B16F10 melanoma cells. Co-delivery of *mi*RNA and *si*RNA by using LPH nanoparticles was successful in significant inhibition of tumor growth and controlling the malignancy (Chen et al. 2010b). The USFDA has also approved PLGA/PEG nanoparticles for clinical purposes as these protect encapsulated drugs from degradation and allow the slow release of the drugs to provide prolonged action. They can also be used for the delivery of the therapeutic *mi*RNAs into tumor cells. The penetration of these nanoparticles into the tumor cells can be enhanced using ultrasound to increase the permeability of tumor cells through sonoporation. Studies have proved that PLGA/PEG nanoparticles encapsulating miR-122 can be successfully delivered into human colon cancer xenografts through an optimized ultrasound-microbubble strategy (Wang et al. 2015).

1.7.3 Nanobots

Nanobots (also called nanorobots) are robots in a nanometer-scale made up of organic materials rather than any mechanical parts, which can be programmed to perform specific biological tasks employing genetic manipulations or biological modifications like integration with aptamers. The concept of nanobots made up of DNA was introduced by Douglas et al. in 2012. Nanobots with embedded chemical biosensors can detect tumor cells in the early stages of development in vivo. These DNA nanobots can also be used for the successful delivery of the drugs (payloads) to specific tumor cells without any significant side-effects. DNA nanobots appear like open-ended barrels with two halves connected by molecular hinges that can be opened and closed. The interior of the nanobots has binding sites for the payloads and aptamer on the surface of nanobots, providing target specificity to cancer cells. When these aptamers bind to their respective cancer cell surface receptors, the payloads are released from the nanobots and come into action. The team also tested these nanobots in vitro lymphoma and leukemia models (Douglas et al. 2012). Although nanobots are complicated structures and expensive to design, they provide controlled drug release at desired sites with fewer side-effects. More experimentation and research are required for nanobots to overcome immune responses. In the same year, scientists at the Wyss Institute of Biologically Inspired Engineering at Harvard University loaded fluorescent-labeled antibodies against human leukocyte antigens (HLAs) into nanobots to make them bind to cancer cells specifically (Tolikas 2012). On detecting the target proteins, the bots would release the payload. Bacteria like

Salmonella typhi are genetically modified to target cancer cells and carry nanobots (bacteriobots) to these cells for specific drug delivery. Bacteriobots can specifically detect malignant cancers, such as breast and colorectal cancers (Park et al. 2013).

1.8 Concluding Remarks

Nanoparticle research in the field of medicine has indeed opened a new door for advanced "magical" therapeutic and imaging applications. Due to their nanosize and ability to target cells specifically, nanoparticles can be used in many areas of medicine where drug-based or conventional physio-surgical treatments are difficult to administer. With a wide range of nanoparticles, starting from simple micelles to specialized multimodal nanoparticles, the developing field of nanomedicine has the edge over the latest-available free drug formulations. Nanoparticles are also used as delivery vehicles for genes, *si*RNAs and *mi*RNAs which act as key therapeutic molecules in gene therapeutic strategies. Similarly, by the development of specialized and less-toxic QDs, the scope of in vivo real-time imaging has strengthened over time. Modern nanotechnological interventions such as nanobots and nano-fortified surfaces are the future's promises for a toxicity-free targeted therapy, with improving recognition of personalized medicine. Cancer, one of the conditions that outlive human medical interventions, has shown surrendering feat to nanoparticle-based targeted delivery systems. The major limitation is the high cost of technology for commercial uses and few works on understanding toxicological profiles. With many ingenious inventions and discoveries in biotechnological and nanotechnological fields, it is just a matter of inputting creativity, perseverance, and resources for combining these two theoretically diverse fields into a novel and feasible cancer therapeutic or imaging strategy.

References

Abdifetah O, Na-Bangchang K (2019) Pharmacokinetic studies of nanoparticles as a delivery system for conventional drugs and herb-derived compounds for cancer therapy: a systematic review. Int J Nanomedicine 14:5659–5677

Agarwal A et al (2009) Dextran conjugated dendritic nanoconstructs as potential vectors for anti-cancer agent. Biomaterials 30(21):3588–3596

Agostinis P et al (2011) Photodynamic therapy of cancer: an update. CA Cancer J Clin 61 (4):250–281

Ahmad N et al (2019) Daunorubicin oral bioavailability enhancement by surface coated natural biodegradable macromolecule chitosan based polymeric nanoparticles. Int J Biol Macromol 128:825–838

Ainslie Lab, The University of North Carolina at Chapel Hill (n.d.) Timeline of therapeutic nanoparticles. https://ainslielab.web.unc.edu/support/timeline-of-nanoparticles/. Accessed 28 Aug 2020

Akakuru OU et al (2018) Utility of nanomedicine for cancer treatment. J Nanomed Nanotechnol 09:481

Amdursky N et al (2010) Elementary building blocks of self-assembled peptide nanotubes. J Am Chem Soc 132(44):15632–15636
Andey T et al (2015) Lipid nanocarriers of a lipid-conjugated estrogenic derivative inhibit tumor growth and enhance cisplatin activity against triple-negative breast cancer: pharmacokinetic and efficacy evaluation. Mol Pharm 12(4):1105–1120
Astruc D (2015) Introduction to nanomedicine, in molecules. p E4
Austin Birmingham Court (n.d.) Nanotechnology. https://austincourt.theiet.org/engineering-exhibits-at-austin-court/100-ideas/nanotechnology/. Accessed 28 Aug 2020
Babu A et al (2014) Nanodrug delivery systems: a promising technology for detection, diagnosis, and treatment of cancer. AAPS PharmSciTech 15(3):709–721
Batrakova EV et al (2006) Polymer Micelles as Drug Carriers. In: Nanoparticulates as Drug Carriers. Imperial College Press, London, pp 57–93
Bernabeu E et al (2014) Paclitaxel-loaded PCL-TPGS nanoparticles: in vitro and in vivo performance compared with Abraxane®. Colloids Surf B Biointerfaces 113:43–50
Berners-Price SJ, Norman RE, Sadler PJ (1987) The autoxidation and proton dissociation constants of tertiary diphosphines: relevance to biological activity. J Inorg Biochem 31(3):197–209
Bhattacharya R, Mukherjee P (2008) Biological properties of "naked" metal nanoparticles. Adv Drug Deliv Rev 60(11):1289–1306
Bhattacharyya S et al (2011) Inorganic nanoparticles in cancer therapy. Pharm Res 28(2):237–259
Bisht S et al (2007) Polymeric nanoparticle-encapsulated curcumin ("nanocurcumin"): a novel strategy for human cancer therapy. J Nanobiotechnol 5:3
Blanco MD et al (2012) Targeted nanoparticles for cancer therapy. In: Recent advances in novel drug carrier systems. InTech, Rijeka
Bolhassani A et al (2014) Polymeric nanoparticles: potent vectors for vaccine delivery targeting cancer and infectious diseases. Hum Vaccin Immunother 10(2):321–332
Buzea C, Pacheco II, Robbie K (2007) Nanomaterials and nanoparticles: sources and toxicity. Biointerphases 2(4):Mr17–Mr71
Campolongo MJ et al (2010) DNA nanomedicine: engineering DNA as a polymer for therapeutic and diagnostic applications. Adv Drug Deliv Rev 62(6):606–616
Chao Y et al (2017) Biodegradable polymersomes as nanocarriers for doxorubicin hydrochloride: enhanced cytotoxicity in MCF-7/ADR cells and prolonged blood circulation. Pharm Res 34 (3):610–618
Chaudhari VS, Murty US, Banerjee S (2020) Lipidic nanomaterials to deliver natural compounds against cancer: a review. Environ Chem Lett 18:1803–1812
Chen YH et al (2007) Methotrexate conjugated to gold nanoparticles inhibits tumor growth in a syngeneic lung tumor model. Mol Pharm 4(5):713–722
Chen F-H et al (2010a) Synthesis of a novel magnetic drug delivery system composed of doxorubicin-conjugated Fe3O4 nanoparticle cores and a PEG-functionalized porous silica shell. Chem Commun 46(45):8633–8635
Chen Y et al (2010b) Nanoparticles modified with tumor-targeting scFv deliver siRNA and miRNA for cancer therapy. Mol Ther 18(9):1650–1656
Chen J et al (2014) Reducible polyamidoamine-magnetic iron oxide self-assembled nanoparticles for doxorubicin delivery. Biomaterials 35(4):1240–1248
Chen JF et al (2016) Clinical applications of NanoVelcro rare-cell assays for detection and characterization of circulating tumor cells. Theranostics 6(9):1425–1439
Chen T et al (2018) DNA nanotechnology for cancer diagnosis and therapy. Int J Mol Sci 19 (6):1671
Cho K et al (2008) Therapeutic nanoparticles for drug delivery in cancer. Clin Cancer Res 14 (5):1310
Chou CY et al (2013) Investigation of the spatiotemporal responses of nanoparticles in tumor tissues with a small-scale mathematical model. PLoS One 8(4):e59135
Contributors W (n.d.-a) Colloidal gold-history. https://en.wikipedia.org/wiki/Colloidal_gold#History. Accessed 28 Aug 2020

Contributors W (n.d.-b) Chemotherapy. https://en.wikipedia.org/w/index.php?title=Chemotherapy&oldid=974974356. Accessed 28 Aug 2020
Contributors W (n.d.-c) Radiation therapy. https://en.wikipedia.org/w/index.php?title=Radiation_therapy&oldid=972018541. Accessed 28 Aug 2020
Contributors W (n.d.-d) Radiofrequency ablation. https://en.wikipedia.org/w/index.php?title=Radiofrequency_ablation&oldid=967230894. Accessed 28 Aug 2020
Contributors W (n.d.-e) Immunotherapy. https://en.wikipedia.org/w/index.php?title=Immunotherapy&oldid=975216053. Accessed 28 Aug 2020
Contributors W (n.d.-f) Sipuleucel-T. https://en.wikipedia.org/w/index.php?title=Sipuleucel-T&oldid=971415889. Accessed 28 Aug 2020
Contributors W (n.d.-g) Arsphenamine. https://en.wikipedia.org/w/index.php?title=Arsphenamine&oldid=964109444. Accessed 28 Aug 2020
Contributors W (n.d.-h) Alexey Ekimov. https://en.wikipedia.org/w/index.php?title=Alexey_Ekimov&oldid=889227335. Accessed 28 Aug 2020
Contributors W (n.d.-i) Louis E. Brus. https://en.wikipedia.org/w/index.php?title=Louis_E._Brus&oldid=959407673. Accessed 28 Aug 2020
Contributors W (n.d.-j) Rubitecan. https://en.wikipedia.org/w/index.php?title=Rubitecan&oldid=962990736. Accessed 28 Aug 2020
Contributors W (n.d.-k) Vitronectin. https://en.wikipedia.org/w/index.php?title=Vitronectin&oldid=951200820. Accessed 28 Aug 2020
Contributors W (n.d.-l) Hyaluronic acid. https://en.wikipedia.org/w/index.php?title=Hyaluronic_acid&oldid=973183009. Accessed 28 Aug 2020
Cunha F et al (2018) Development of nanoparticulate systems with action in breast and ovarian cancer: nanotheragnostics. J Drug Target 27:1–23
Daldrup-Link HE et al (2003) Quantification of breast tumor microvascular permeability with feruglose-enhanced MR imaging: initial phase II multicenter trial. Radiology 229(3):885–892
Das S, Chaudhury A (2011) Recent advances in lipid nanoparticle formulations with solid matrix for oral drug delivery. AAPS PharmSciTech 12(1):62–76
de Lussanet QG et al (2003) Gadopentetate dimeglumine versus ultrasmall superparamagnetic iron oxide for dynamic contrast-enhanced MR imaging of tumor angiogenesis in human colon carcinoma in mice. Radiology 229(2):429–438
Derakhshandeh K, Erfan M, Dadashzadeh S (2007) Encapsulation of 9-nitrocamptothecin, a novel anticancer drug, in biodegradable nanoparticles: factorial design, characterization and release kinetics. Eur J Pharm Biopharm 66(1):34–41
DeVita VT, Lawrence TS, Rosenberg SA (2008) DeVita, Hellman, and Rosenberg's cancer: principles & practice of oncology. Cancer: principles & practice (2 Vol). Wolters Kluwer/Lippincott Williams & Wilkins, Philadelphia
Ding Y et al (2008) Poly-L-lysine/hydroxyapatite/carbon nanotube hybrid nanocomposite applied for piezoelectric immunoassay of carbohydrate antigen 19-9. Analyst 133(2):184–190
Dobson J (2006) Magnetic nanoparticles for drug delivery. Drug Dev Res 67(1):55–60
Douglas SM, Bachelet I, Church GM (2012) A logic-gated nanorobot for targeted transport of molecular payloads. Science 335(6070):831
Düzgüneş N, Gregoriadis G (2005) Introduction: the origins of liposomes: Alec Bangham at Babraham. In: Methods in enzymology. Academic Press, Cambridge, MA, pp 1–3
Elzoghby AO et al (2013) Ionically-crosslinked milk protein nanoparticles as flutamide carriers for effective anticancer activity in prostate cancer-bearing rats. Eur J Pharm Biopharm 85(3 Pt A):444–451
Ernsting MJ et al (2012) Preclinical pharmacokinetic, biodistribution, and anti-cancer efficacy studies of a docetaxel-carboxymethylcellulose nanoparticle in mouse models. Biomaterials 33(5):1445–1454
Estelrich J, Busquets MA (2018) Iron oxide nanoparticles in photothermal therapy. Molecules 23(7):1567

Estrada CR et al (2006) Behavioral profiling of human transitional cell carcinoma ex vivo. Cancer Res 66(6):3078–3086
European Inventor Award-European Patent Office (2017) Fighting cancer with nanotechnology. https://www.epo.org/news-events/events/european-inventor/finalists/2013/couvreur/feature.html. Accessed 28 Aug 2020
European Science Foundation policy briefing-ESF scientific forward look on nanomedicine. 2005. http://archives.esf.org/fileadmin/Public_documents/Publications/Nanomedicine_01.pdf
Fan Z et al (2014) Theranostic nanomedicine for cancer detection and treatment. J Food Drug Anal 22(1):3–17
Fang M et al (2012) Quantum dots for cancer research: current status, remaining issues, and future perspectives. Cancer Biol Med 9(3):151–163
Farokhzad OC et al (2004) Nanoparticle-Aptamer Bioconjugates. Cancer Res 64(21):7668
Farrer NJ, Salassa L, Sadler PJ (2009) Photoactivated chemotherapy (PACT): the potential of excited-state d-block metals in medicine. Dalton Trans 48:10690–10701
Feng S-S et al (2007) Chemotherapeutic engineering: vitamin E TPGS-emulsified nanoparticles of biodegradable polymers realized sustainable paclitaxel chemotherapy for 168h in vivo. Chem Eng Sci 62(23):6641–6648
Ferrari M (2005) Cancer nanotechnology: opportunities and challenges. Nat Rev Cancer 5 (3):161–171
Gálisová A et al (2020) Glycogen as an advantageous polymer carrier in cancer theranostics: straightforward in vivo evidence. Sci Rep 10(1):10411
Gao Y et al (2016) Nanoemulsion enhances α-tocopherol succinate bioavailability in rats. Int J Pharm 515(1–2):506–514
Gradishar WJ (2006) Albumin-bound paclitaxel: a next-generation taxane. Expert Opin Pharmacother 7(8):1041–1053
Grange JM, Stanford JL, Stanford CA (2002) Campbell De Morgan's 'Observations on cancer', and their relevance today. J R Soc Med 95(6):296–299
Gulfam M et al (2012) Anticancer drug-loaded gliadin nanoparticles induce apoptosis in breast cancer cells. Langmuir 28(21):8216–8223
Guo Y et al (2014) Chitosan-g-TPGS nanoparticles for anticancer drug delivery and overcoming multidrug resistance. Mol Pharm 11(1):59–70
Haiduc I, Silvestru C (1989) Rhodium, iridium, copper and gold antitumor organometallic compounds (review). In vivo (Athens, Greece) 3(4):285–293
Han J et al (2014) Cationic bovine serum albumin based self-assembled nanoparticles as siRNA delivery vector for treating lung metastatic cancer. Small 10(3):524–535
Han L et al (2016) A facile route to form self-carried redox-responsive vorinostat nanodrug for effective solid tumor therapy. Int J Nanomedicine 11:6003–6022
Hanessian S et al (2008) Synthesis of chemically functionalized superparamagnetic nanoparticles as delivery vectors for chemotherapeutic drugs. Bioorg Med Chem 16(6):2921–2931
He H et al (2019) Survey of clinical translation of cancer nanomedicines—lessons learned from successes and failures. Acc Chem Res 52:2445–2461
Ho KS et al (2012) Amphiphilic micelles of poly(2-methyl-2-carboxytrimethylene carbonate-co-D, L-lactide)-graft-poly(ethylene glycol) for anti-cancer drug delivery to solid tumours. Biomaterials 33(7):2223–2229
Hofheinz R-D et al (2005) Liposomal encapsulated anti-cancer drugs. Anti-Cancer Drugs 16 (7):691–707
Hong S et al (2020) Protein-based nanoparticles as drug delivery systems. Pharmaceutics 12(7):604
Hossen S et al (2019) Smart nanocarrier-based drug delivery systems for cancer therapy and toxicity studies: a review. J Adv Res 15:1–18
Ibrahim MA, Hazhirkarzar B, Dublin AB (2020) Magnetic Resonance Imaging (MRI) Gadolinium. In: StatPearls. StatPearls Publishing, Treasure Island, FL
Jacob J et al (2018) Biopolymer based nanomaterials in drug delivery systems: a review. Mater Today Chem 9:43–55

Jain RK (1999) Transport of molecules, particles, and cells in solid tumors. Annu Rev Biomed Eng 1(1):241–263
Jain A et al (2010) Mannosylated solid lipid nanoparticles as vectors for site-specific delivery of an anti-cancer drug. J Control Release 148(3):359–367
Janko C et al (2019) Functionalized superparamagnetic iron oxide nanoparticles (SPIONs) as platform for the targeted multimodal tumor therapy. Front Oncol 9:59
Jiang XH et al (1995) The antihepatoma effect of lyophilized aclacinomycin a polyisobutylcyanoacrylate nanoparticles in vitro and in vivo. Yao Xue Xue Bao 30(3):179–183
Jiang X et al (2020) Preparation and evaluation of novel emodin-loaded stearic acid-g-chitosan oligosaccharide nanomicelles. Nanoscale Res Lett 15(1):93
Jokerst JV et al (2009) Nano-bio-chips for high performance multiplexed protein detection: determinations of cancer biomarkers in serum and saliva using quantum dot bioconjugate labels. Biosens Bioelectron 24(12):3622–3629
Jordan A et al (2006) The effect of thermotherapy using magnetic nanoparticles on rat malignant glioma. J Neuro-Oncol 78(1):7–14
Jose J et al (2020) Magnetic nanoparticles for hyperthermia in cancer treatment: an emerging tool. Environ Sci Pollut Res 27(16):19214–19225
Kalaria DR et al (2009) Design of biodegradable nanoparticles for oral delivery of doxorubicin: in vivo pharmacokinetics and toxicity studies in rats. Pharm Res 26(3):492–501
Karra N et al (2013) Antibody conjugated PLGA nanoparticles for targeted delivery of paclitaxel palmitate: efficacy and biofate in a lung cancer mouse model. Small 9(24):4221–4236
Khare V et al (2016) Long-circulatory nanoparticles for gemcitabine delivery: development and investigation of pharmacokinetics and in-vivo anticancer efficacy. Eur J Pharm Sci 92:183–193
Khosa A, Reddi S, Saha RN (2018) Nanostructured lipid carriers for site-specific drug delivery. Biomed Pharmacother 103:598–613
Khurana RK et al (2017) Enhancing biopharmaceutical performance of an anticancer drug by long chain PUFA based self-nanoemulsifying lipidic nanomicellar systems. Eur J Pharm Biopharm 121:42–60
Kircher MF et al (2003) In vivo high resolution three-dimensional imaging of antigen-specific cytotoxic T-lymphocyte trafficking to tumors. Cancer Res 63(20):6838
Kobayashi H et al (2003) Micro-magnetic resonance lymphangiography in mice using a novel dendrimer-based magnetic resonance imaging contrast agent. Cancer Res 63(2):271–276
Koizumi F et al (2006) Novel SN-38-incorporating polymeric micelles, NK012, eradicate vascular endothelial growth factor-secreting bulky tumors. Cancer Res 66(20):10048–10056
Krishna Sailaja A, Amareshwar P, Chakravarty P (2011) Current pharma research formulation of solid lipid nanoparticles and their applications. Curr Pharma Res 1:197–203
Kumar D et al (2020) Antibody-targeted nanoparticles for cancer treatment. In: Saxena SK, Khurana SMP (eds) NanoBioMedicine. Springer, Singapore, pp 35–65
Kunjiappan S et al (2018) Design graph theoretical analysis and in silico modeling of Dunaliella Bardawil biomass encapsulated N-Succinyl chitosan nanoparticles for enhanced anticancer activity. Anti Cancer Agents Med Chem 18(13):1900–1918
Langley RR, Fidler IJ (2011) The seed and soil hypothesis revisited--the role of tumor-stroma interactions in metastasis to different organs. Int J Cancer 128(11):2527–2535
Lawaczeck R et al (1997) Magnetic iron oxide particles coated with carboxydextran for parenteral administration and liver contrasting. Pre-clinical profile of SH U555A. Acta Radiol 38(4 Pt 1):584–597
Lee JY et al (2014) Poly(styrene)-b-poly(DL-lactide) copolymer-based nanoparticles for anticancer drug delivery. Int J Nanomedicine 9:2803–2813
Lee BK, Yun YH, Park K (2015) Smart nanoparticles for drug delivery: boundaries and opportunities. Chem Eng Sci 125:158–164
Lee JY et al (2016) Polyethylene glycol-conjugated chondroitin sulfate A derivative nanoparticles for tumor-targeted delivery of anticancer drugs. Carbohydr Polym 151:68–77

Li S et al (2008) Pharmacokinetic characteristics and anticancer effects of 5-fluorouracil loaded nanoparticles. BMC Cancer 8:103
Lin M et al (2014) Nanostructure embedded microchips for detection, isolation, and characterization of circulating tumor cells. Acc Chem Res 47(10):2941–2950
Liu D et al (2016) The smart drug delivery system and its clinical potential. Theranostics 6 (9):1306–1323
Lohcharoenkal W et al (2014) Protein nanoparticles as drug delivery carriers for cancer therapy. Biomed Res Int 2014:180549
Lombardo D, Kiselev MA, Caccamo MT (2019) Smart nanoparticles for drug delivery application: development of versatile nanocarrier platforms in biotechnology and nanomedicine. J Nanomater 2019:26
Ma YY et al (2017) Molecular imaging of cancer with nanoparticle-based theranostic probes. Contrast Media Mol Imaging 2017:1026270
Madhwi et al (2017) In vivo pharmacokinetic studies and intracellular delivery of methotrexate by means of glycine-tethered PLGA-based polymeric micelles. Int J Pharm 519(1–2):138–144
Markman M (2006) Pegylated liposomal doxorubicin in the treatment of cancers of the breast and ovary. Expert Opin Pharmacother 7(11):1469–1474
Medarova Z et al (2006) In vivo imaging of tumor response to therapy using a dual-modality imaging strategy. Int J Cancer 118(11):2796–2802
Medical and Editorial Content Team, American Cancer Society (2014) History of cancer. https://www.cancer.org/cancer/cancer-basics/history-of-cancer
MG K et al (2015) History and possible uses of nanomedicine based on nanoparticles and nanotechnological progress. J Nanomed Nanotechnol. https://doi.org/10.4172/2157-7439.1000336
Mikhaylova M et al (2009) Imaging of cationic multifunctional liposome-mediated delivery of COX-2 siRNA. Cancer Gene Ther 16(3):217–226
Mineo C, Anderson RG (2001) Potocytosis. Robert Feulgen lecture. Histochem Cell Biol 116 (2):109–118
Mitra A et al (2006) Nanocarriers for nuclear imaging and radiotherapy of cancer. Curr Pharm Des 12(36):4729–4749
Mosbach K, Schröder U (1979) Preparation and application of magnetic polymers for targeting of drugs. FEBS Lett 102(1):112–116
Mottaghitalab F et al (2017) Targeted delivery system based on gemcitabine-loaded silk fibroin nanoparticles for lung cancer therapy. ACS Appl Mater Interfaces 9(37):31600–31611
Nano.gov-US National Nanotechnology Initiative (n.d.) Nanotechnology timeline. https://www.nano.gov/timeline. Accessed 28 Aug 2020
Nanotechnology panel-American Chemistry Council (n.d.) The NANO timeline-a BIG history of the very SMALL. https://nanotechnology.americanchemistry.com/Nanotechnology-Timeline/. Accessed 28 Aug 2020
Nardelli F et al (2018) Succinimide-based conjugates improve IsoDGR cyclopeptide affinity to α(v)β(3) without promoting integrin allosteric activation. J Med Chem 61(17):7474–7485
Nisha CK et al (2004) Complexes of poly(ethylene glycol)-based cationic random copolymer and calf thymus DNA: a complete biophysical characterization. Langmuir 20(6):2386–2396
Noble GT et al (2014) Ligand-targeted liposome design: challenges and fundamental considerations. Trends Biotechnol 32(1):32–45
Nyman DW et al (2005) Phase I and pharmacokinetics trial of ABI-007, a novel nanoparticle formulation of paclitaxel in patients with advanced nonhematologic malignancies. J Clin Oncol 23(31):7785–7793
Observatory GC (2018) Cancer tomorrow. International Agency for Research on Cancer, World Health Organization. https://gco.iarc.fr/tomorrow/home
Ohtani S et al (2007) Tumor suppressor 101F6 and ascorbate synergistically and selectively inhibit non-small cell lung cancer growth by caspase-independent apoptosis and autophagy. Cancer Res 67(13):6293–6303

Oliveira AM et al (2013) Nano spray drying as an innovative technology for encapsulating hydrophilic active pharmaceutical ingredients (API). J Nanomed Nanotechnol 4(6):1–6
Onoue S, Yamada S, Chan HK (2014) Nanodrugs: pharmacokinetics and safety. Int J Nanomedicine 9:1025–1037
Park SJ et al (2013) New paradigm for tumor theranostic methodology using bacteria-based microrobot. Sci Rep 3(1):3394
Patra HK, Dasgupta AK (2012) Cancer cell response to nanoparticles: criticality and optimality. Nanomedicine 8(6):842–852
Patra CR et al (2008) Application of gold nanoparticles for targeted therapy in cancer. J Biomed Nanotechnol 4(2):99–132
Patra JK et al (2018) Nano based drug delivery systems: recent developments and future prospects. J Nanobiotechnol 16(1):71
Peer D et al (2007) Nanocarriers as an emerging platform for cancer therapy. Nat Nanotechnol 2 (12):751–760
Pirollo KF et al (2007) Materializing the potential of small interfering RNA via a tumor-targeting nanodelivery system. Cancer Res 67(7):2938–2943
Pisanic Ii T, Zhang Y, Wang T (2014) Quantum dots in diagnostics and detection: principles and paradigms. Analyst 139:2968–2981
Porcel E et al (2010) Platinum nanoparticles: a promising material for future cancer therapy? Nanotechnology 21(8):085103
Qiao H et al (2013) Synthesis and characterization of multi-functional linear-dendritic block copolymer for intracellular delivery of antitumor drugs. Int J Pharm 452(1–2):363–373
Qu QL et al (2006) Intraperitoneal chemotherapy with mitomycin C bound to activated carbon nanoparticles for nude mice bearing human gastric carcinoma. Zhonghua Zhong Liu Za Zhi 28 (4):257–260
Rafiei P, Haddadi A (2017) Docetaxel-loaded PLGA and PLGA-PEG nanoparticles for intravenous application: pharmacokinetics and biodistribution profile. Int J Nanomedicine 12:935–947
Ramazanov M, Karimova A, Shirinova H (2020) Magnetism for drug delivery, MRI and hyperthermia applications: a review. Biointerface Res Appl Chem 11(2):14
Ramesh R et al (2004) Local and systemic inhibition of lung tumor growth after nanoparticle-mediated mda-7/IL-24 gene delivery. DNA Cell Biol 23(12):850–857
Rivera E (2003) Current status of liposomal anthracycline therapy in metastatic breast cancer. Clin Breast Cancer 4:S76–S83
Rosenthal E et al (2002) Phase IV study of liposomal daunorubicin (DaunoXome) in AIDS-related Kaposi sarcoma. Am J Clin Oncol 25(1):57–59
Rothemund PW (2006) Folding DNA to create nanoscale shapes and patterns. Nature 440 (7082):297–302
Ruoslahti E (2012) Peptides as targeting elements and tissue penetration devices for nanoparticles. Adv Mater 24(28):3747–3756
Sahay G, Alakhova DY, Kabanov AV (2010) Endocytosis of nanomedicines. J Control Release 145 (3):182–195
Sanhai WR et al (2008) Seven challenges for nanomedicine. Nat Nanotechnol 3(5):242–244
Sapra P, Allen TM (2003) Ligand-targeted liposomal anticancer drugs. Prog Lipid Res 42 (5):439–462
Saremi S et al (2013) Enhanced oral delivery of docetaxel using thiolated chitosan nanoparticles: preparation, in vitro and in vivo studies. Biomed Res Int 2013:150478
Sargazi A et al (2018) Hyaluronan magnetic nanoparticle for mitoxantrone delivery toward CD44-positive cancer cells. Colloids Surf B Biointerfaces 171:150–158
Sawant RR, Torchilin VP (2012) Challenges in development of targeted liposomal therapeutics. AAPS J 14(2):303–315
Schneider YJ et al (1984) Drug targeting in human cancer chemotherapy. In: Gregoriadis G et al (eds) Receptor-mediated targeting of drugs. Springer, Boston, MA, pp 1–25
Seeman NC (2003) DNA nanotechnology. Mater Today 6(1):24–29

Seeman NC (2010) Nanomaterials based on DNA. Annu Rev Biochem 79:65–87
Senthilkumar M, Mishra P, Jain NK (2008) Long circulating PEGylated poly(D,L-lactide-co-glycolide) nanoparticulate delivery of docetaxel to solid tumors. J Drug Target 16(5):424–435
Senyei A, Widder K, Czerlinski G (1978) Magnetic guidance of drug-carrying microspheres. J Appl Phys 49(6):3578–3583
Seo S-J et al (2015) Tumor-targeting co-delivery of drug and gene from temperature-triggered micelles. Macromol Biosci 15(9):1198–1204
Shalaby KS et al (2016) Nanoparticles based on linear and star-shaped poly(ethylene glycol)-poly (ε-caprolactone) copolymers for the delivery of antitubulin drug. Pharm Res 33(8):2010–2024
Sharma AK et al (2018) Chitosan engineered PAMAM dendrimers as nanoconstructs for the enhanced anti-cancer potential and improved in vivo brain pharmacokinetics of temozolomide. Pharm Res 35(1):9
Shavi GV et al (2015) Nanomedicine of anastrozole for breast cancer: physicochemical evaluation, in vitro cytotoxicity on BT-549 and MCF-7 cell lines and preclinical study on rat model. Life Sci 141:143–155
Shi J et al (2010) Nanotechnology in drug delivery and tissue engineering: from discovery to applications. Nano Lett 10(9):3223–3230
Shi J et al (2017) Cancer nanomedicine: progress, challenges and opportunities. Nat Rev Cancer 17 (1):20–37
Shidhaye SS et al (2008) Solid lipid nanoparticles and nanostructured lipid carriers – innovative generations of solid lipid carriers. Curr Drug Deliv 5(4):324–331
Singh N et al (2010) Potential toxicity of superparamagnetic iron oxide nanoparticles (SPION). Nano Rev 1(1):5358
Sturesson C, Carlfors J (2000) Incorporation of protein in PLG-microspheres with retention of bioactivity. J Control Release 67(2–3):171–178
Sumer B, Gao J (2008) Theranostic nanomedicine for cancer. Nanomedicine 3(2):137–140
Sun D-X et al (2012) Nanoparticle-mediated local delivery of an antisense TGF-β1 construct inhibits intimal hyperplasia in autogenous vein grafts in rats. PLoS One 7(7):e41857
Sun T et al (2014) Engineered nanoparticles for drug delivery in cancer therapy. Angew Chem Int Ed 53(46):12320–12364
Sutton D et al (2007) Functionalized micellar systems for cancer targeted drug delivery. Pharm Res 24(6):1029–1046
Takakura Y et al (1990) Disposition characteristics of macromolecules in tumor-bearing mice. Pharm Res 7(4):339–346
Tan W et al (2011) Molecular aptamers for drug delivery. Trends Biotechnol 29(12):634–640
Thevenot P et al (2008) Surface chemistry influences cancer killing effect of TiO2 nanoparticles. Nanomed Nanotechnol Biol Med 4(3):226–236
Tian XX, Groves MJ (1999) Formulation and biological activity of antineoplastic proteoglycans derived from Mycobacterium vaccae in chitosan nanoparticles. J Pharm Pharmacol 51 (2):151–157
Tolikas M (2012) Researchers at Harvard's Wyss Institute develop DNA Nanorobot to trigger targeted therapeutic response. Wyss Institute, Boston, MA
Tran S et al (2017) Cancer nanomedicine: a review of recent success in drug delivery. Clin Transl Med 6(1):44
Tréhin R et al (2006) Fluorescent nanoparticle uptake for brain tumor visualization. Neoplasia 8 (4):302–311
Tseng C-L et al (2008) Targeting efficiency and biodistribution of biotinylated-EGF-conjugated gelatin nanoparticles administered via aerosol delivery in nude mice with lung cancer. Biomaterials 29(20):3014–3022
Turetschek K et al (2001) MR imaging characterization of microvessels in experimental breast tumors by using a particulate contrast agent with histopathologic correlation. Radiology 218 (2):562–569
University of Montreal (2013) Nanomedicine: DNA clamp to grab cancer before it develops

Unsoy G et al (2014) Synthesis of doxorubicin loaded magnetic chitosan nanoparticles for pH responsive targeted drug delivery. Eur J Pharm Sci 62:243–250
Vafadar A et al (2020) Quercetin and cancer: new insights into its therapeutic effects on ovarian cancer cells. Cell Biosci 10:32
Varallyay P et al (2002) Comparison of two superparamagnetic viral-sized iron oxide particles ferumoxides and ferumoxtran-10 with a gadolinium chelate in imaging intracranial tumors. AJNR Am J Neuroradiol 23(4):510–519
Vardhan H et al (2017) Development of long-circulating docetaxel loaded poly (3-hydroxybutyrate-co-3-hydroxyvalerate) nanoparticles: optimization, pharmacokinetic, cytotoxicity and in vivo assessments. Int J Biol Macromol 103:791–801
Varghese SE et al (2016) Lecithin and PLGA-based self-assembled nanocomposite, Lecithmer: preparation, characterization, and pharmacokinetic/pharmacodynamic evaluation. Drug Deliv Transl Res 6(4):342–353
Veiseh O, Gunn JW, Zhang M (2010) Design and fabrication of magnetic nanoparticles for targeted drug delivery and imaging. Adv Drug Deliv Rev 62(3):284–304
Ventola CL (2012) The nanomedicine revolution: part 1: emerging concepts. 37(9):512–525
Verma RK, Garg S (2001) Current status of drug delivery technologies and future directions. Pharm Technol 25(2):1–14
Wang G, Uludag H (2008) Recent developments in nanoparticle-based drug delivery and targeting systems with emphasis on protein-based nanoparticles. Expert Opin Drug Deliv 5(5):499–515
Wang R, Billone PS, Mullett WM (2013) Nanomedicine in action: an overview of cancer nanomedicine on the market and in clinical trials. J Nanomater 2013:629681
Wang T-Y et al (2015) Ultrasound-guided delivery of microRNA loaded nanoparticles into cancer. J Control Release 203:99–108
Wang S et al (2016) Nanoparticle-mediated inhibition of survivin to overcome drug resistance in cancer therapy. J Control Release 240:454–464
Wang D et al (2018) Nucleoside analogue-based supramolecular nanodrugs driven by molecular recognition for synergistic cancer therapy. J Am Chem Soc 140(28):8797–8806
Web Team, Weekly Technology Times (2016) Magnetic hyperthermia. https://www.technologytimes.pk/2016/02/21/magnetic-hyperthermia-2/. Accessed 28 Aug 2020
Wissing SA, Kayser O, Müller RH (2004) Solid lipid nanoparticles for parenteral drug delivery. Adv Drug Deliv Rev 56(9):1257–1272
Woo HN et al (2012) Preclinical evaluation of injectable sirolimus formulated with polymeric nanoparticle for cancer therapy. Int J Nanomedicine 7:2197–2208
World Health Organization (2018) Cancer. https://www.who.int/news-room/fact-sheets/detail/cancer. Accessed 29 Aug 2020
Wu Y et al (2009) Fabrication of elastin-like polypeptide nanoparticles for drug delivery by electrospraying. Biomacromolecules 10(1):19–24
Xing Y et al (2006) Molecular profiling of single cancer cells and clinical tissue specimens with semiconductor quantum dots. Int J Nanomedicine 1(4):473–481
Xu Z, Kleinstreuer C (2018) Direct nanodrug delivery for tumor targeting subject to shear-augmented diffusion in blood flow. Med Biol Eng Comput 56(11):1949–1958
Xu Z, Kleinstreuer C (2019) Heterogeneous blood flow in microvessels with applications to nanodrug transport and mass transfer into tumor tissue. Biomech Model Mechanobiol 18 (1):99–110
Yang K et al (2001) Preparation of cucurbitacinBE polylactic acid nano-particles for targeting cervical lymph nodes. Hua Xi Kou Qiang Yi Xue Za Zhi 19(6):347–350
Yang L et al (2007) Preparation, characterization and biodistribution of the lactone form of 10-hydroxycamptothecin (HCPT)-loaded bovine serum albumin (BSA) nanoparticles. Int J Pharm 340(1–2):163–172
Yang L et al (2009) Receptor-targeted nanoparticles for in vivo imaging of breast cancer. Clin Cancer Res 15(14):4722–4732

Ye M et al (2013) Targeted biodegradable dendritic MRI contrast agent for enhanced tumor imaging. J Control Release 169(3):239–245
Yigit MV, Moore A, Medarova Z (2012) Magnetic nanoparticles for cancer diagnosis and therapy. Pharm Res 29(5):1180–1188
Yin PT, Shah BP, Lee K-B (2014) Combined magnetic nanoparticle-based MicroRNA and hyperthermia therapy to enhance apoptosis in brain cancer cells. Small 10(20):4106–4112
Yu JM et al (2009) Polymeric nanoparticles of cholesterol-modified glycol chitosan for doxorubicin delivery: preparation and in-vitro and in-vivo characterization. J Pharm Pharmacol 61 (6):713–719
Yu MK et al (2011) Image-guided prostate cancer therapy using aptamer-functionalized thermally cross-linked superparamagnetic iron oxide nanoparticles. Small 7(15):2241–2249
Yu Y et al (2013) Antitumor activity of docetaxel-loaded polymeric nanoparticles fabricated by Shirasu porous glass membrane-emulsification technique. Int J Nanomedicine 8:2641–2652
Yuan ZP et al (2006) Nanoliposomal quercetin inhibits formation of malignant ascites of hepatocellular carcinoma. Ai Zheng 25(8):941–945
Zabaleta V et al (2012) Oral administration of paclitaxel with pegylated poly(anhydride) nanoparticles: permeability and pharmacokinetic study. Eur J Pharm Biopharm 81(3):514–523
Zhang H et al (2016) Chitosan-based nanoparticles for improved anticancer efficacy and bioavailability of mifepristone. Beilstein J Nanotechnol 7:1861–1870
Zhao J, Stenzel MH (2018) Entry of nanoparticles into cells: the importance of nanoparticle properties. Polym Chem 9(3):259–272
Zhao Z, Li Y, Xie MB (2015a) Silk fibroin-based nanoparticles for drug delivery. Int J Mol Sci 16 (3):4880–4903
Zhao Y et al (2015b) Nanodrug formed by coassembly of dual anticancer drugs to inhibit cancer cell drug resistance. ACS Appl Mater Interfaces 7(34):19295–19305
Zhen X et al (2013) Cellular uptake, antitumor response and tumor penetration of cisplatin-loaded milk protein nanoparticles. Biomaterials 34(4):1372–1382
Zheng J et al (2015) A multimodal nano agent for image-guided cancer surgery. Biomaterials 67:160–168
Zuany-Amorim C et al (2002) Long-term protective and antigen-specific effect of heat-killed *Mycobacterium vaccae* in a murine model of allergic pulmonary inflammation. J Immunol 169(3):1492
Zununi Vahed S et al (2017) Liposome-based drug co-delivery systems in cancer cells. Mater Sci Eng C 71:1327–1341

Strategies for Improving the Efficiency of Nanomaterials

2

Sukhendu Maity, Madhuchhanda Adhikari, Rajkumar Guchhait, Ankit Chatterjee, Ajishnu Roy, and Kousik Pramanick

Abstract

The complexities associated with spatiotemporal delivery of drugs in disease therapy from the biomedical viewpoint, gradual increase in pollution level in the mother environment, and the quest for renewable energy sources as an alternative to the use of fossil fuels make it highly anticipated the development of technologies averting the therapeutic complexities and providing a better way of environmental remediation and energy production. The advent of nanotechnologies and its recent progress could provide opportunities for dwindling the aforementioned problem. In this chapter, we tried to summarize different technological advancements for improving the efficiency of nanoparticles, especially in the field of nanomedicine. The crucial points to be emerged from this study are the physicochemical parameters, most importantly the size, shape, crystallinity, and surface chemistry which would be manipulated for qualitative functional improvement of nanoparticles; and also modifying the nanoparticles surface with molecules (peptide, antibody, protein, lipid, surfactant, small molecules, ligands, polyethylene glycol, etc.) tackling a particular therapeutic concern like cellular internalization, stability, solubility, immune clearance, drug targeting, etc. would be of immense therapeutic values.

Keywords

Nanoparticles · Nanomedicine · Physicochemical parameters · Therapeutics · Qualitative improvements

S. Maity · M. Adhikari · R. Guchhait · A. Chatterjee · A. Roy · K. Pramanick (✉)
Integrative Biology Research Unit (IBRU), Department of Life Sciences, Presidency University, Kolkata, India
e-mail: kousik.dbs@presiuniv.ac.in

A. Malik et al. (eds.), *Nanomedicine for Cancer Diagnosis and Therapy*,
https://doi.org/10.1007/978-981-15-7564-8_2

2.1 Introduction

The release of different pollutants, including organic pollutants, into the environment from various sources represents the caveat connected to their environmental monitoring and risks evaluation (Jing et al. 2013). The designing and successful implementation of different remedial measures could be considered as a promising challenge for a healthy environment. Employment of traditional remediation techniques in removing the environmental contaminants is still not competent enough to stop their emissions into the environment completely. The extensive use of fossil fuels might lead to the exhaustion of their natural sources in the near future. In order to deal with the relevant problems of the environment, energy conservation, and disease therapy, the advancement of nanotechnologies has attracted much attention. The particles measuring a size of less than 100 nm are defined as nanoparticles. In this regard, the development of new technologies should be eco-friendly, inexpensive, and sustainable.

In many cases, the clinical improvements or successful implications of therapeutics in order to treat or decrease the symptoms of some ailments (cancer, Alzheimer's, autoimmune diseases, diabetes, etc.) require the tissue/organelle-specific targeting of therapeutic species/agents in a spatiotemporal manner (Sakhrani and Padh 2013). The biomedical implication of nanotechnologies has enabled us to bypass the problems of intracellular drug delivery as the nanoparticles in the form of nanocarriers are capable of crossing the physiological barriers reaching to the specific targets. Nanoparticles enabled the therapeutic agents to be delivered into the target organelles in a controlled way and thereby minimizing the side effects or mistargeting and also increasing the functional efficiency through the qualitative enrichment at target sites. Different molecular targets for a given therapeutic agent may be distributed throughout the entire cellular space, including cytoplasm and different organelles. The low pH and the abundance of proteolytic enzymes in lysosomes and endosomes might influence the chemical degradation or nonspecific distribution of drugs. The advancement of nanobiotechnology enabled the engineering of nanoparticles with desired attributes required to circumvent the major impediments for the successful treatment of diseases , including cancer. High bioavailability, stability, longer half-life, permeability, and target specificity are the key properties to be determined carefully while designing a drug with greater therapeutic efficiency. The fascinating, unique surface chemistry, composition, small size, and high surface to volume ratio of nanoparticles have attracted much attention for designing and synthesis of nanomedicines having high pharmacokinetics, pharmacodynamics, and therapeutic index. The remodeling of nanoparticles through the fine-tuning of their key surface properties may ameliorate the therapeutic values of nanomedicines by means of their high drug loading capacity, increasing circulation time, and enhanced permeation and retention effects (EPR). The evolution of nanomedicine has enabled us to tackle the associated problems of target specific drug delivery and their controlled release. The qualitative enrichment of nanomedicines requires their strategic modulations, and here, we addressed different strategies used to increase the efficiency of nanoparticles especially from therapeutic viewpoints.

The enhanced accumulation of nanomedicine is required for cancer therapy. Naturally, the angiogenesis in neoplastic cells is accompanied by aberrant blood vessels formation having pores and fenestrations. This unique property of angiogenic blood vessels together with the poor drainage system leads to the accumulation of extravasated nanoparticles in tumors but it is the type of tumors and disease progression status that determine the permeability, accumulation of nanoparticles in tumor cells. So nanotherapy of tumors requires the strategic development of nanomedicine with enhanced permeability and retention effects (Villaverde and Baeza 2019).

The size and shape are the two attributes of nanoparticles to be determined meticulously for the acceleration of EPR effects as the too small (<5 nm) or too large (>200 nm) nanoparticles are subject for renal clearance and hampered extravasation from aberrant vasculature system in tumors, respectively. The non-spherical nanorods experience better frictional resistance (tumbling and rolling motions) than the spherical ones with similar hydrodynamic diameter. This phenomenon facilitates the longer interaction of nanoparticles with vessel wall and, therefore, their extravasation. Usually the size range 12–60 nm and non-spherical (elongated) nanoparticles show increased EPR effects (Stylianopoulos and Jain 2015). The size of the nanodrugs also affects their half-life in the circulatory system as the larger particles are relatively facile to recognize and engulf for liver and phagocytic cells. Polymer doping of nanodrugs like PEGylation of 200 nm nanoliposome enhances their longevity in blood but it is still not to the level of 100 nm liposome with the same coating (Chow and Ho 2013; Woodle et al. 1992).

So, it is clear that the size and surface structures are the two intriguing properties of nanomedicines affecting their EPR effects mediated passive targeting to the sites of tumors although the angiogenic aberrant vasculature system and the tumor types are known to regulate the passive targeting (Mattheolabakis et al. 2012). But this passive targeting often lacks the target specificity, consistency, and sometimes the desired therapeutic level of nanomedicine is not achieved at the site of their action. So, in order to overcome the concerned problems of passive targeting nanoparticles are formulated in a way to conjugate specific ligand molecules having elevated expression of cognate receptors at target sites (tumor cells or microenvironment). The process of active targeting of nanomedicines comprises a wide range of molecules including antibodies or engineered fragment of antibody, aptamers, peptides, small molecules, proteins, etc. (Mattheolabakis et al. 2012).

A suite of rewarding physical and chemical properties of nanomaterials has enabled us to use them as a remedial tool for resolving the critical issues of ecology, environment, and human health. Based on the available literatures the size, shape, material type, and surface properties including optical property, charge separation would be considered to be the key elemental properties of nanoparticles to be tuned with aim to increase the qualitative and functional efficiencies. The small-sized nanoparticles excerpt the high surface to volume ratio signifying the abundance of interaction centers on their surface. Crystals of nanoparticles (nanocrystals) adopt three crystalline phases—anatase (stable at high temperature), rutile, and brookite phases (metastable). Among these three phases anatase is considered to be the most active one. Under high temperature nanocrystals undergo phase transformation and agglomeration which eventually result in particle growth. So, the basic criteria central to the designing of efficient nanoparticles are the small size, high thermal stability, high crystallinity with minimum surface defects.

2.2 Strategies for the Improvement of Nanomaterials

2.2.1 Photocatalytic Efficiency

Use of metal oxide nanoparticles as semiconductor photocatalysis is thought of as the emerging and one of the most promising technologies in the near future for environmental remediation of organic pollutants from air and water, and renewable energy production. Semiconductor photocatalysis utilizes the solar energy catalyzing redox reactions on the surface of semiconductors and is being potentially used in the photocatalytic (1) synthesis of organic substances, (2) degradation of organic pollutants, (3) splitting of water, and (4) reduction of CO_2 (Jing et al. 2013; Yang et al. 2017). The peculiar band arrangement (electronic structure) on the surface of a semiconductor, i.e., the valence band (high energy electronic band; VB) and the conductance band (low energy electronic band; CB) separated by a band gap make it function as a photoactive material which upon photon incidence causes the photoexcitation of surface electron-hole pairs and subsequent separation of electron and hole (charge separation) catalyzes the oxidation-reduction reaction. So, the optical absorption, photoexcitation, and charge separation or simply absorption-excitation-separation form the underlying basis of photocatalytic performance of a photocatalyst. The size reduction or increase in surface area of photocatalyst, being the most widely used strategy to enhance the catalytic performance, has been adopted to develop more useful and efficient nanoscale photocatalyst. But the successful employment of nanosemiconductors suffers from some surface defects which could greatly impair the desired surface properties and in order to peter out the surface defects choosing suitable molecules for the structural and functional alteration(s) of nanosemiconductor is indispensable. Several oxide-based nanoparticles are in use as photocatalyst and superior performance requires minimum surface defects. Treatment of nanocrystals with elevated temperature is considered to be a good strategy to minimize the surface defects through enhanced surface crystallinity but following this strategy might cause the phase reversal from anatase to rutile, which is undesirable because of particle growth and hence the reduction of surface area. In this regard, increasing the thermal stability of nanocrystals is considered to be a suitable approach for enhanced surface properties with quality performance. This can be achieved by metal ion doping and surface binding of oxide, carbon, inorganic acid anion, and amine and ammonia surface (Yang et al. 2011; Jing et al. 2013). It is worth mentioning that the crystalline phase of nanocrystals depends on the ratio of O to H atoms on the surface of nanocrystals.

For example, the preponderance of O atoms stabilizes rutile phase while the H atoms stabilizes the anatase phase.

2.2.2 Therapeutic Efficiency

2.2.2.1 Strategic Improvement of Nanomaterials for Enhanced Permeability and Retention (EPR) Effects

Different physical-chemical properties, including size, shape, elasticity and stability, surface composition, and charge, greatly affect the cellular internalization of nanomaterials, and several strategies have been evolved for more efficient cellular uptake taking the modulation of these properties under consideration. The employment of nanotechnology in designing improved intracellular drug delivery systems requires the vigilance on fundamental issues to escape the modification or degradation of drugs induced by the robust environment of GIT, macrophage-mediated phagocytic pathway, nonspecific delivery of drugs and drug efflux pumps, and to retain the pharmacokinetics with original bioavailability during the course of transportation to the specific target cells. Once come in contact with the target cell nanomaterials follow the path of pre-adsorption, cellular uptake, translocation, and eventually interaction with target molecules.

The intracellular transport of nanoparticles is mainly achieved by paracellular and endocytic pathways. The paracellular pathway mediates the transport of hydrophilic drugs that in turn are regulated by the opening of tight junctions (TJs). In general, TJs restrict nanoparticle transport, so the chemical modification of nanocarriers in order to make them hydrophilic using permeation enhancer can be considered as a suitable approach to keep TJs reversibly open allowing transport of nanocarriers. A set of enhancers of high molecular weight (PPS-dimethyl palmitoyl ammonio propanesulfonate, lectin, self-assembling lipid-like peptides, chitosan, polyacrylate, and phytic acid) could be linked on the surface of nanocarriers to increase their cellular uptake through opening of TJs (paracellular routes). These enhancers keep TJs open as a consequence of the downregulation of TJs proteins (occludin and claudin) and enzymatic inhibition. Polyacrylate derivatives bind more strongly with cations (Ca+) regulating the opening of TJs. Thiomers (thiolated anionic and cationic polymers), chitosan, polyacrylate are the commonly used permeation enhancer. Thiomers conjugated nanoparticles appear to have enhanced mucosal adhesion and the ability to inhibit the enzymatic activity of protein tyrosine phosphatase (PTP) on the absorption surface. Disulfide bonds (–S–S–), which are formed by the reduction of thiol groups (–SH) present in mucosal glycoproteins, help in the adsorption of glycoproteins onto the surface of nanoparticles. On the other hand, the concomitant reduction of glutathione during the formation of disulfide bonds in mucosal glycoproteins, inhibits the function of protein tyrosine phosphatase (PTP) by binding to their cysteine containing active sites. These molecular events lead to an increase in the concentration of phosphorylated tyrosine in TJs, which keep them open (Clausen et al. 2002; Chen et al. 2013). This is an effective way to improve the permeation property of nanomaterials. Sodium orthovanadate could also function to improve the permeability through TJs as it is the case in bovine corneal epithelial cells. Polyethylenimine (PEI) enhances the membrane permeability for the cellular uptake of nanocarriers (Fig. 2.1a).

The blood–brain barrier (BBR) represents a special type of physiological barrier that sequesters the cerebrospinal compartment from the systemic circulation system. The passing of drugs through blood–brain barrier that usually hampers the movement of larger molecules or particles is indispensable for the treatment of many diseases, including tumor. So it is a promising challenge in the field of nanotechnology to design nanomedicine so as to confirm their passage through blood–brain barrier and arrival to the specific site. Tethering peptides having the ability to enter the central nervous system to nanoparticles, coating with surfactants, and the mechanical disruption of BBR using techniques like ultrasound are the major technological advancements in this regard (von Roemeling et al. 2017; Carpentier et al. 2016). But most of the strategic improvements are still at their experimental stage and thus would be considered a big deal to be determined (Fig. 2.1b).

Once the nanoparticles come into the blood stream, several plasma proteins called opsonins (serum albumin, apolipoproteins, immunoglobulins, etc.) are adsorbed to the surface of nanoparticles. These surface opsonins (linked by opsonization) serve as molecular markers to be recognized by the receptors of phagocytic cells, which causes the immune clearance of nanoparticles effectively reducing their circulation time (Jiang et al. 2017). In order to increase the time of residence in the blood that could help the nanocarriers to reach and interact with their specific target cells, and also to mitigate the rate of nanoparticles engulfment by macrophages reducing the emission of toxic byproducts and redistribution to liver and spleen, the nanoparticles have been designed strategically.

The PEGylation (encapsulation of nanoparticles with Polyethylene glycol) of nanoparticles is considered to be the most suited strategic improvement of nanoparticles avoiding their immune clearance and increasing the residency time in blood. The PEGylation interferes with the adsorption of proteins to the surface of nanoparticles through the formation of a hydrating layer on the surface of nanoparticles. So, the macrophage-mediated uptake of nanoparticles through serum absorption is the only way that we can avoid using PEGylation of nanoparticles (Tong and Kohane 2016; Jiang et al. 2017). The stealth effects of PEG functionalized nanoparticles vary with their size and surface charge and also depend more on the type of opsonin markers adsorbed on the surface of nanoparticles than the effects of PEG on opsonin adsorption (Jiang et al. 2017; Schottler et al. 2016) (Fig. 2.1c).

The asymmetric shape enables nanoparticles to avoid the immune clearance by macrophages. On the contrary, the spherical (symmetrical) shape of nanoparticles facilitates their easy internalization through biological membranes. As the shape of nanoparticles can be changed over time upon stimulus so selecting an asymmetric shape initially and then changing it into a symmetric one upon stimulus is considered as a good strategy for intracellular delivery of drugs. Synthesizing more elastic nanoparticles is thought to be of more improved quality than the less elastic ones for efficient drug delivery. This is due to the fact that more elastic nanoparticles

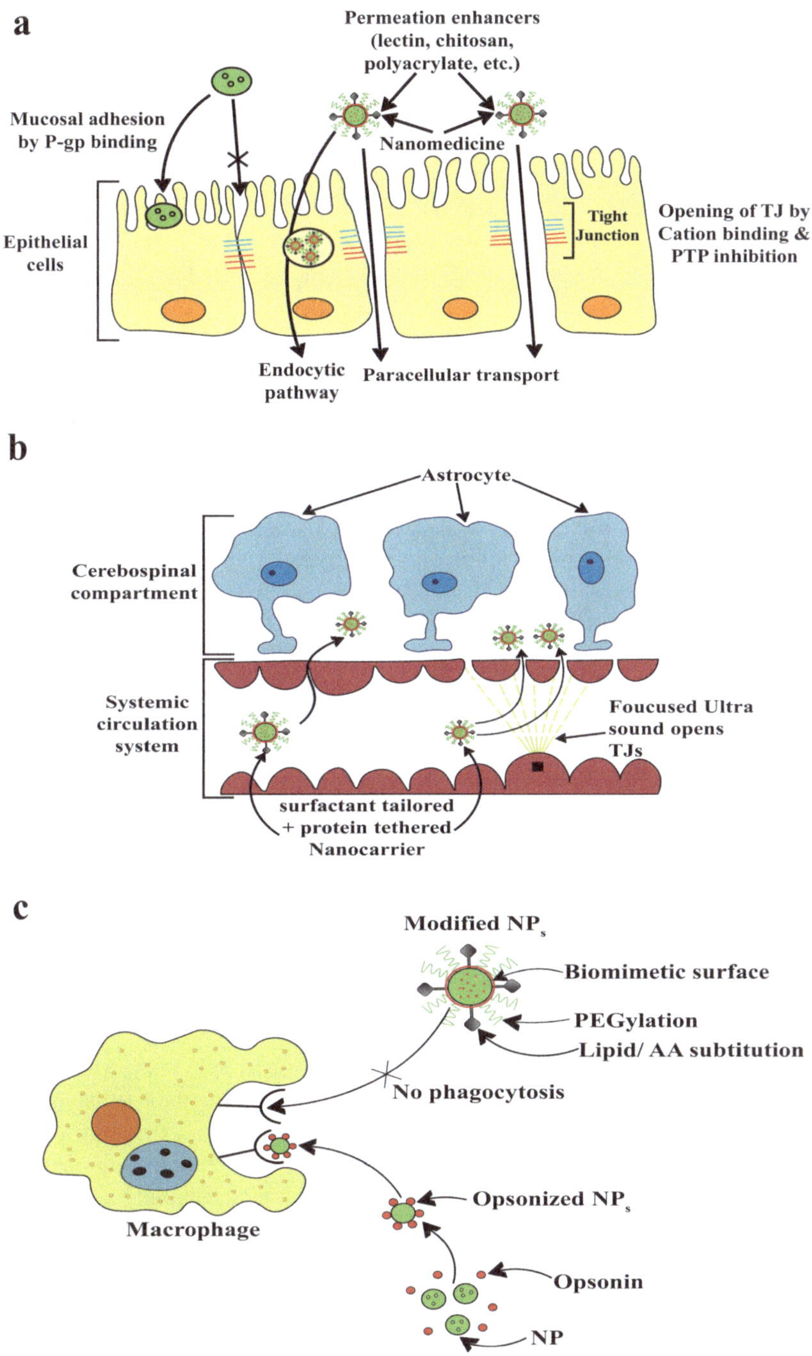

Fig. 2.1 Active-targeting for enhanced EPR effects. (**a**) Overcoming of transcellular barrier. (**b**) Crossing of blood-brain barrier. (**c**) Overcoming macrophage clearance for longer circulation

retain good circulation time and able to escape the immune clearance. Increasing the solubility of nanomaterials through the addition of fatty acids or substitutions of amino acids is desirable for enhanced drug delivery. Linoleic acid, capric acid, oleic acid, and lauric acid can increase the solubility of nanomaterials significantly. The surface composition of nanocarriers affecting the hydro-phobicity or -philicity is a good attribute to be tuned for better drug delivery. The hydrophilic surface is of superior quality in terms of escaping the immune clearance and increasing circulation time but poor in terms of cellular internalization than the hydrophobic surface. Conjugating PEG-polyethylene glycol chains can make the surface of nanomaterials hydrophilic.

Engineering the surface of nanoparticles with molecular ligands (like CD47, leukocytes, erythrocytes, self-recognizing peptides) having the potential to be recognized as self is another way to improve circulation time evading the immune clearance. Modulating the dynamic behavior of cytoskeletal network forms the underlying basis of phagocytosis. The CD47 interacts with signal recognition protein of macrophages and dendritic cells inhibiting remodeling of the cytoskeleton and thereby phagocytosis (Jiang et al. 2017; Takizawa and Manz 2007). So, the nanomaterials mimicking biomembrane such as coating surface with CD-47 markers leukocytes prevent their immune clearance. The nanocarriers with charged surfaces are more easily taken up by the target cells. This is the case especially for positively charged nanomaterials. The neutral or slightly negatively charged particles have long residence time than highly positively or negatively charged nanomaterials because latters are affected by macrophages.

The nanoparticles that are less than 6 nm are effectively filtered through renal filtration, but this is not the scenario for larger particles. In many cases of cancer therapy, especially for those patients who suffer from kidney disorders or nephropathy or nephrotoxicity, the glomerular filtration of nanoparticles that depends on the size and charge of nanoparticles is not competent enough due to renal inefficiency (Schrier 2002).

2.2.2.2 Strategic Improvement of Nanomedicine for Improved Drug Delivery Systems

Liposome Based Nanoformulation

The low molecular weight of chemotherapeutants may lead to their facile excretion causing serious side effects because of their high concentration (beyond the therapeutic level) required for the effective treatment. Besides the aforementioned problem, the nonspecificity, low solubility, and bioavailability of current chemotherapeutic agents are the challenges to be dealt with carefully (Bharali et al. 2009). The nanoformulation of chemotherapeutic agents allows to get rid of many problems linked to conventional chemotherapeutic agents. For example, paclitaxel linked to the albumin-bound nanoparticle used for the treatment of breast cancer does not initiate the hypersensitivity that would be the case if paclitaxel with cremophor EL (a solvent for paclitaxel) would be used. Nanoformulation formulation of doxorubicin using liposome represents another example. The nanoformulation of liposome in nanomedicine helps to circumvent several problems of drug delivery such as short half-life, enroute degradation, low biocompatible, nonspecific delivery, and toxicity. Encapsulation of drugs with liposome safeguards forms degradation and ensures arrival to targets with original bioavailability therefore enhancing their half-life, reducing toxicity and side effects. Myocet and Caelyx represent the liposomal nanoformulation of doxorubicin, with uncoated liposome and PEG-coated liposome, respectively. Caelyx has high half-life, circulation time, and area under curve than the Myocet which in turn has high half-life, circulation time than the doxorubicin alone. The surface of drug containing liposome in nanomedicine could further be engineered in order to achieve many well-being attributes. For example, modifying the surface of liposome with homing molecules (called targeted liposomes) like peptides or antibodies that are directly incorporated into the lipid bilayer or linked to the distal end of PEG or a composite liposome with both types of surface modifications is a nice strategy for targeted delivery, high circulation time, increased internalization (Allen et al. 1995; Torchilin et al. 1979; Sawant et al. 2006). The incorporation of pH-sensitive linkages on the surface of liposome increases the therapeutic efficiency through the enhanced release of drugs in the environment of PH sufficiently lower than the PH for liposome formulation (PH 7.4). One strategy for the synthesis of PH sensitive linkers is the inclusion of orthoesters and hydrazone bonds in lipids between phosphatidylethanolamine and PEG (Huang et al. 1987; Masson et al. 2004).

Polymerosomes are like liposomes but consist of graft, dendritic copolymers, amphiphilic diblock, and triblock, and have surface characters to be modulated for the formulation of polymerosomes with enhanced therapeutic efficiency. The implication of polymerosomes in cancer therapy especially for drug delivery needs to be determined as it is more stable and biocompatible than liposomes being synthesized from natural or semisynthetic lipids. The polymerosomes that are engineered with polylactic (PLA)- PEG and contain doxorubicin and paclitaxel showed acculturation and slow release of drugs in tumors (Ahmed et al. 2006).

The nucleic acids like siRNA or others having short half-life may be loaded with lipid nanocarriers in order to increase their half-life and therapeutic efficiency (Wicki et al. 2015; Coelho et al. 2013). Doxorubicin linked with squalene self-assembled into nanocarriers and persists for long-term in the circulatory system and showed high clinical efficiency in the pancreatic cancer of mice. So squalenoylation might be a suitable approach for designing nanocarriers loaded with anticancer drugs (Maksimenko et al. 2014) (Fig. 2.2).

Nanoemulsions

Nanoemulsions are the small nanosized (usually 30–300 nm) droplets of water in oil or oil in water that are formed via the disruption of the balance between two phases through high energy (stirring, homogenization, and ultrasound) and low energy (using system's energy) emulsification steps (Wang et al. 2009). The instabilities of nanoemulsions bestowed by Ostwald ripening could be avoided or reduced by the addition of polymeric surfactants or a less soluble oil phase. The nanoemulsions have been implicated in drug delivery due to its long perpetuity in the circulatory

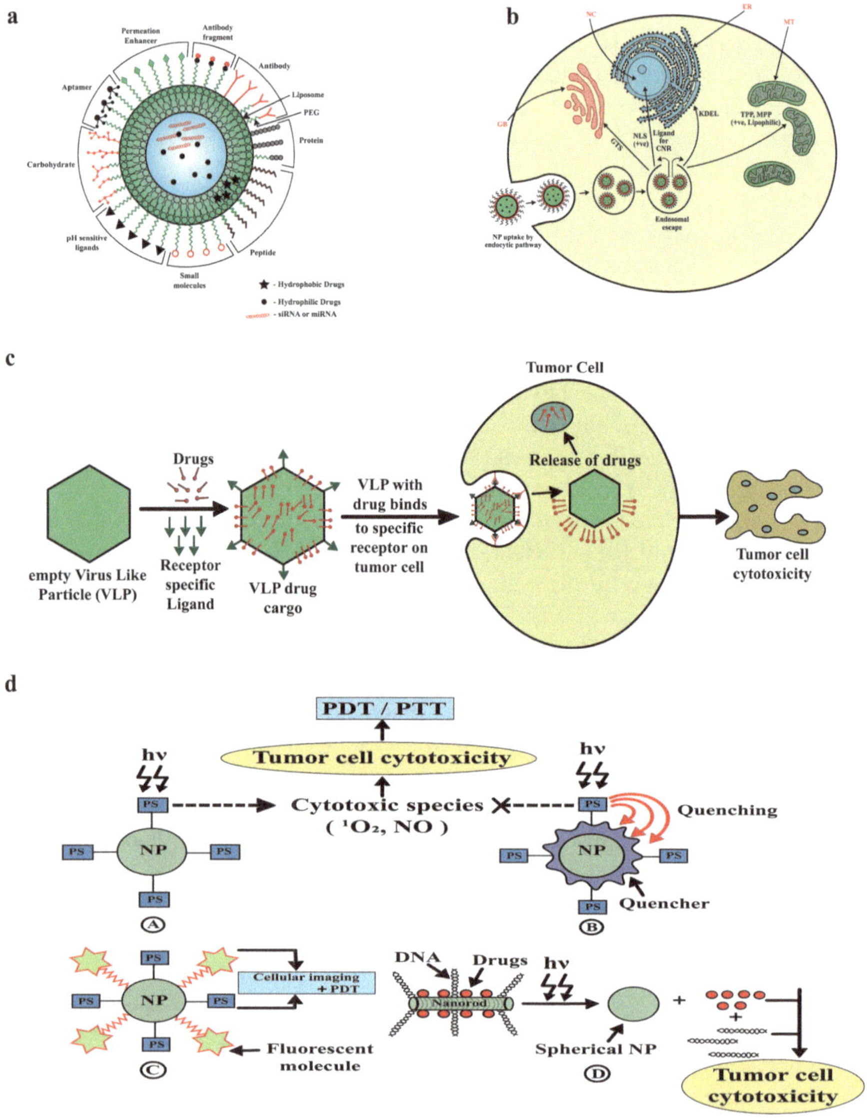

Fig. 2.2 Active-targeting for enhanced drug delivery. (**a**) Liposome-based drug delivery. (**b**) Organalle specific drug delivery. (**c**) Virus-based drug delivery. (**d**) Photocatalytic strategy based drug delivery

system, ability to be filtered sterilized and slow release of drugs. Nanoemulsion formulation of paclitaxel (TOCOSOL paclitaxel) showed the increased efficacy (Mattheolabakis et al. 2012; Bogdanova et al. 2003).

Solid Lipid Nanoparticles (SLN)

SLN is the lipid-based formulations of nanomedicine and shows high stability in body temperature due to added surfactants. SLN comprises different lipids, including glycerides, fatty acids (stearic acid, palmitic acid), sterols/waxes, and surfactants (Schwarz et al. 1994). SLN contributes to the field of nanomedicine by preventing drug degradation and enhancing target-specific drug delivery but sometimes has to compromise with drug loading capacity due to its ordered crystalline structure when formed from one type of molecules (Wissing et al. 2004). Several lipids-based nanoformulation incorporating the drugs (such as doxorubicin and paclitaxel) acting on P-glycoprotein (P-gp) that is amenable for multidrug resistance has got attractive results in preclinical trials (Dong et al. 2009).

Strategies for Organelles Specific Targeting of Nanodrugs

The therapeutic success of many drugs depends on their target-specific delivery. Different cellular organelles and the cytoplasm represent the potential target sites for drugs used in the treatment of diseases derived from the malfunctioning at these sites. Nanomedicine conjugation with signaling molecules destined for the organelle-specific localization or function would be considered to be the major strategy for organelle-specific drug delivery.

Many suitable approaches for cytoplasmic delivery of drugs have been evolved and most notably pH sensitive liposomes or fusogen containing liposomes, cationic nanomaterials, CPP conjugated nanoparticles, and polyampholyte nanoparticles (Kim et al. 2015). Endosomal release of drugs into cytoplasm forms the underlying basis for these aforementioned designing of nanomedicine.

So far, the best way to design nanomedicine for mitochondrial delivery is their nanoformulation with mitochondrial targeting sequence (MTS) or peptides like triphenylphosphine (TPP) and mitochondrial processing proteinases (MPP). Gold nanostar doped with triphenylphosphine modified a-helical pro-apoptotic peptide (TPP-KLA) represents a suitable example. The lipophilic molecules having a positive charge are suitable for mitochondrial targeting (Chen et al. 2017).

Nuclear pore complex (NPC) measuring the central pore diameter about 10 nm restricts the free diffusion of larger molecules (>9 nm diameter and MW > 40). In this case, tagging nanoparticles with nuclear localization signal (NLS) or molecules having a strong affinity for DNA (such as C60-ser, TAT peptide) or molecules recognized by cytosolic nuclear receptor-like dexamethasone enabled the nucleus-specific drug delivery (Parodi et al. 2015; Tammam et al. 2016). The PH sensitive modulation of NP size could provide another important means of drug delivery to the nucleus. PEG-benzoic imine-oligo-L-lysine/iridium (III) metallodrug complex of NP when encounters the acidic pH of endosomes undergoes the size reduction through the shedding of PEG coating and subsequently, oligolysine directs the NP movement into the nucleus (Fan et al. 2016a, b).

Coating nanoparticles with signal peptides like beta-hairpin structural motif (golgi localization signal), and KDEL peptide recognized by ER resident KDEL receptor or antibodies binding organelle-specific proteins represent the possible strategy for targeted delivery of drugs into golgi body and endoplasmic reticulum (Cohen et al. 2011; Parodi et al. 2015) (Fig. 2.2b).

Virus Based Nanoformulation

Another important strategy of employing nanoparticles in cancer therapy is by using engineered tumor-homing viruses, (such as species of pox viruses like myxoma and vaccinia), which are able to replicate specifically in tumor cells and express therapeutic proteins. JX594 is an engineered oncolytic poxvirus that replicates using tumor cells and in turn activates EGFR Ras MAPK pathway to destroy them as well as express granulocyte colony stimulating factor (G-CSF) promoting cancer immunotherapy. It has shown promising results in phase 1 trial with primary or metastatic hepatocarcinoma, when intravenously administered, JX594 homed to tumor tissue and displayed dose-dependent antitumoral activity (Park et al. 2008; Breitbach et al. 2011). Cancer therapy using oncolytic virus achieved first successful result in phase 3 trial by using T-Vec in advanced non-visceral melanoma patients. T-Vec, a Herpes simplex virus type 1 derived and GM-CSF expressing virus, showed a durable response in 16.3% non-visceral melanoma patients when injected in multiple doses, while 2.1% remained in the control arm.

Besides animal virus, plant viruses are also used as nanocarrier in cancer therapy as their protein shell has large cargo capacity and ability to protect the sequestered chemotherapeutic agents better than other nanocarriers, so the plant virus-based nanoparticles are effectively used as carriers of therapeutic and imaging agents to melanoma, breast, ovarian, prostate cancer, and other malignancies. Studies on Red Clover Necrotic Mosaic virus have reported that it is well suited for reversible loading of therapeutic agents to the target site and can carry a payload of about 1000 molecules of Doxorubicin to the tumor site by passively diffusing across the membrane (Loo et al. 2008). Tobacco Mosaic Virus (TMV) is also used as a nanocarrier of cisplatin in the therapy of platinum resistant (PR) ovarian cancer cells. It exhibits a loading capacity of 1900 cisplatin/TMV and superior cytotoxicity by DNA strand breakage in PS and PR ovarian cancer cells, as compared to free cisplatin (Franke et al. 2018). TMV has promising results as nanotheranostic agents in PC-3 prostate cancer cells, where they are loaded with gadolinium particles and coated with a biocompatible polymer, polydopamine (PDA). It facilitates photothermal therapy along with multimodal (magnetic resonance/photoacoustic) imaging of cancer cells (Hu et al. 2019) (Fig. 2.2c).

Apart from cancer therapy and diagnostic purposes, plant virus NPs are used as potential cancer immunotherapeutic agents, where they modulate the tumor microenvironment and coordinate downstream antitumor immune responses. Studies showed that inhalation of self-assembling virus-like nanoparticles from empty cowpea mosaic virus (CPMV) effectively reduces lung melanoma and activates Ly6G+ neutrophils, associated with antitumor immune response. Such viral NPs not only enhances cancer treatment efficacy but generates an immune response in ovarian, colon, breast, and other metastases (Lizotte et al. 2016).

2.2.2.3 Photoactivated Nanomaterials for Photodynamic and Photothermal Therapy (PDT/PTT)

Nanomedicine is the most promising and emerging field of nanotechnology destined for designing and synthesizing nanoparticles having desired attributes of clinical of relevance for the sake of diagnosis, treatment, and prevention of many diseases (http://pubs.acs.org/page/ancac3/vi/2). The spatiotemporal release of therapeutics at their desired concentration to achieve a good therapeutic index is a challenging concern in nanomedicine to be determined or properly addressed. Among several factors regulating the release of drug, the light is the fascinating one as it acts biofriendly and also due to easily manipulating photochemical reactions. So, photochemistry plays a crucial role in the strategic synthesis and delivery of nanoconjugated drugs.

Singlet oxygen, nitric oxide, and heat are the major cytotoxic agents produced by photosensitizers (PS) under the control of light. These cytotoxic agents are of great importance for photodynamic and photothermal mode of non-invasive cancer therapy. So careful regulation of timing and site of illumination may define the type of cytotoxic species produced upon photon absorption. The transfer of energy from PS to nearby molecular oxygen is responsible for the generation of singlet oxygen and thereby oxidizing the biomolecules like protein, lipid, etc. leading to the cytotoxicity or cell death. So, the cellular uptake of photosensitizers and their potentiality to form singlet oxygen upon illumination form the underlying basis of photodynamic therapy (PDT).

The phenomenon of hyperthermia-heating cancer cells with a certain temperature (41–47 °C) for a certain time (10 min) leads to the irreversible cell death which may confine the surrounding healthy cells as well and this is a problem of hyperthermia based photothermal cancer therapy. Selection of suitable PS which upon absorption of light is excited but then comes to the ground state through the non-radiative decay losing heat into the surrounding environment and this is the fundamental basis of photothermal therapy (PTT). The unique properties of several nanomaterials including high thermal stability, absorption coefficient and conversion of light to heat, and biocompatibility have attracted their application in PTT.

The function of NO is highly dose dependent and site specific and its synthesis under light results in the breakdown of photoactive center. The incorporation of photodonor giving rise to NO into the suitable material forms a potential NO reservoir and enhances the light harvesting ability of PS. A combinatorial approach of PTT or PDT with the photoactive center releasing NO could provide a new way of multimodal therapy.

Three excellent light-based drug delivery systems have evolved recently, viz. photocaging, photochemical internalization, and photo triggered mechanized system. Combination of each of these approaches with photothermia could present more effective way to the controlled release of drugs.

Different nanoparticles like nanoshell, quantum dots, nanorods have led to the development of nanohybrids that are designed by surface modification and functionalization to improve their therapeutic index through photoactive release of cytotoxic species. High thermal stability, biocompatibility, non-toxic, water solubility, and photoresponse to the lights of higher wavelength are the desirable characteristics of nanohybrids. Synthesis of thiol stabilized metal nanoparticles in order to release NO under light activation is achieved by different approaches:

1. Nanoformulation involving the linking of NO photodonor (e.g., nitroaniline) to the surface of carboxy-terminated PtNP which upon light absorption release NO and cause cell death.
2. Adding both the NO photodonor and a fluorescence molecule such as porphyrin to the PtNP combines the photodynamic therapy to their cellular detection.
3. Supramolecular approach in which Pt core is replaced with Au gives rise to the bifunctional molecule having PTT property of Au and PDT property of surface dwelling NO photodonor. This is exemplified by the surface modification of AuNP with NO donor and alpha cyclodextrin, where cyclodextrin connects NO donor to the surface of AuNP and increases the solubility in polar solvents and biocompatibility.
4. Another way to design NPs having both PTT/PDT potential is to combine the quenching ability of metal surface to the excited state of PS. Anionic phthalocyanine electrostatically attached to the PEG modified positively charged surface of AuNP, cannot produce the singlet oxygen due to energy transfer from excited PS to metal surface but upon irradiation, PS gets detached from AuNP surface photogenerating singlet oxygen and therefore enabling combined approach of PTT/PDT therapy.
5. Photoinduction of shape transformation of NPs is a suitable way of drug delivery. The thiolated DNA molecules having fluorescent markers for their cellular localization could be conjugated to the surface of differently shaped AuNP such as nanocapsules or nanobones. These nanobones/capsules upon light irradiation transform into the spherical shapes releasing the surface linked DNA molecules (Fig. 2.2d).

2.2.2.4 Mesoporous Silica Nanoparticles (MSNP)

Tunable pore size, optical transparency, and excellent biocompatibility of MSNP make them suitable for drug delivery. The pores of negatively charged MSNP containing paclitaxel are photocapped by AuNP that, in turn, photocaged with positively charged by o-nitrobenzyl. Light illumination liberates the photocage through the cleavage of photosensitive cationic linkers and thereby leaving only the anionic AuNP with MSNP but the electrostatic repulsion leads to the opening of pores and the release of loaded drug. The inner wall of MSNP could be functionalized with photoresponsive azobenzene derivatives that upon irradiation undergo *cis-trans* isomerization via wagging motion resulting in the release of anticancer drugs.

Reversible photoinduced cleavage and dimerization of coumarin derivatives linked to the pores of MSNP provide another way of controlled release of drugs. The basic principle in this strategy is that light of >320 nm leads to the coumarin dimerization preventing the drug release, while the light of 250 nm breaks the dimers into monomers and cause the drug release.

2.2.2.5 Dendrimers

Dendrimers are highly branched polymeric macromolecules having a 3D structure and three structural components, viz. initiator core monomer from which released the branching molecules (second, third generation molecules, and so on) and terminal groups. These terminal groups could be functionalized to have desired attributes for biomedical implications like drug delivery. DOXdendrimer nanoformulation of doxorubicin in which doxorubicin was linked to polyethylene oxide dendrimer appeared to have reduced cytotoxicity (in vitro), low bioaccumulation in liver and heart, and increased half-life (43). The 3D dendrimer of polyamidoamine (PAMAM) linked to the doxorubicin through amide bond or hydrazone bond showed to enhance the therapeutic index of doxorubicin.

2.2.3 Engineering Nanoparticles to Evade the Multidrug Resistance (MDR) in Cancer

At present the development of multi-drug resistance is a big problem as it nullifies the therapeutic potential of many therapeutic agents including chemotherapeutants. So, dealing with multidrug resistance with regard to avoid multidrug resistance is an astonishing challenge. P-gp, a transporter protein encoded by MDR1 gene mediates the multidrug resistance to most of the chemotherapeutic agents used for cancer therapy through effluxing them out of the cells. Direct administration of P-gp inhibitors in order to inhibit P-gp arise the problems of serious side effects. The ability of nano-based drug delivery systems to inhibit P-gp demolished the problems of multidrug resistance. Some technological advancements with aim to mitigate the multidrug resistance through enhanced endocytosis and cellular uptake ate formulation of nanoliposome with P-gp inhibitor or surface modification (Wu et al. 2007), nanocapsules made of polymer or lipid or both nanoparticles (Wong et al. 2006a, b; Colin de Verdiere et al. 1997), lipid nanoparticles with surfactants like brij (Dong et al. 2009), polymer drug conjugation (Omelyanenko et al. 1998), pluronic micelles (Alakhov et al. 1996).

The use of liposomes in circumventing the multidrug resistance benefits from the facts that liposomes may deliver the loaded drugs through endocytic pathway thereby escaping P-gp or the targeted therapeutic agent and a P-gp inhibitor are entrapped in the same liposomes or ligand conjugation of drug loaded liposomes (Ford and Hait 1990; Rahman et al. 1992). Linking transferrin on the surface of liposome co-loaded with doxorubicin and verapamil showed elevated therapeutic efficiency in K562-resistant leukemia cells (Wu et al. 2007).

Designing nanocapsules through the encapsulation of drugs with lipid or polymer nanoparticles or both (hybrid polymer and lipid nanoparticles-PLN) would be a suitable approach to increase the therapeutic efficiency of drugs against multidrug resistance. The nanocapsule made of polyisohexylcyanoacrylate (PIHCA) nanoparticles and containing doxorubicin appeared to have better cytotoxicity than the doxorubicin alone has in resistant cell line-C6. Nanoformulation of doxorubicin containing nanocapsule with highly biodegradable polymers like PIBCA accelerates its cytotoxicity (therapeutic potential) in resistant cell line through P-gp saturation as the doxorubicin is readily available in close proximity to the cell surface. The biodegradation of nanocapsule encapsulating doxorubicin gives rise to cyanoacrylate that forms ion pairs with doxorubicin neutralizing the surface charge and thus promoting their internalization by free diffusion (Colin De Verdiere et al. 1997). The hybrid nanocapsule escapes P-gp mediated efflux of doxorubicin by following phagocytosis (Wong et al. 2006a, b).

Synthesis of lipid nanoparticles with surfactants such as brij 78 on their surface increases the cellular concentration and therapeutic efficiency of drug in multidrug resistant cells by means of ATP depletion as in case of brij or by P-gp inhibition. Covalent attachment of Poly(N-[2-hydroxypropyl] methacrylamide) (polyHPMA) or HPMA copolymers to drugs is known to overcome the P-gp mediated multidrug resistance by controlling the molecular events such as gene expression and apoptosis (Minko et al. 2001). Pluronic copolymers are amphiphilic in nature and their surfactant property self-assembles them into micelles. The nanoassembles of pluronic copolymers into micelles entrapping drugs promote the therapeutic potential by virtue of energy depletion through the inhibition of efflux pumps and their cognate ATPase (Alakhov et al. 1996; Batrakova et al. 2001).

2.2.4 Nanoparticle-Based Combination Therapy

In many cases, tumors show the resistance to chemotherapeutic agent due to mutations rendering selective advantages to the survival of tumors against chemotherapeutic agents. In that sense, administration of multiple drugs each having a specific target, at a time and in an optimized ratio is supposed to be more effective than using one drug at a time. But the major caveat connected to the combination therapy is their varying rate of metabolic processes, in turn, make their pharmacokinetics and biodistribution patterns complicated. These complications would be resolved by the implication of nanomedicine in which multiple drugs are encapsulated or linked with single nanoliposome or other nanocarriers maintaining optimized ratio, pharmacokinetic and pharmacodynamic behavior of each different drug and therefore enhancing the efficacy of combination therapy (Xu et al. 2015).

2.3 Conclusion

Normalization of tumor microenvironment enhances NP efficacy. Engineering the nanoparticles in order to increase the therapeutic efficacy of chemotherapeutants is not the whole story to appreciate. Several pathophysiological features of cancer may represent the obstacles to their chemotherapeutants underscoring their therapeutic values and interestingly the modulation of tumor microenvironment in order to normalize them such as vascular normalization, matrix normalization, and stress normalization may enhance the effectiveness of nanomedicines used to treat cancer (Chauhan and Jain 2013). So a combinatorial approach for normalizing tumor microenvironment on the one hand and increasing the therapeutic potential of drugs on the other hand might be considered as a suitable strategy to treat cancer and in this respect designing nanomedicines for serving dual purpose may be considered to be a great challenge in near future.

References

Ahmed F, Pakunlu RI, Srinivas G et al (2006) Shrinkage of a rapidly growing tumor by drug-loaded polymersomes: pH-triggered release through copolymer degradation. Mol Pharm 3(3):340–350

Alakhov VY, Moskaleva E, Batrakova EV, Kabanov AV (1996) Hypersensitization of multidrug resistant human ovarian carcinoma cells by Pluronic P85 block copolymer. Bioconjug Chem 7 (2):209–216

Allen TM, Brandeis E, Hansen CB, Kao GY, Zalipsky S (1995) A new strategy for attachment of antibodies to sterically stabilized liposomes resulting in efficient targeting to cancer cells. Biochim Biophys Acta 1237(2):99–108

Batrakova EV, Li S, Vinogradov SV, Alakhov VY, Miller DW, Kabanov AV (2001) Mechanism of pluronic effect on P-glycoprotein efflux system in blood–brain barrier: contributions of energy depletion and membrane fluidization. J Pharmacol Exp Ther 299(2):483–493

Bharali DJ, Khalil M, Gurbuz M, Simone TM, Mousa SA (2009) Nanoparticles and cancer therapy: a concise review with emphasis on dendrimers. Int J Nanomedicine 4:1–7

Bogdanova N, Lissianskaya A, Gorelov A, Moiseyenko V, Golubev A, Weiden P (2003) TOCOSOL (TM) paclitaxel (paclitaxel injectable emulsion): Phase 1–2 study of weekly administration in patients with non-small cell lung, ovarian, urothelial future science group transitional cell or colorectal carcinoma. Clin Cancer Res 9(16):6136S–6137S

Breitbach CJ, Burke J, Jonker D, Stephenson J, Haas AR, Chow LQM et al (2011) Intravenous delivery of a multi-mechanistic cancer-targeted oncolytic poxvirus in humans. Nature 477:99–102

Carpentier A et al (2016) Clinical trial of blood-brain barrier disruption by pulsed ultrasound. Sci Transl Med 8:343re2

Chauhan VP, Jain RK (2013) Strategies for advancing cancer nanomedicine. Nat Mater 12 (11):958–962

Chen YM, Tu IH, Hu FR, Lin CT, Chen WL (2013) The role of protein tyrosine phosphorylation in the cell-cell junctions and intercellular permeability of post-confluent bovine corneal epithelial cells. Taiwan J Ophthalmol 3:37–41

Chen K, Guo L, Zhang J et al (2017) A gene delivery system containing nuclear localization signal: increased nucleus import and transfection efficiency with the assistance of RanGAP1. Acta Biomater 48:215–226

Chow EK, Ho D (2013) Cancer nanomedicine: from drug delivery to imaging. Sci Transl Med 5 (216):216rv4

Clausen AE, Cast CE, Bernkop-Schnürch A (2002) The role of glutathione in the permeation enhancing effect of thiolated polymers. Pharm Res 19:602–608

Coelho T, Adams D, Silva A, Lozeron P, Hawkins PN, Mant T et al (2013) Safety and efficacy of RNAi therapy for transthyretin amyloidosis. N Engl J Med 369:819–829

Cohen JR, Lin LD, Machamer CE (2011) Identification of a Golgi complex-targeting signal in the cytoplasmic tail of the severe acute respiratory syndrome coronavirus envelope protein. J Virol 85:5794–5803

Colin De Verdiere A, Dubernet C, Nemati F et al (1997) Reversion of multidrug resistance with polyalkylcyanoacrylate nanoparticles: towards a mechanism of action. Br J Cancer 76 (2):198–205

Dong X, Mattingly CA, Tseng MT et al (2009) Doxorubicin and paclitaxel-loaded lipid-based nanoparticles overcome multidrug resistance by inhibiting P-glycoprotein and depleting ATP. Cancer Res 69(9):3918–3926

Fan W, Xia D, Zhu Q, Hu L, Gan Y (2016a) Intracellular transport of nanocarriers across the intestinal epithelium. Drug Discov Today 21:856–863

Fan Y, Li C, Li F, Chen D (2016b) pH-activated size reduction of large compound nanoparticles for in vivo nucleus-targeted drug delivery. Biomaterials 85:30–39

Ford JM, Hait WN (1990) Pharmacology of drugs that alter multidrug resistance in cancer. Pharmacol Rev 42(3):155–199

Franke CE, Czapar AE, Patel RB, Steinmetz NF (2018) Tobacco mosaic virus-delivered cisplatin restores efficacy in platinum-resistant ovarian cancer cells. Mol Pharm 15(8):2922–2931

Hu H, Yang Q, Baroni S, Yang H, Aime S, Steinmetz NF (2019) Polydopamine-decorated tobacco mosaic virus for photoacoustic/magnetic resonance bimodal imaging and photothermal cancer therapy. Nanoscale 11(19):9760–9768

Huang L, Connor J, Wang CY (1987) pH-sensitive immunoliposomes. Methods Enzymol 149:88–99

Jiang W, Von Roemeling CA, Chen Y, Qie Y, Liu X, Chen J, Kim YSB (2017) Designing nanomedicine for immuno-oncology. Nat Biomed Eng 1(2):1–11

Jing L, Zhou W, Tian G, Fu H (2013) Surface tuning for oxide-based nanomaterials as efficient photocatalysts. Chem Soc Rev 42:9509–9549

Kim JH, Moon JS, Yu JS, Lee SK (2015) Intracellular cytoplasm-specific delivery of SH3 and SH2 domains of SLAP inhibits TcR-mediated signaling. Biochem Biophys Res Commun 460:603–608

Lizotte PH, Wen AM, Sheen MR et al (2016) In situ vaccination with cowpea mosaic virus nanoparticles suppresses metastatic cancer. Nat Nanotechnol 11(3):295–303

Loo L, Guenther RH, Lommel SA, Franzen S (2008) Infusion of dye molecules into Red clover necrotic mosaic virus. Chem Commun 2008:88–90

Maksimenko A, Dosio F, Mougin J, Ferrero A, Wack S, Reddy LH et al (2014) A unique squalenoylated and nonpegylated doxorubicin nanomedicine with systemic longcirculating properties and anticancer activity. Proc Natl Acad Sci 111:E217–E226

Masson C, Garinot M, Mignet N et al (2004) pH-sensitive PEG lipids containing orthoester linkers: new potential tools for nonviral gene delivery. J Control Release 99(3):423–434

Mattheolabakis G, Rigas B, Constantinides PP (2012) Nanodelivery strategies in cancer chemotherapy: biological rationale and pharmaceutical perspectives. Nanomedicine 7(10):1577–1590

Minko T, Kopeckova P, Kopecek J (2001) Preliminary evaluation of caspases-dependent apoptosis signaling pathways of free and HPMA copolymer-bound doxorubicin in human ovarian carcinoma cells. J Control Release 71(3):227–237

Omelyanenko V, Kopeckova P, Gentry C, Kopecek J (1998) Targetable HPMA copolymer-adriamycin conjugates. Recognition, internalization and subcellular fate. J Control Release 53 (1–3):2537

Park BH, Hwang T, Liu TC, Sze DY, Kim JS, Kwon HC (2008) Use of a targeted oncolytic poxvirus, JX-594, in patients with refractory primary or metastatic liver cancer: a phase I trial. Lancet Oncol 9:533–542

Parodi A, Corbo C, Cevenini A, Pandolfi L, Tasciotti E et al (2015) Enabling cytoplasmic delivery and organelle targeting by surface modification of nanocarriers. Nanomedicine 10:1923–1940

Rahman A, Husain SR, Siddiqui J et al (1992) Liposome-mediated modulation of multidrug resistance in human HL-60 leukemia cells. J Natl Cancer Inst 84(24):1909–1915

Sakhrani NM, Padh H (2013) Organelle targeting: third level of drug targeting. Drug Des Devel Ther 7:585–599

Sawant RM, Hurley JP, Salmaso S et al (2006) SMART drug delivery systems: double targeted pH-responsive pharmaceutical nanocarriers. Bioconjug Chem 17(4):943–949
Schottler S, Becker G, Winzen S, Steinbach T et al (2016) Protein adsorption is required for stealth effect of poly(ethyleneglycol)- and poly(phosphoester)-coated nanocarriers. Nat Nanotechnol 11:372–377
Schrier RW (2002) Cancer therapy and renal injury. J Clin Invest 110:743–745
Schwarz C, Mehnert W, Lucks JS, Muller RH (1994) Solid lipid nanoparticles (Sln) for controlled drug-delivery. 1. Production, characterization and sterilization. J Control Release 30(1):83–96
Stylianopoulos T, Jain RK (2015) Design considerations for nanotherapeutics in oncology. Nanomedicine 11(8):1893–1907
Takizawa H, Manz MG (2007) Macrophage tolerance: CD47–SIRP-α-mediated signals matter. Nat Immunol 8:287–1289
Tammam SN, Azzazy HME, Lamprecht A (2016) How successful is nuclear targeting by nanocarriers? J Control Release 229:140–153
Tong R, Kohane DS (2016) New strategies in cancer nanomedicine. Annu Rev Pharmacol Toxicol 56:41–57
Torchilin VP, Khaw BA, Smirnov VN, Haber E (1979) Preservation of antimyosin antibody activity after covalent coupling to liposomes. Biochem Biophys Res Commun 89(4):1114–1119
Villaverde G, Baeza A (2019) Targeting strategies for improving the efficacy of nanomedicine in oncology. Beilstein J Nanotechnol 10:168–181
Von Roemeling C, Jiang W, Chan CK, Weissman IL, Kim BYS (2017) Breaking down the barriers to precision cancer nanomedicine. Trends Biotechnol 35(2):159–171
Wang L, Tabor R, Eastoe J, Li X, Heenan RK, Dong J (2009) Formation and stability of nanoemulsions with mixed ionic-nonionic surfactants. Phys Chem Chem Phys 11 (42):9772–9778
Wicki A, Witzigmann D, Balasubramanian V, Huwyler J (2015) Nanomedicine in cancer therapy: challenges, opportunities, and clinical applications. J Control Release 200:138–157
Wissing SA, Kayser O, Muller RH (2004) Solid lipid nanoparticles for parenteral drug delivery. Adv Drug Deliv Rev 56(9):1257–1272
Wong HL, Bendayan R, Rauth AM, Xue HY, Babakhanian K, Wu XY (2006a) A mechanistic study of enhanced doxorubicin uptake and retention in multidrug resistant breast cancer cells using a polymer-lipid hybrid nanoparticle system. J Pharmacol Exp Ther 317(3):1372–1381
Wong HL, Rauth AM, Bendayan R et al (2006b) A new polymer–lipid hybrid nanoparticle system increases cytotoxicity of doxorubicin against multidrug-resistant human breast cancer cells. Pharm Res 23(7):1574–1585
Woodle MC, Matthay KK, Newman MS, Hidayat JE, Collins LR, Redemann C, Martin FJ, Papahadjopoulos D (1992) Versatility in lipid compositions showing prolonged circulation with sterically stabilized liposomes. Biochim Biophys Acta 1105(2):193–200
Wu J, Lu Y, Lee A et al (2007) Reversal of multidrug resistance by transferrin-conjugated liposomes co-encapsulating doxorubicin and verapamil. J Pharm Pharm Sci 10(3):350–357
Xu X, Ho W, Zhang X, Bertrand N, Farokhzad O (2015) Cancer nanomedicine: from targeted delivery to combination therapy. Trends Mol Med 21(4):223–232
Yang L, Jiang X, Yang M (2011) Improvement of surface enhanced Raman scattering performance for broad band gap semiconductor nanomaterial (TiO2): strategy of metal doping. Appl Phys Lett 99:111114
Yang Y, Niu S, Han D, Liu T et al (2017) Progress in developing metal oxide nanomaterials for photoelectrochemical water splitting. Adv Energy Mater 7:1700555

Bioinspired Nanoparticles in Cancer Theranostics

3

Abhilash Rana and Seema Bhatnagar

Abstract

In recent years, numerous nanomaterials have emerged as an exciting platform for cancer theranostic applications due to their multifunctional properties and intrinsic molecular properties that enable efficient diagnosis, imaging, and effective therapy. This field is associated with a variety of clinical applications, especially in cancer treatment. More recently, efforts to create nanoparticles using biological materials have gained growing interest in overcoming the drawbacks of drug delivery systems, such as biocompatibility, toxicity, and targeting. This chapter summarized the detailed overview of the applications of various bioinspired cancer therapies, which includes the recent examples of lipid nanoparticles, liposomes, protein nanoparticles, viral nanoparticles, and inorganic nanoparticles. Finally, the difficulties and future scope of these NPs in cancer therapy and diagnostic applications are illustrated.

Keywords

Cancer nanotechnology · Bioinspired Nanoparticles · Theranostics · Cancer diagnosis · Molecular Imaging · Nanomedicine

3.1 Introduction

The quest for targeted cancer treatment has led scientists to explore several advanced treatment modalities. However, achieving optimal drug delivery by steering them to their required target site by specific drug delivery vehicles at concentrations that

A. Rana · S. Bhatnagar (✉)
Amity Institute of Biotechnology, Amity University, Noida, India
e-mail: sbhatnagar1@amity.edu

A. Malik et al. (eds.), *Nanomedicine for Cancer Diagnosis and Therapy*,
https://doi.org/10.1007/978-981-15-7564-8_3

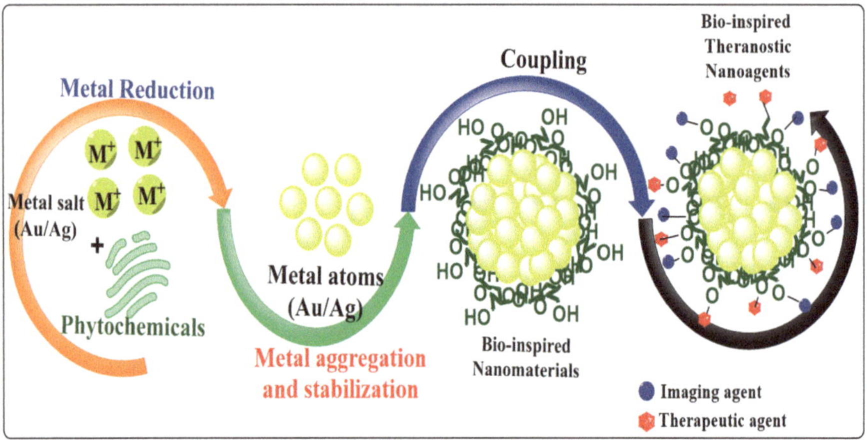

Fig. 3.1 Diagrammatic representation of bioinspired synthesis and surface functionalization of the theranostics nanoagents

have minimal toxicity and monitoring the success of treatment is a formidable challenge (Neubi et al. 2018). Nanotechnology has the potential as an emerging field that can provide a new range of products for such applications. Nanomaterials have gained prominence due to their unique ability to interact with biological systems at the atomic level, which in turn contributes to a wide range of applications in the biological system (Sharmila et al. 2018). Imaging combined with diagnostics using a nanotechnology approach has emerged as an exciting opportunity for researchers across the world for targeted delivery of drugs to cancer (Madamsetty et al. 2019). Nanocarriers have proved to be highly efficacious to ferry cargo with the ability of simultaneously loading both imaging and therapeutic agents (Madamsetty et al. 2019). A plethora of newly generated nanoparticles (NPs) within the impressive collage of nanocarriers that have dual capacity of therapeutic delivery and diagnosis have accelerated the dominion of personalized medicine (Madamsetty et al. 2019). Significantly, nanocarriers within the size range of 1–100 nm have been majorly employed in biomedical applications (Bhaumik et al. 2015; Lin et al. 2012; Mittal et al. 2013; Narayanan and Sakthivel 2010). Bioinspired routes for synthesis of nanoparticles are considered to be superior, cost-effective, and sustainable routes as they avoid the use of toxic chemicals (Lin et al. 2012; Madamsetty et al. 2019; Narayanan and Sakthivel 2010).

The emerging field of "theranostics" refers to single nanoplatforms that can ferry cargo comprising of both therapeutics and diagnostic agents (Gou et al. 2018; Pene et al. 2009). It not only enables simultaneous diagnosis and treatment response monitoring but also encompasses high accuracy and specificity (Bardhan et al. 2011; Janib et al. 2010) (Fig. 3.1).

Bioinspired theranostic nanoagents can be designed by taking into consideration four crucial aspects: (1) selection of effective therapeutic agent; (2) optimization of stable carrier; (3) implementation of a targeting and sustainable drug release approach; (4) cautious selection of an imaging agent (Chi et al. 2017; Chowdhury et al. 2017; Cong et al. 2018; Madamsetty et al. 2019). Numerous types of theranostic platforms have been reported in the literature which includes viral NPs, protein NPs, aptamers, apoferritin, solid lipid NPs, etc. (Sivarajakumar et al. 2018). Biosynthesized multifunctional nanoparticles with noble metal centers that encapsulate both the therapeutic and imaging also have tremendous scope in the treatment of cancer (Duan et al. 2015; Madamsetty et al. 2019; Ovais et al. 2018). Several synthetic strategies have been employed for the development of bioinspired theranostic nanoagents:

1. Selection and screening of plant extracts for the synthesis of nanoparticles;
2. Optimization of several physicochemical parameters for biosynthesis;
3. Conjugation of the synthesized nanoparticles with therapeutics and imaging agents;
4. Characterization of synthesized nanocarriers by analytical techniques (Bhaumik et al. 2015; Duan et al. 2015; Madamsetty et al. 2019).

3.2 Novelty of Bioinspired Nanoparticles Based Theranostics

Essentially nanotheranostics are nanocarriers, which will serve a dual purpose by allowing both diagnosis and treatment to be contained in an "all in one" package (Chen et al. 2014). An imaging agent introduced into their design permits them to be tracked in the body and the therapeutic drug that is carried together with the imaging agents will be released when the nanocarrier binds to the cell. This saves valuable time as therapy and diagnosis of the treatment can be instantaneous (Chapman and Pascu 2012; Chen et al. 2014). Nanotheranostics can be classified based on the type of nanoplatform delivery system employed or by the agents coupled with drugs to provide imaging functions, including liposomal nanoparticles, metal nanoparticles, viral nanoparticles, protein nanoparticles, and lipid nanoparticles (Chapman and Pascu 2012; Madamsetty et al. 2019). An overview of the different types of nanotheranostics is discussed below with their schematic diagram (Figs. 3.2 and 3.3).

3.2.1 Liposomes in Cancer Theranostics

The repository of nanocarriers that can be used for cancer theranostics includes a plethora of lipid-based nano-arsenals, of which liposomes are the most widely investigated nanomaterials for cancer therapy. Liposomes are lipid vesicles comprising of a hydrophilic head group and lipophilic tail that have the unique ability to spontaneously form spheres at critical concentrations. These can be used to encapsulate therapeutics and diagnostics for delivery to the target site (Chapman and Pascu 2012). In addition, they offer various advantages, namely ease of synthesis, ability to incorporate both hydrophilic and hydrophobic chemotherapeutic compounds, low

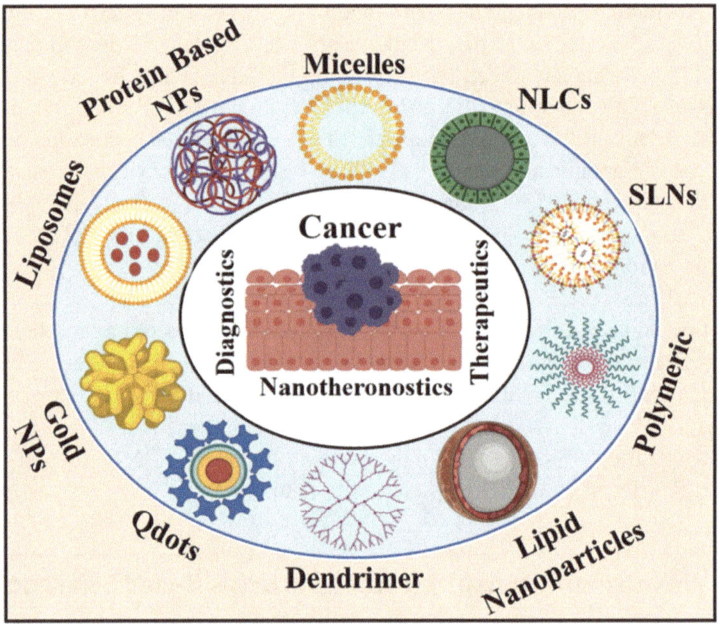

Fig. 3.2 Various theranostic nanomedicine approaches

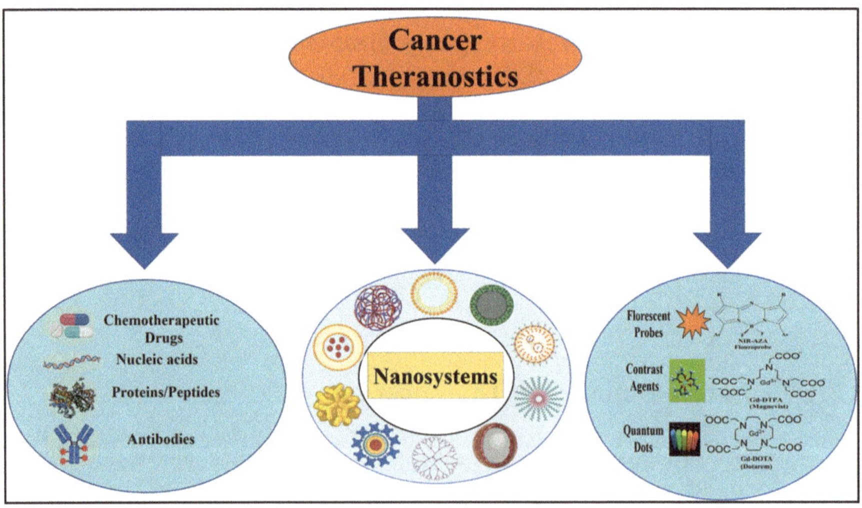

Fig. 3.3 Nanotheranostics: polymeric, lipid-based, and metallic nanomaterials for cancer theranostics

toxicity, biodegradability, biocompatibility, and sustained release of the therapeutics that is significant in achieving optimal efficacy (Silva et al. 2019). Liposomes are spherical vesicles composed of phospholipids, phosphatidylcholine, and cholesterol and the characteristics depend on the nature of the ingredients (Sivarajakumar et al. 2018). Several liposomal drugs have been clinically approved and many are under clinical trials. Presently two USFDA approved liposomal products are available in the market, namely (a) DOXIL for ovarian cancer and (b) Marqibo for lymphoblastic leukemia (Babu et al. 2013). Multimodal imaging agents such as fluorescent probes, radio-isotopes (^{64}Cu and ^{14}C), and nanoparticles like magnetic nanoparticles or quantum dots (QDs), gadolinium (Gd)-based contrast agents, and SPIONs along with small molecule therapeutics have been used in liposomal theranostics (Madamsetty et al. 2019; Sivarajakumar et al. 2018).

3.2.2 Lipid Nanoparticles in Cancer Theragnostic

Lipid nanoparticles (LNP) comprise a lipid monolayer that is enclosed in a solid lipid core. Natural lipids such as phospholipids and cholesterol have been used that can encapsulate molecules in a hydrophilic or hydrophobic core (Bromma et al. 2019). LNPs are one of the most productive platforms for cancer theranostics as they are biocompatible and can be easily upscaled (Tang et al. 2018). Dyes such as near-infrared (NIR) irradiated cyanine fluorescent dyes have been used for both imaging and thermal ablation of tumor cells (Feng et al. 2017). 1,1-dioctadecyl-3,3,3,3-tetramethylindotricarbocyanine iodide (DiR) dyes have been investigated. DiR displayed extended absorption wavelength, resulting in condensed autofluorescence and enhanced tissue penetration and highly efficacious antitumor activity (Pansare et al. 2012). In another study, targeting ligand *apolipoprotein E3* (apoE3) fabricated porphyrin loaded-LNPs have been reported to display encouraging therapeutic efficacy in glioblastoma (Rajora et al. 2017). In another study, Lin et al. synthesized a co-loaded NIR dye and siRNA. These LNPs demonstrated highly sensitive NIR imaging, non-invasive and real-time monitoring of drug delivery and its response in an orthotopic prostate tumor model (Lin et al. 2014). The following sub-categories of LNPs with their respective applications in cancer theranostics are discussed below.

3.2.2.1 Solid Lipid Nanoparticles (SLNs)

SLNs are spherical colloidal nanocarriers that have a size ranging between 50 and 100 nm. The solid lipid core of SLNs is made up of fatty acids, triglycerides, etc. alleviated by an interfacial surfactant layer (Lopes et al. 2014; Madamsetty et al. 2019). The unique feature of SLNs as compared to other colloidal carriers is that liquid lipid is replaced by solid lipid. SLNs comprise lipid (0.1–30% (w/w)) dispersed in an aqueous solution of surfactant (0.5–5% (w/w)) as stabilizing agent. The use of solid lipid as a matrix material for drug delivery is well known from lipid pellets for oral drug delivery such as Mucosolvan® (Müller et al. 2000). Recently Kuang and coworkers developed $\alpha_v\beta_3$ integrin targeted IR-780 iodide loaded tumor vasculature targeted SLNs to monitor photo-thermal therapy (PTT) by imaging, which was selectively accumulated at glioblastoma tissue (Kuang et al. 2017).

3.2.2.2 Nano-Structured Lipids (NLCs)

NLC are drug delivery systems that are composed of physiological and biocompatible lipids, surfactants, and co-surfactants in a mixture. Their core matrix is made up of both solid and liquid lipids. As drug delivery systems, they offer many advantages, including increased solubility, the ability to enhance storage stability, improved permeability and bioavailability, reduced adverse effects, prolonged half-life, and tissue-targeted delivery. Literature reports suggest that NLC display increased entrapment efficiency of drug payload. This can be attributed to the structural parity of two lipids in NLCs that results in imperfections in their structure, while solidification provides space for the accommodation of drug payload (Mittal et al. 2013). Another factor that contributes to the higher entrapment efficiency is due to higher solubility of drugs in liquid lipids in comparison to solid lipids (Chowdhury et al. 2017). Higher payload capacity and long shelf storage stability make NLCs as attractive option for oral drug delivery. NLCs also offer the dual advantage of incorporating both hydrophilic and lipophilic drugs. In addition to this, they may provide sustained release of drugs and target them to the site of action. A higher ratio of lipids up to 95% can be used in NLCs (Han et al. 2016). In 2017, Li et al. developed a simple and multifunctional nanosystem of NIR dye-loaded CXCR4-targeted NLCs and was able to impede tumor progression and prevent metastasis (Li et al. 2017). In another study, co-loaded NLCs with quantum dots (CdTe/CdS/ZnS) and paclitaxel were prepared, which detected tumor by imaging and improved antitumor activity in a murine tumor model of hepatocellular carcinoma (Olerile et al. 2017).

3.2.2.3 Lipid Nanocapsules (LNCs)

LNCs are biomimetic nanocarriers that have a hybrid structure between polymeric nanoparticles and liposomes. The central core comprises medium-chain triglycerides, surrounded by a shell of surfactants (Aparicio-Blanco and Torres-Suárez 2015). Their size range from 20 to 100 nm and LNCs are prepared by phase inversion technique (PIT), a solvent-free, soft-energy procedure with physical stability up to 18 months (Aparicio-Blanco and Torres-Suárez 2015; Huynh et al. 2009). In 2013, Balzeau and team developed LNCs for treating glioblastoma that comprised of neurofilament derived-peptide (NFLTBS.40-63 peptide) as targeting ligand co-encapsulated with paclitaxel and far-red fluorochrome (Chen et al.). These targeted LNCs preferentially accumulated by glioblastoma cells in mice (Balzeau et al. 2013). In other studies, LNCs were used for gene delivery like long-circulating DNA, DNALNCs, or plasmid DNA (Balzeau et al. 2013). Scientists have an optimistic view of the future applications of this platform.

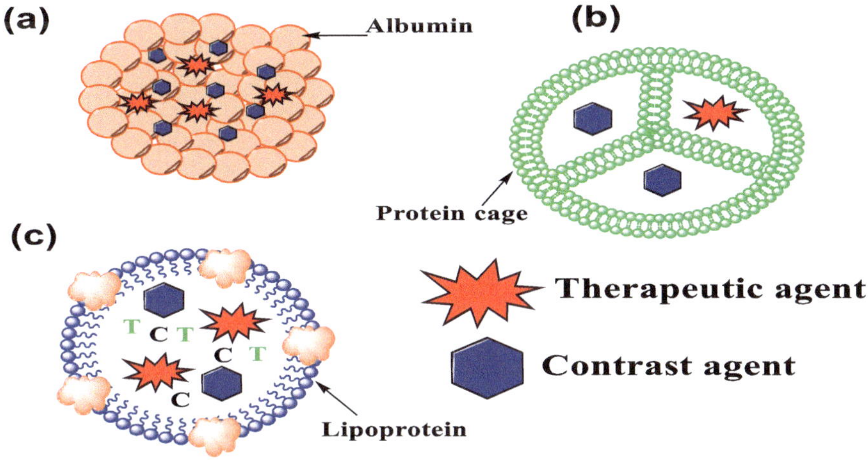

Fig. 3.4 Structural representation of protein-based theranostic nanoplatforms: (**a**) albumin nanoparticle, (**b**) protein cage, and (**c**) lipoprotein. T: triacylglycerol, C: cholesterol

3.2.3 Protein-Based Nanoparticles for Cancer Theranostics

Proteins are promising delivery materials as they offer greater biocompatibility and biodegradability coupled with minimal toxicity that is key to the success of any drug delivery system. Protein-based NPs have raised expectations in the minds of scientists due to their natural availability and compatibility with human physiology. Protein-based delivery platforms have been used for cancer therapy with drug payloads comprising of doxorubicin (DOX) and paclitaxel (Madamsetty et al. 2019; Rosenberg et al. 1990). Albumin can be used as a biocompatible carrier for delivering imaging/anticancer agents to tumor microenvironments. Accordingly, abraxane which is albumin-bound paclitaxel has been approved by FDA (Madamsetty et al. 2019; Rosenberg et al. 1990) (Fig. 3.4).

Recently, Kolluru et al. developed theranostic albumin nanoparticles loaded with a dye indocyanine green (NIR dye) and doxorubicin. The in vivo NIRF imaging of tumor-bearing mice after intravenous injection indicated enhanced accumulation of the albumin nanoparticles in the tumor target site (Kolluru et al. 2013). Yang et al. developed albumin nanoparticles modified with a photodynamic therapy agent hematoporphyrin (HP) and functionalized with gamma-emitting nuclides (99mTc) for scintigraphic imaging (Yang et al. 2010).

Chen et al. produced ultra-small gold nanoclusters coated with bovine serum albumin (BSA), which were simultaneously conjugated with a NIR fluorescent dye MPA, targeting ligand folic acid and doxorubicin, which exhibited low toxicity in normal tissues, selective affinity, and antitumor activity in folate receptor-positive tumors (Chen et al. 2012). Human serum albumin (HSA) has been explored as a natural transporter of IR825, IR780, organic/inorganic oxides, super-paramagnetic iron oxide, and chlorin e6 (Ce6) for effective theranostics construction (Gou et al.

2018). Xie et al. developed an HSA-coated iron oxide nanoparticle (IONP) for multimodal imaging and drug delivery and these HAS-coated IONPs were dually labeled with Cy5.5 and ^{64}Cu-DOTA and could be easily loaded with different drugs, such as paclitaxel and exhibited prolonged circulation half-life, massive accumulation in lesion sites, high extravasation rate, and low uptake by macrophages (Xie et al. 2010). Chen et al. developed an HSA based theranostic nano-complex (HSA-Gd-IR825) for dual-modal imaging-guided PTT to inhibit lymphatic metastasis of cancer post-surgery (Chen et al. 2014). In another study, Yu et al. developed a multifunctional nanoparticle using gemcitabine and pheophorbide-A (P@) loaded HSA (P@-Gem-HSA-NP) for the treatment of lymphatic metastases of PDAC (Yu et al. 2017).

Most recently in 2019, Gao et al. developed HSA based tumor microenvironment-responsive NPs containing both gambogic acid (GA) (heat shock protein (HSP90) inhibitor and an anticancer agent) and dc-IR825 (Gao et al. 2019). These nano-complexes (HSA/dc-IR825/GA) performed well in diagnosis and PTT-mediated inhibition of tumor growth. To date, numerous other protein-based NPs, including legumin, gelatine, transferrin, elastin, ferritin, milk proteins, gliadin, silk, zein, and soy proteins, were developed and their efficacies in various preclinical models were evaluated (Gou et al. 2018; Madamsetty et al. 2019).

Apoferritin/ferritin is a naturally derived vacant protein nanocage made of self-assembling 24 polypeptide units and containing 14 channels without the iron core. Out of 14 channels, 8 channels are of hydrophilic nature, while the remaining channels are hydrophobic nature, allowing the potential for the transport of both hydrophobic and hydrophilic drugs and imaging agents as well. Since apoferritin can endure changes in pH it can be utilized towards the encapsulation of therapeutic agents and imaging probes in different nanoparticles in cancer theranostics (Dostalova et al. 2017; Uchida et al. 2007). Kang et al. developed a multifunctional ferritin based theranostic (F5M-Thr-Pf_Fn-NPB) nanoplatform that can hold cargo molecules securely, deliver them to the targeted sites, and release them to the targeted (MDA MB 231) cells line triggered by thrombin (protease) induced cleavage (Kang et al. 2012).

Luo et al. reported the synthesis of apoferritin based hyaluronic acid (HA)-conjugated nanocages for pH-responsive controlled delivery of an anticancer drug daunomycin (DN), encapsulated into the core of apoferritin for the selective targeting and killing of cancer cells upon binding to the CD44 receptor (Luo et al. 2015). In another study Li et al. developed a multifunctional hybrid nanostructure of ferritin that demonstrated the diagnosis of lung cancer using MR and fluorescence imaging of a multifunctional apoferritin nanostructure (Li et al. 2012). Additionally, ferrimagnetic Fe_3O_4 nanoparticles presence in the hollow ferritin cavity was critical for the MR imaging of $\alpha v\beta_3$ integrin upregulated cancer cells (Madamsetty et al. 2019). Liang et al. demonstrated that natural H-ferritin (HFn) nanocages could carry higher doses of doxorubicin (Dox) for tumor-specific targeting and killing without any targeting ligand functionalization (Liang et al. 2014). The author developed DOX-loaded HFn (HFn-Dox) nanocarrier for the tumor-specific targeted delivery of DOX to tumorous cells causing significant inhibition of tumor growth with a single-dose treatment in various subcutaneous murine cancer models (HT-29, A375, or MDA-MB-231) (Liang et al. 2014).

3.2.4 Virus like Nanoparticles in Cancer Theranostics

Virus like nanoparticles (VLP) are prefabricated nanoscaffolds. The interiors of VLP can be used to protect sensitive compounds, whereas the exterior of virus particles can be functionalized with a wide array of small molecules. As viruses are biocompatible they can be uniquely positioned as natural vehicles to deliver the specific payload to target cells (Yoo et al. 2011). VNPs can be re-engineered with the targeted ligand, chemotherapeutic drugs, and imaging reagents (Madamsetty et al. 2019). For example, the visualization of the flow of blood and vasculature in living chick-embryos was done by using fluorescent *Cowpea mosaic virus* (CPMV) sensors for up to 500μm depths, which has been further exploited in tumor angiogenesis imaging (Suci et al. 2007). Recently, VNPs were also acknowledged as components for non-invasive imaging applications, namely MRI and PET (Shukla and Steimetz 2015). Flexman et al. examined the biodistribution of a viral envelope frequently used as a nanoscale gene delivery vehicle using PET and investigated the magnetic alteration of its biodistribution. ^{18}F-fluoride and iron oxide particles were encapsulated into packets resulting from hemagglutinating virus of Japan (HVJ) and accomplished high signal-to-noise imaging resolution in PET (Flexman et al. 2008).

3.2.5 Inorganic and Bionanoparticles in Cancer Theranostics

Silica, gold, silver, zinc oxide, iron oxides, and rare earth oxides have been widely used for cancer theranostics, diagnostics, drug delivery, bioimaging, bio-sensing, and nucleic acid delivery. These NPs possess exciting physicochemical properties (Madamsetty et al. 2019; Silva et al. 2019). Recently, the biosynthesis of inorganic nanoparticles utilizing green synthesis has gained enormous attention. Green synthesis has been found to be a simple, fast, economical, and eco-friendly method. A large pool of bio-reducing agents, including plants, algae, bacteria, etc. are easily available for green synthesis. Additionally, the use of environmentally friendly solvents such as water makes this technique very sustainable.

Biosynthesized NPs of gold and silver have displayed potential application in the delivery of anticancer drugs in vitro and in vivo studies (Mukherjee et al. 2016; Patra et al. 2015). Gold nanoparticles (AuNPs) surface-functionalized with PEG, biotin, paclitaxel and rhodamine B linked b-cyclodextrin (b-CD) (Heo et al. 2012) have been prepared. Paclitaxel formed an inclusion complex with b-CD conjugated to AuNPs. On similar lines, biosynthesized AuNPs, (b-Au-PP)-based drug-delivery system (DDS) using DOX (b-Au-PP-Dox) (Mukherjee et al. 2016) were studied. The b-AuNPs were synthesized using the aqueous leaf extract of *Peltophorum pterocarpum* to deliver DOX (Madamsetty et al. 2019, Mukherjee et al. 2016). Similarly, mono-dispersed gold nanoparticles (PAuNPs) were prepared by mixing the gold solution with fruit peel extract of *Punica granutum* without using any surfactant or external energy (Ganeshkumar et al. 2013). The same research group also studied the delivery of 5-fluorouracil using folic acid conjugated b-AuNPs in breast cancer cells in a targeted manner (Ganeshkumar et al. 2013; Madamsetty et al. 2019). In another study fluorescence-based bioimaging of in situ b-AuNPs for the detection of Human leukemia cells (K562) and human hepato-carcinoma cells (HepG2) in xenograft tumor mouse models (Wang et al. 2013) were studied. The b-AuNPs were synthesized using the Lantana montevidensis leaf extract (Mukherjee et al. 2015).

In vitro studies indicate that AuNPs have a high affinity towards cancer cells such as A549, HeLa and MG63 in comparison to NIH3T3 cell lines (Heo et al. 2012). b-AuNPs theranostics exhibited excellent biocompatibility when the C57BL6/J mice were treated with b-AuNPs compared to the mice treated with chemically synthesized AuNPs after seven consecutive intraperitoneal injections of 10 mg/kg/ b.w. of dose (Madamsetty et al. 2019, Mukherjee et al. 2016). Treatment with b-AuNPs conjugated DOX caused a significant reduction of melanoma tumor growth in mice compared to DOX (Madamsetty et al. 2019). b-NPs were exploited as anti-cancer agents due to the presence of therapeutically active phytochemicals (Taxol, polyphenols, flavonoids and isoflavons).

Similarly, Bio-synthesized silver nanoparticles using methanolic extract of *Olax scandens* leaves (Heo et al. 2012), anisotropic b-AuNPs using seed extract of *Theobroma cacao* [cocoa] having photo-thermal ablation activities of towards epidermoid carcinoma A431 cells upon laser exposure (Fazal et al. 2014).

3.3 Conclusions and Future Perspectives

Nanomedicine is a niche area that can be visualized as the next dimension for the ongoing development of cancer theranostic systems. New strategies encompassing the use of functionalized nanomaterials can deliver therapeutics and assist in the early detection, diagnosis, and therapy of the disease. The main objective of efficient nano-structured delivery systems is the reduction of a drug dose to attain and achieve an efficient therapeutic effect, thereby causing cost reduction and decreasing the side effects. Developments have been made in the arena of nanomaterials along with their intended applications in the field of cancer theranostics but various challenges are still there limiting widespread clinical translation. One of the most significant challenges in this field is to have nanoparticles embellished with complex multifunctional agents. In most cases, the exciting results of theranostics nanomedicines in the literature are available only from in vitro studies. The path to preclinical, clinical translation and industrial scale-up is challenging and arduous. This field is being explored by researchers, yet more efforts are needed to improve ligand conjugation, drug encapsulation and colloidal stability of nanoparticles. Additionally, increasing their efficiency in biological milieu as well as the use of economical and biocompatible biomaterials is required for future applications. The accumulation of NPs in the spleen and the liver is a barrier in clinical translation and requires careful consideration for translation from bench to clinics. Accordingly, a deeper understanding of bio-nano interactions, especially with lipids, proteins and immune system following their clearance from the human body should be pursued in detail, along with more studies on pharmacokinetics and pharmacodynamics of such revolutionary delivery systems is required. In addition, long-term safety/toxicity-related studies of nano-formulation, selection of the appropriate imaging and contrast modalities for the exact clinical circumstance as well as limitations related to fluorescence and photo-bleaching is the key for successful application of cancer theranostics in nanomedicine.

In conclusion, nanomedicine will be the future of medicine, and nanoparticle-based theranostics will be undoubtedly at the heart of these endeavors. Though inspiring evidences sprouted from recent discoveries is evident but the significant ground needs to be covered and requires a concerted interdisciplinary approach for translation and clinical application of these platforms. The positive outlook for bioinspired nanotheranostics and its clinical translation is encouraging and holds promise to modernizing cancer therapy in the future.

References

Aparicio-Blanco J, Torres-Suárez AI (2015) Glioblastoma multiforme and lipid nanocapsules: a review. J Biomed Nanotechnol 11:1283–1311

Babu A, Templeton AK, Munshi A et al (2013) Nanoparticle-based drug delivery for therapy of lung cancer: progress and challenges. J Nanomater 2013:14

Balzeau J, Pinier M, Berges R et al (2013) The effect of functionalizing lipid nanocapsules with NFL-TBS. 40-63 peptide on their uptake by glioblastoma cells. Biomaterials 34:3381–3389

Bardhan R, Lal S, Joshi A et al (2011) Theranostic nanoshells: from probe design to imaging and treatment of cancer. Acc Chem Res 44:936–946

Bhaumik J, Thakur NS, Aili PK et al (2015) Bioinspired nanotheranostic agents: synthesis, surface functionalization, and antioxidant potential. ACS Biomater Sci Eng 1:382–392

Bromma K, Rieck K, Kulkarni J et al (2019) Use of a lipid nanoparticle system as a Trojan horse in delivery of gold nanoparticles to human breast cancer cells for improved outcomes in radiation therapy. Cancer Nanotechnol 10:1

Chapman M, Pascu SI (2012) Nanomedicines design: approaches towards the imaging and therapy of brain tumours. J Nanomed Nanotechnol 4:006

Chen H, Li S, Li B et al (2012) Folate-modified gold nanoclusters as near-infrared fluorescent probes for tumor imaging and therapy. Nanoscale 4:6050–6064

Chen Q, Liang C, Wang X et al (2014) An albumin-based theranostic nano-agent for dual-modal imaging guided photothermal therapy to inhibit lymphatic metastasis of cancer post surgery. Biomaterials 35:9355–9362

Chi Y-H, Hsiao J-K, Lin M-H et al (2017) Lung cancer-targeting peptides with multi-subtype indication for combinational drug delivery and molecular imaging. Theranostics 7:1612

Chowdhury SR, Mukherjee S, Das S et al (2017) Multifunctional (3-in-1) cancer theranostics applications of hydroxyquinoline-appended polyfluorene nanoparticles. Chem Sci 8:7566–7575

Cong Y, Xiao H, Xiong H et al (2018) Dual drug backboned shattering polymeric theranostic nanomedicine for synergistic eradication of patient-derived lung cancer. Adv Mater 30:1706220

Dostalova S, Vasickova K, Hynek D et al (2017) Apoferritin as an ubiquitous nanocarrier with excellent shelf life. Int J Nanomed 12:2265

Duan H, Wang D, Li Y (2015) Green chemistry for nanoparticle synthesis. Chem Soc Rev 44:5778–5792

Fazal S, Jayasree A, Sasidharan S et al (2014) Green synthesis of anisotropic gold nanoparticles for photothermal therapy of cancer. ACS Appl Mater Interface 6:8080–8089
Feng L, Cheng L, Dong Z et al (2017) Theranostic liposomes with hypoxia-activated prodrug to effectively destruct hypoxic tumors post-photodynamic therapy. ACS Nano 11:927–937
Flexman JA, Cross DJ, Lewellen BL et al (2008) Magnetically targeted viral envelopes: a PET investigation of initial biodistribution. IEEE Trans Nanobioscience 7:223–232
Ganeshkumar M, Sathishkumar M, Ponrasu T et al (2013) Spontaneous ultra fast synthesis of gold nanoparticles using Punica granatum for cancer targeted drug delivery. Colloids Surf B Biointerfaces 106:208–216
Gao G, Jiang YW, Sun W et al (2019) Molecular targeting-mediated mild-temperature photothermal therapy with a smart albumin-based nanodrug. Small 15:1900501
Gou Y, Miao D, Zhou M et al (2018) Bio-inspired protein-based nanoformulations for cancer theranostics. Front Pharmacol 9:421
Han Y, Li Y, Zhang P et al (2016) Nanostructured lipid carriers as novel drug delivery system for lung cancer gene therapy. Pharm Dev Technol 21:277–281
Heo DN, Yang DH, Moon H-J et al (2012) Gold nanoparticles surface-functionalized with paclitaxel drug and biotin receptor as theranostic agents for cancer therapy. Biomaterials 33:856–866
Huynh NT, Passirani C, Saulnier P et al (2009) Lipid nanocapsules: a new platform for nanomedicine. Int J Pharm 379:201–209
Janib SM, Moses AS, Mackay JA (2010) Imaging and drug delivery using theranostic nanoparticles. Adv Drug Deliv Rev 62:1052–1063
Kang YJ, Park DC, Shin H-H et al (2012) Incorporation of thrombin cleavage peptide into a protein cage for constructing a protease-responsive multifunctional delivery nanoplatform. Biomacromolecules 13:4057–4064
Kolluru LP, Rizvi SA, D'souza M et al (2013) Formulation development of albumin based theragnostic nanoparticles as a potential delivery system for tumor targeting. J Drug Target 21:77–86
Kuang Y, Zhang K, Cao Y et al (2017) Hydrophobic IR-780 dye encapsulated in cRGD-conjugated solid lipid nanoparticles for NIR imaging-guided photothermal therapy. ACS Appl Mater Interface 9:12217–12226
Li H, Wang K, Yang X et al (2017) Dual-function nanostructured lipid carriers to deliver IR780 for breast cancer treatment: anti-metastatic and photothermal anti-tumor therapy. Acta Biomater 53:399–413
Li K, Zhang Z-P, Luo M et al (2012) Multifunctional ferritin cage nanostructures for fluorescence and MR imaging of tumor cells. Nanoscale 4:188–193
Liang M, Fan K, Zhou M et al (2014) H-ferritin–nanocaged doxorubicin nanoparticles specifically target and kill tumors with a single-dose injection. Proc Natl Acad Sci 111:14900–14905
Lin N, Huang J, Dufresne A (2012) Preparation, properties and applications of polysaccharide nanocrystals in advanced functional nanomaterials: a review. Nanoscale 4:3274–3294
Lin Q, Jin CS, Huang H et al (2014) Nanoparticle-enabled, image-guided treatment planning of target specific RNAi therapeutics in an orthotopic prostate cancer model. Small 10:3072–3082
Lopes R, Gaspar M, Pereira J et al (2014) Liposomes versus lipid nanoparticles: comparative study of lipid-based systems as oryzalin carriers for the treatment of leishmaniasis. J Biomed Nanotechnol 10:3647–3657
Luo Y, Wang X, Du D et al (2015) Hyaluronic acid-conjugated apoferritin nanocages for lung cancer targeted drug delivery. Biomater Sci 3:1386–1394
Madamsetty VS, Mukherjee A, Mukherjee S (2019) Recent trends of the bio-inspired nanoparticles in cancer theranostics. Front Microbiol 10:1264
Mittal AK, Chisti Y, Banerjee UC (2013) Synthesis of metallic nanoparticles using plant extracts. Biotechnol Adv 31:346–356

Mukherjee S, Dasari M, Priyamvada S et al (2015) A green chemistry approach for the synthesis of gold nanoconjugates that induce the inhibition of cancer cell proliferation through induction of oxidative stress and their in vivo toxicity study. J Mater Chem B 3:3820–3830

Mukherjee S, Sau S, Madhuri D et al (2016) Green synthesis and characterization of monodispersed gold nanoparticles: toxicity study, delivery of doxorubicin and its bio-distribution in mouse model. J Biomed Nanotechnol 12:165–181

Müller RH, Maèder K, Gohla SJ et al (2000) Solid lipid nanoparticles (SLN) for controlled drug delivery–a review of the state of the art. Eur J Pharm Biopharm 50:161–177

Narayanan KB, Sakthivel N (2010) Biological synthesis of metal nanoparticles by microbes. Adv Colloid Interface Sci 156:1–13

Neubi GMN, Opoku-Damoah Y, Gu X et al (2018) Bio-inspired drug delivery systems: an emerging platform for targeted cancer therapy. Biomater Sci 6:958–973

Olerile LD, Liu Y, Zhang B et al (2017) Near-infrared mediated quantum dots and paclitaxel co-loaded nanostructured lipid carriers for cancer theragnostic. Colloids Surf B Interfaces 150:121–130

Ovais M, Khalil AT, Ayaz M et al (2018) Biosynthesis of metal nanoparticles via microbial enzymes: a mechanistic approach. Int J Mol Sci 19:4100

Pansare VJ, Hejazi S, Faenza WJ et al (2012) Review of long-wavelength optical and NIR imaging materials: contrast agents, fluorophores, and multifunctional nano carriers. Chem Mater 24:812–827

Patra S, Mukherjee S, Barui AK et al (2015) Green synthesis, characterization of gold and silver nanoparticles and their potential application for cancer therapeutics. Mater Sci Eng C Mater Biol Appl 53:298–309

Pene F, Courtine E, Cariou A et al (2009) Toward theragnostics. Crit Care Med 37:S50–S58

Rajora M, Ding L, Valic M et al (2017) Tailored theranostic apolipoprotein E3 porphyrin-lipid nanoparticles target glioblastoma. Chem Sci 8:5371–5384

Rosenberg SA, Aebersold P, Cornetta K et al (1990) Gene transfer into humans—immunotherapy of patients with advanced melanoma, using tumor-infiltrating lymphocytes modified by retroviral gene transduction. N Engl J Med 323:570–578

Sharmila C, Ranjith Kumar R, Chandar Shekar BJ et al (2018) Psidium guajava: a novel plant in the synthesis of silver nanoparticles for biomedical applications. Asian J Pharm Clin Res 11:341–345

Shukla S, Steinmetz NF (2015) Virus-based nanomaterials as positron emission tomography and magnetic resonance contrast agents: from technology development to translational medicine. Wiley Interdiscp Rev Nanomed Nanobiotechnol 7:708–721

Silva CO, Pinho JO, Lopes JM et al (2019) Current trends in cancer nanotheranostics: metallic, polymeric, and lipid-based systems. Pharmaceutics 11:22

Sivarajakumar R, Mallukaraj D, Kadavakollu M et al (2018) Nanoparticles for the treatment of lung cancers. Adv Exp Med Biol 890:137–147

Suci PA, Varpness Z, Gillitzer E et al (2007) Targeting and photodynamic killing of a microbial pathogen using protein cage architectures functionalized with a photosensitizer. Langmuir 23:12280–12286

Tang W-L, Tang WH, Li SD (2018) Cancer theranostic applications of lipid-based nanoparticles. Dug Discov Today 23:1159–1166

Uchida M, Klem MT, Allen M et al (2007) Biological containers: protein cages as multifunctional nanoplatforms. Adv Mater 19:1025–1042

Wang J, Zhang G, Li Q et al (2013) In vivo self-bio-imaging of tumors through in situ biosynthesized fluorescent gold nanoclusters. Sci Rep 3:1157

Xie J, Chen K, Huang J et al (2010) PET/NIRF/MRI triple functional iron oxide nanoparticles. Biomaterials 31:3016–3022

Yang S-G, Chang J-E, Shin B et al (2010) 99mTc-hematoporphyrin linked albumin nanoparticles for lung cancer targeted photodynamic therapy and imaging. J Mater Chem 20:9042–9046

Yoo J-W, Irvine DJ, Discher DE et al (2011) Bio-inspired, bioengineered and biomimetic drug delivery carriers. Nat Rev Drug Discov 10:521–535

Yu X, Zhu W, Di Y et al (2017) Triple-functional albumin-based nanoparticles for combined chemotherapy and photodynamic therapy of pancreatic cancer with lymphatic metastases. Int J Nanomed 12:6771

Nanomedicines for Solid Tumors: Current Status, Challenges, and Future Prospects

4

Janani Gopi, Madhumala Gopinath, Antara Banerjee, Secunda Rupert, Rosy Vennila, and Surajit Pathak

Abstract

Cancer is considered to be a dreadful disease affecting a wide array of populations that are acquired by sedentary lifestyle changes or through an inherited condition. There is large documentation of drugs that are administered to the cancer treatment and the trouble in selectively destroying all the cancer cells is a complicated one. Even though there are several FDA approved drugs which are utilized for cancer treatment, but the drug resistance and other biological barriers like renal, hepatic, and immune clearances are the pitfalls to triumph over for efficient drug delivery. Nanomedicine is known to emerge as a new therapeutic application which might guide as active pharmaceutical constituent engineered within the nanoparticles. Nanocarrier is considered to be a tumor-targeted vector wherein the liposomes, dendrimers, micelles, etc. are doped along with adjuvant and other essential components to accomplish the targeted delivery by not only devastating the solid tumor but also the tumor microenvironment to prevent the recurrence of cancer at that site. Focusing keenly on the synthesizing biocompatible nanoparticles and fabrication techniques are employed in order to avoid immune rejection. Moreover, the photodynamic therapy targeting the solid tumor along with imaging agents also emphasizes on the tumor heterogeneity in the tumor microenvironment. Theranostic nanoparticles act as multifunctional nanosystems which aids in both the diagnostic and medical applications in a single nanoparticle for better therapeutic efficiency in cancer therapy. With an increasing clinical

J. Gopi · M. Gopinath · A. Banerjee · S. Pathak (✉)
Faculty of Allied Health Sciences, Chettinad Academy of Research, and Education, Chettinad Hospital and Research Institute (CHRI), Chennai, India
e-mail: drsurajitpathak@chettinadhealthcity.com

S. Rupert · R. Vennila
Stanley Medical College Hospital, Chennai, India

A. Malik et al. (eds.), *Nanomedicine for Cancer Diagnosis and Therapy*,
https://doi.org/10.1007/978-981-15-7564-8_4

trial with FDA approved cancer drugs to be doped along with the nanoparticles for efficient delivery to the targeted tumor site, which is highly heterogeneous and continuously evolving nature of the tumor microenvironment altogether concentrates on the optimal design of nanoparticles which are likely to be disease-specific by the construction of nanotherapeutics based on approaches that reduce tumor heterogeneity treatment.

Keywords

Cancer · Solid tumor · Nanomedicine · Tumor microenvironment · Nanoparticle

4.1 Introduction

Growth and development are a primary progressions in any given system. The body includes an organization of a regulated network of interactions to control the gene expression of mRNA, proteins, and other epigenetic factors, which guide the development of the organism towards growth and a disease-free system. This allows us to also understand how to combat diseases with the help of different therapies which are involved in maintaining the system. National cancer institute states cancer to be a disease in which abnormal cells divide uncontrollably and invade the body tissue. Our human body has two types of outcomes of dysregulation that leads to abnormal cell division which are categorized into malignant and benign in case of cancer detection. Tumors are groups of abnormal cells that form lumps or growths which can start in any one of the trillions of cells in our bodies. Tumors develop and behave differently, depending on whether they are cancerous, non-cancerous, or precancerous. Generally, the tumor builds up a pathological environment like abnormal vasculature, increased interstitial fluid pressure as well as intense extracellular matrix which inherently hamper the migration of nanomedicine aided nanoparticles to the tumor parenchyma. Solid tumors may be benign or malignant depending upon the severity of the tumor mass and they are classified into different types of tumor depending on the residence of the tumor cell population. Based on the literature search, colorectal cancer is third most commonly diagnosed cancer globally, with a cumulative lifetime risk of approximately 5–6% (William 2003). While the enhanced permeability and retention effect have emerged as a key rationale for using nanoparticles to treat solid tumors, it does not ensure uniform delivery of these particles to all regions of tumors in sufficient quantities. This heterogeneous distribution of therapeutics is a result of physiological barriers existing by the abnormal tumor vasculature and interstitial matrix and strategies that have been exploited to overcome these barriers for optimizing the delivery of nanoparticles to the tumors site.

4.2 Possible Factors that Initiate Cancer Growth

4.2.1 Age

Age plays a significant risk factor for the distinct cancer types based on their site and it adverse as the aging occurs significantly. At some stage in cancer diagnosis, information has revealed that somatic mutations, as well as germ line variation, are encumbered by the cancer genes significantly.

4.2.2 Cancer Causing Elements

Cancer is instigated at the genetic level due to their exposure of nucleic acids such as DNA and RNA to harmful substances. As suggested by the National Toxicology Program, some of the detrimental substances such as nickel, asbestos, formaldehyde, vinyl chloride, trichloroethylene, arsenic, beryllium, cadmium, ethylene oxide, benzene, and aflatoxin are known to be the key attributes of developing cancer. Consumption of alcohol can habitually intensify the possibility of causing cancer in other body parts such as the mouth, pharynx, larynx, esophagus, liver, and breast. On the other hand, tobacco smoking and mainly second hand smoking pave the way to advanced risk factors of cancer like lung cancer, larynx, mouth cancer, digestive tract cancer, throat cancer, and so forth. Tobacco smoking contains the toxic element nicotine that damages the genetic material such as the deoxyribonucleic acid which leads to mutation of cancer causing genes at their molecular level that down-regulates to the protein level for interference.

4.2.3 Immunosuppression

Repression of the immune system in the case of organ transplantation acts as a major possibility of acquiring cancer in immunodeficient patients. The immunodeficient patients are easily susceptible to cancer due to their consumption of immunosuppressive drugs that in turn let down the immune system to sense the cancer cells and devastate them due to weakened immune surveillance to recruit the immune cells at the site of tumor mass which would have been a promising factor in a healthy person. Individuals who are suffering from the human immunodeficiency virus or acquired immune-deficiency syndrome heighten the risk of acquiring cancer which is also obtained from viral infections and other co-morbidities.

4.2.4 Infectious Agents

Some of the infectious agents mostly involve bacteria, parasites, and viruses which lead to a higher risk of developing cancer. Generally, viruses are transmitted easily from an infected person to a healthy person through blood and other body fluids.

4.2.5 Radiation

Emission of the high energy ionizing radiation such as gamma rays, X-rays, α-particles, β-particles, and neutrons can cause the impairment of the genetic material, deoxyribonucleic acid that causes mutation of the genes. Over exposure of people working in nuclear power plants with radioactive elements and also in radiation therapy with computed tomography scan, positron emission tomography scans might lead to cancer progression.

4.3 Tumor Classification Based on Tissue of Origin

Classification of the tumor as in Figure 4.1 which can occur in distinct body tissues namely connective tissue, muscle, epithelial tissue, endothelium and mesothelium, gonadal tumor invading germ cells, neural as well as the blood and lymphoid cells precisely. Molecular testing methods such as DNA methylation array profiling and next-generation sequencing analysis have paved their way to diagnose cancer genes at their molecular levels through the recent sophisticated technology based tools for better diagnosis at their genetic level more precisely. Array analysis has revealed that CpG acts as a biomarker which is more than enough for precise diagnosis of cancer which is examined by quantitative polymerase chain reaction and targeted next-generation sequencing (Xia et al. 2020).

4.4 Existing Treatment Options Available for Cancer

The preliminary treatment methods availed in cancer diagnosis are surgery, whereas the adjuvant treatment options include chemotherapy, targeted drug therapy, immunotherapy, radiation therapy, hormone therapy, cryoablation, and radiofrequency ablation which are to be endured after the primary treatment of cancer. Among the above palliative treatment methods, the conventional therapies include chemotherapy and radiation therapy to be undergone routinely. For instance, the transitory explanation of few cancer therapies listed above involves cryoablation, targeted drug delivery, and radiofrequency ablation. In cryoablation, the procedure involves the insertion of a cryoprobe through the epidermis and unswervingly into the tumor site. Then, the gas is impelled into the cancerous tissue via cryoprobe which in turn freeze the tissue followed by thawing, the same procedure is reiterated several times until the tumor tissue is completely eradicated. At the same time, explaining the radiofrequency ablation procedure requires the cryoprobe to be introduced into the skin followed by the deliverance of high frequency energy to the tumor site via the probe that destroys the cancer cells by process of heating (Gavhane et al. 2011). Therefore, the recurrence of tumors at the site and also concentrating on the side effects endured by the patient are known to be excruciating during cancer treatment. Thus, the researchers have turned their focus towards the recent emerging technology based methods in nanomedicine paves the way for a better therapeutic

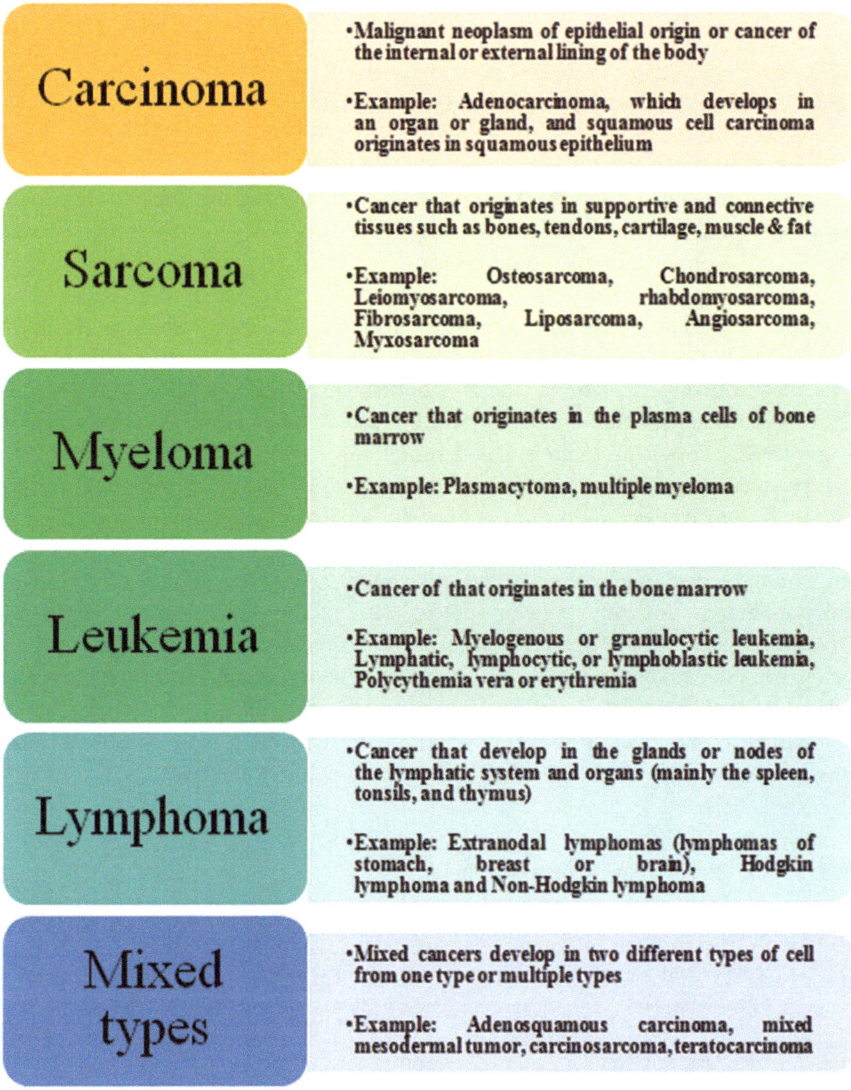

Fig. 4.1 Tumor classification based on their tissue of origin

application due to their particle size, feasibility, and other factors contributing to targeted drug delivery methods whilst overcoming adversities of the standard treatment options available for cancer therapy. The recent emerging technique involves the targeted drug delivery to the cancer site using nanotechnology based methods.

4.5 Description of Solid Tumor

Solid tumors are characterized by aberrant tumor vasculature along with increased tumor extracellular matrix paves the way for an intense delivery mechanism to be designed for the eradication at the tumor site. Solid tumors are classified into different types based on their tissue of origin as depicted in Table 4.1. Categorization of cancers through the tissue of origin is the primary feature for the diagnostic pathology of neoplasia. Solid tumors consist of two components, namely parenchyma and stroma which play a diverse role in tumor development. So, the parenchyma is comprised of cancerous cells and tissues, whereas stroma encompasses neoplastic cells which stimulate and spread diversely. Tumors which arise from the epithelial tissue possess basal lamina that delineates stroma from the mass of tumor cells. Consequently, the stroma is known to be located adjacent between the normal and cancerous cells which indirectly pave the way for the progression of the tumor. Angiogenesis, tumor promoting genes, tumor suppressor genes, and other inflammatory mediators such as cytokines, chemokines are the foremost factors contributing to cancer. Solid tumors majorly fall into two categories as benign or malignant depending on the severity and progression of cancer at the targeted site. The prototypical classification of solid tumors widely includes sarcoma, carcinoma, and lymphomas precisely (Gavhane et al. 2011). Thus, the extracellular matrix encompasses of elastin fibers, collagen, proteoglycans, and glycosaminoglycan which are a dense matrix which deeply hinders the dissemination of nanoparticles in the tumor interstitium. Therefore, overcoming the pitfalls of the deliverance of nanoparticles and selecting the appropriate vector, and fabricating according to the tumor type to be effective at their site of action (Parodi et al. 2014).

Table 4.1 Solid tumor based on tissue of origin

S. No	Solid tumor based on tissue of origin	Example of solid tumor	
		Benign	Malignant
1	Smooth muscle	Leiomyoma	Leiomyosarcoma
2	Stratified squamous	Papilloma	Squamous cell carcinoma
3	Glandular epithelium	Adenoma	Adenocarcinoma
4	Striated muscle	Rhabdomyoma	Rhabdomyosarcoma
5	Placenta	Hydatidiform mole	Choriocarcinoma
6	Nerve cells	Ganglioneuroma	Neuroblastoma
7	Nerve sheath	Neurofibroma	Neurofibrosarcoma
8	Breast	Fibroadenoma	Cystosarcoma phylloides
9	Parathyroid	Parathyroid adenoma	Parathyroid carcinoma
10	Stomach and intestine	Carcinoid	Malignant carcinoid

4.6 Nanomedicine

At the molecular level, the resistance of drugs is known to be a physiological hindrance to the deliverance of anti-cancer medicine. The major negative aspect of chemotherapy is their intricate permeability into the solid tumor due to their pathological features such as abnormal tumor vasculature, interstitial hypertension, and dilated angiogenesis. Ideal nanocarriers should possess the following characteristics such as the biodegradability and biocompatibility, effective homing accommodating the therapeutic agent localized within the tumor site, fabricated with optimal physiochemical features for enhanced drug loading, circulation half-life, the liberation of drugs at the site precisely and lastly acquiescent to cost-effective scale up for commercialization (Xiaoyang Xu et al. 2015). Thus, nanomedicine has revolutionized with the help of nanoparticles loaded with the appropriate drug deliverance to the targeted tumor site to surmount the restriction associated with cytotoxic side effects during chemotherapy (El-Readi and Althubiti 2019).

4.6.1 Unlocking Novel Cancer Applications Exploited in the Field of Nanomedicine

Nanomedicine has the potential to transfigure cancer diagnosis and therapy by advancing in protein engineering and materials science which have contributed to novel nanoscale level targeting approaches to cancer patients. Several therapeutic nanocarriers such nanoliposomes, dendrimers, and several other carriers have been approved for clinical use (Peer et al. 2007). Cell multiplication, immigration, and differentiation are unswervingly restrained by the targeted therapies at the site of the tumor. Thus, targeted therapies are intended to take control over the tumor microenvironment for tackling the alterations caused by the cancerous cells and other types of cells which engage in designing of the nanoparticle (Parodi et al. 2014). Miniature molecules such as monoclonal antibodies with a molecular weight of less than 900 Daltons are favorable for their infiltration into the tumor mass and impede their uncontrolled cell proliferation as well as other related mechanisms. The food and drug administration has approved some of the targeted agent for cancer, including the cetuximab and bevacizumab which have underwent the phase IV of the clinical trial successfully. For instance, the biomarker such as Programmed Death Ligand 1 (PD-L1) is involved in assessing colorectal cancer by analyzing the levels of PD-L1 marker in the affected cancer individual (Xia et al. 2020). Nanomedicine is variedly classified into different types based on their source of fabrication of nanoparticle which is comprised of the lipid derived nanoparticle, polymer derived nanoparticle and inorganic based nanoparticle as shown in Table 4.2 (Rizwanullah et al. 2018).

Table 4.2 Types of nanoparticles for targeted drug delivery in nanomedicine

S. No	Types of nanocarrier in nanomedicine	Features of nanoparticles in nanomedicine
(1)	*Lipid-based nanomedicine* • Liposome • Solid lipid nanoparticle • Nanostructured lipid carrier • Lipid micelle	Lipid-based nanomedicines provide promising possibilities to assure a specific drug accumulation intrinsically into the tumor site, improving the pharmacokinetic profile such as short biological plasma half-life, non-uniform oral absorption, and also the safety of the reduced formation of toxic degradation compounds and localized activity of such molecules
(2)	*Polymer-based nanomedicine* • Polymeric nanoparticle • Polymeric micelle • Polymer drug conjugate • Dendrimer	Polymeric based nanomedicines are solid colloidal systems in which anticancer drug is dissolved, encapsulated onto the constituent polymer matrix. Several polymers, such as poly (lactide-co-glycolide)(PLGA), polylactide (PLA), polycaprolactone(PCL), polyglycolide, poly(d,l-lactide), and chitosan, have been developed for passive and active delivery of therapeutic moieties
(3)	*Inorganic nanomedicine* • Iron oxide nanoparticle • Gold nanoparticle • Carbon nanotube	Inorganic nanomedicine has been extensively studied as therapeutic agents for cancer treatment due to their unique physicochemical properties, versatile development strategies, easy surface engineering, and biocompatibility

4.7 Fabrications of Nanocarrier for Drug Delivery

Particles of size less than 100 nm are characterized as nanoparticles and among the various nanomaterials metal-based nanoparticles are the most equipped nanomaterials, in therapeutics of anticancer dealt with nanomedicine precisely. (Borowik et al. 2019). Polymer-based vectors include nanoliposomes as in Fig. 4.2, dendrimers and the covalent conjugation of synthetic polymers, particularly poly (ethylene glycol) (PEG), encapsulated along with the protein drugs increases their plasma residence, reduces protein immunogenicity and can increase their therapeutic index for cancer therapy (Duncan 2006). Nanotechnology has a significant prospective in the field of medicine by fabricating biocompatible polymers and nanocarriers developed at the nanoscale level for various ailments (Guerrini et al. 2018).

4.8 Targeted Delivery of Nanocarrires to the Tumor Niche as Well as Solid Tumor

Solid tumors are extremely heterogeneous which exist in a complex tumor microenvironment (Banerjee et al. 2011). The tumor niche comprised of numerous cell types such as myofibroblast, adipocytes, immune cells, fibroblast, extracellular matrix as

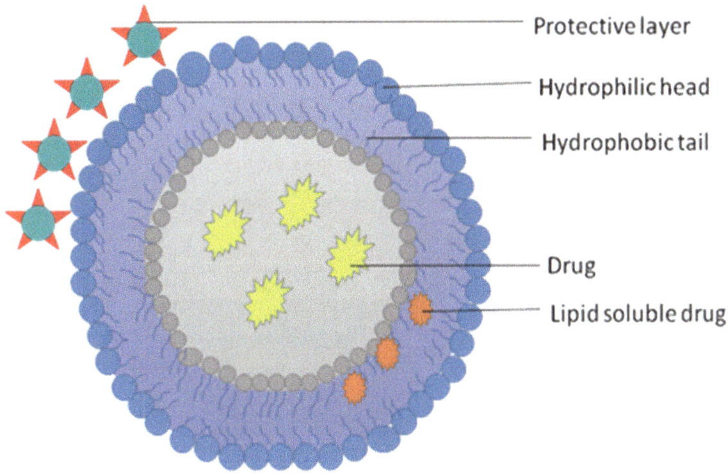

Fig. 4.2 Nano-liposome mediated drug delivery to the tumor site

well as blood and lymphatic vasculature significantly (Albini and Sporn 2007). Previous research articles provide increasing evidence that the tumor microenvironment plays a decisive role in cancer growth, multiplication, and malignancy at the tumor site (Chen et al. 2015). The tumor niche promotes the cessation of the cancer therapies which indirectly exterminate at the tumor site. The emerging field of nanomedicine will facilitate in the fabrication of nanoparticles which might intervene in targeting the tumor microenvironment features, including the vasculature, extracellular matrix, and the immune cells, on altering the immune reaction. The sensitivity of the tumor to cancer therapies such as chemotherapy is mainly persuaded by besieging the tumor vasculature (Klemm and Joyce 2015). Subsequently, intensification of therapeutic efficacy is aided by the nanotherapeutics to distribute drugs via the nanocarriers to inhibit the tumor development and also concentration on the tumor microenvironment. Nanoparticle plays a major role in affecting the immune cells and their alteration inside in the tumor niche. The cytokine encapsulated within the nanocarrier impart sustained liberation and decreased toxicity whilst the systematically delivered is known to induce general immune stimulation. An intense extracellular matrix causes a substantial impediment to effective migration and profound permeability of the nanoparticles inside the tumor tissue. Thus, the eradication of cancer does not aim not only on killing the tumor mass but also destroying the tumor niche by the deliverance of the novel nanocarriers designed appropriately by accommodating other cytokines and anti-cancer drugs for a better therapeutic application at the tumor site (Siegler et al. 2016).

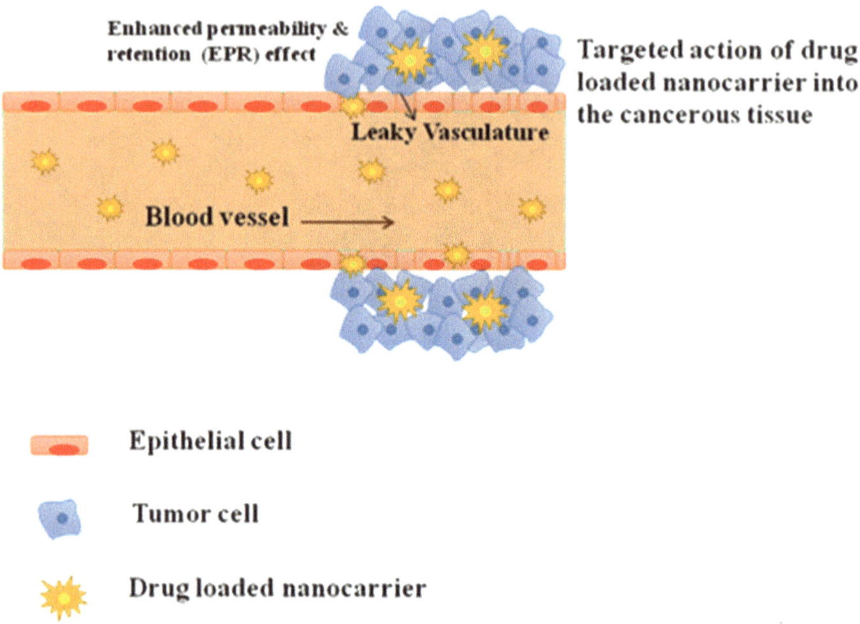

Fig. 4.3 Drug loaded nanocarrier targeted to the tumor tissue

4.8.1 Drug Targeting Mechanisms and Surface Functionalization of Nanocarriers Aiding Nanomedicine Based Technologies in Solid Tumors

Initial detection of cancer site in our body involves the active as well as passive targeting mechanism, higher biocompatibility, and other radiological imaging techniques pave way for a competent therapeutic potential employing nanotechnology in the medical field. The foremost benefit of utilizing nanomaterials is the ease of size which is easily functionalized using specific receptors, antibodies, and biomolecules that facilitate them to definite organelle within certain cells or tissues of the targeted tumor site. Thus, the nanomaterials are fabricated and doped along with cancer drugs at a specific dose range which tends to deliver it to the targeted tumor site for invasion appropriately (Wang et al. 2013). The passive targeting mechanism depends on the pathophysiology as well as immunochemical characteristic of the cancer tissue. The tumor carrying blood vessels are generally seepage in nature which in turn allows the nanocarrier to effortlessly migrate into the interstitial space by traversing the endothelial barrier. Subsequently, normal endothelium measures up to 10 nm, whereas the tumor bearing endothelium is several folds greater measuring from 100 nm to 700 nm distinctively. The solid tumor has a deprived lymphatic drainage network which leads to ineffective circulatory retrieval of the extravasated molecules transpire that directs in the grouping of nanocarriers at the tumor site is known as the enhanced permeability and retention effect as depicted in Fig. 4.3, which is considered as an effective mechanism for targeting the tumor site precisely. Nevertheless, the nanocarrier loaded with small molecular weight drugs which is effective in systemic circulation and reaches the cancer tissue precisely. Encapsulations of the drug inside nanocarrier mainly follow nanotechnology tools that are mainly focused on polymeric-based as well as pH dependent method for withholding the drug for a greater period of time which in turn leads to sustained release at their targeted tumor site. A multitude of nanoparticlulate drug delivery system has acquired massive consideration in tumor treatment, enduring to their interesting accretion at the tumor site through the enhanced permeability and retention effect (Gao 2016).

4.9 Nanoscience Based Imaging Technologies in the Detection of Solid Tumors

Nevertheless, the existing radiological imaging technologies play a vital role as a diagnostic tool in cancer detection along with contrast and other tracers are prevalent in the clinical application which holds intrinsic limitations along with certain drawbacks such as rapid metabolism, nonspecific dissemination all over the body along with detrimental side effects in solid tumor. Nanotechnology has advanced in their non-invasive in-vivo detection as well as enhanced targeted efficiency for tumor the paves way for a better therapeutic application in cancer diagnosis by employing nanoparticles as contrast agents for imaging. Different nanoparticle types have been constructed for molecular imaging like magnetic resonance imaging, computerized tomography, ultrasonography imaging, and positron emission tomography which are diagnostic tools. Multiple components loaded nanostructures called theragnosis or theranostics have been widely analyzed as a strategy to achieve simultaneous cancer diagnosis and treatment. Theranostic nanoparticles act as multifunctional nanosystems by amalgamating the diagnostic and medical possibilities in a single nanoparticle for better therapeutic efficiency in cancer therapy (Ma et al. 2017). Initially, the preclinical manifestation of nanotheranostics was concentrating on the imaging to longitudinally monitor the deposition of nanoparticles into tumor. Ultimately, tumors exhibit heterogeneities in their microenvironment, which ultimately affects the intratumoral delivery of nanoparticles intrinsically into the solid tumor (Petersen et al. 2012).

4.9.1 Photodynamic Nanomedicine in the Treatment of Solid Tumors

Another promising treatment approach is photodynamic therapy, wherein it consists of three components, namely oxygen, photosensitizer drug as well as drug triggering light of specific wavelength accurately. The mechanism behind the photodynamic therapy is the stimulation of photosensitizer drugs at a specific wavelength of light which in turn energy transfer cascade, which end results in cytotoxic reactive oxygen species that render necrotic with apoptotic cell death. Subsequently, photodynamic therapy into deep tissue solid tumor requires optimization of tumor specific delivery of the photosensitizers along with the photo activating light to determine the dosimetric association of light and drug parameters to PDT induced tumor response. Thus, the nanomedicine method shows all the signs for enhanced control of photosensitizer bio-distribution and tumor-specific deliverance via nanoparticles fabricated according to the biocompatibility of solid tumors. Nanoparticles can be fabricated accordingly to enhance their efficacy in tumor-targeted photosensitizer delivery methods include optimal photosensitizer encapsulation, enhanced uptake inside the tumor tissue and cell, selective release of drug in the tumor microenvironment as well as integration of imaging agents can lead to precise photodynamic nanomedicine therapy for tumors of a different category (Master et al. 2013).

4.10 Nanomedicine and Solid Tumor Heterogenecity

Tumor heterogeneity explains about different tumor cells which exhibit distinct tumor cells with varied morphological as well as phenotypic profiles such as cell shape, gene expression, metabolism, motility, proliferation, and metastatic potential. The drawback in the tumor heterogeneity is their inadequate therapeutic effectiveness exhibited by nanomedicine in-vivo. Therefore, the shortcomings such as transport restrictions within the tumor microenvironment and mainly the fabrication of the nanoparticles from bulk to local indices according to their size limitations are to be addressed by the researchers to enhance the deliverance efficacy into the solid tumor. Nanomedicine can establish as a therapeutic modality, unlike other cancer treatments due to their decreased systemic toxicities which is accomplished via the nanoparticle. The nanoparticle impelled pharmacokinetics as well as bio-distribution of effective therapeutic agents. Consequently, the tumor heterogeneity remains to be substantial challenge in cancer treatment. Treatment stratification in the case of a solid tumor should mainly concentrate on the different types of cells and tissues engrossed in the tumor type as well as with the tumor microenvironment so as to design the nanocarrier accurately to target the tumor efficiently by encapsulating with the necessary materials for their biocompatibility and participate competently at the site of action (Ekdawi et al. 2016).

4.11 Nanomedicine in Solid Tumors: PROS and CONS?

Advancement in nanomedicine occurs through the fabrication of novel nanocarriers and technologies for drug delivery. Researchers have turned their limelight towards the limitations of delivery barriers as in solid tumors, which are known to be exceptionally complicated and to exert their focus on the major drawbacks of the nanocarriers accurately.

4.11.1 PROS

The advantages of nanomedicine are as follows: the physiochemical features of nanoparticles include the particle size, shape as well as charges that play a crucial role in the deliverance into their intratumoral dispersion. Various approaches have been exploited to control the release of nanoparticles at their respective site. Subsequently, improvising on the nanoparticles based on many processes among which the stimuli responsive multistage nanocarrier could modify their size in reaction to the tumor niche, which will enhance their tumor permeability. Extracellular matrix disintegrating methods can be recognized by functionalizing the nanoparticles with enzymes that destroy the tumor niche components precisely (Parodi et al. 2014).

4.11.2 CONS

Efficient delivery methods for cancer treatment have quite a lot of impediments to hamper their therapeutic efficacy. One long term blockage leading to an ineffective delivery is the poor permeability of the nanoparticles in the solid tumor, which holds the primary drawback in nanomedicine. So, the solid tumor particularly holds certain features, as shown in Fig. 4.4, which obstructs the effective distribution of the nanoparticle at the tumor site (Zhang et al. 2018).

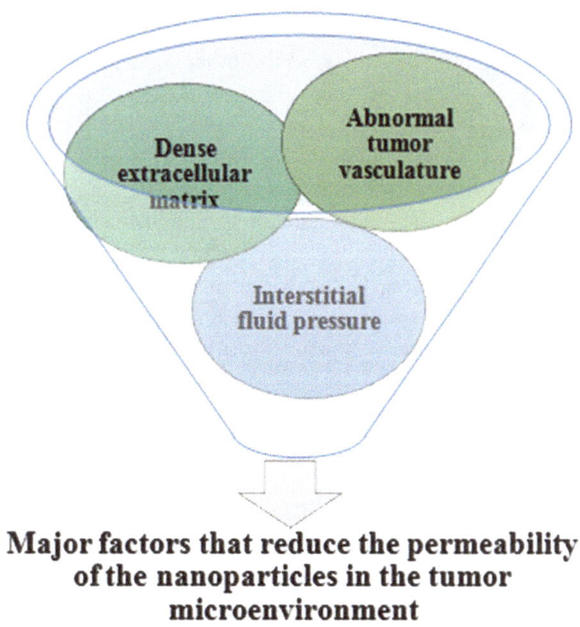

Fig. 4.4 Critical aspects of tumor microenvironment by nanocarrier

4.12 Discussion

As the nanocarrier relies on the slower diffusion to the intratumoral transport as well as the size of the nanoparticle plays a major role in controlling the tumor permeability of nanocarrier with the diffusion rates is inversely proportional towards the particle size. Therefore, the smaller the nanoparticle, the faster they migrate within the tumor. The research article has found out that polymeric micelles of 30 nm in size exhibit much better tumor permeability due to their particle size, whereas the 100 nm nanoparticle is known to be poorly permeable within the tumor. Furthermore, concern towards the small particle size of less than 5 nm is noticed to be eliminated more rapidly by the renal system. Thus, the selection of nanocarrier based on their size that finds equilibrium between extended circulations in the blood vessel moreover improves the tumor permeability in the tumor parenchyma. Thus, nanomedicine aims at designing size switching properties in the tumor niche that generate the endogeneous stimuli include low pH and high matrix metalloproteinases or else involve light as their exogenous stimuli to enhance their delivery efficacy of the nanoparticle (Zhang et al. 2018). There are several anticancer drugs available commercially that are doped inside nanovehicles such as liposomes, micelles, dendrimers for drug delivery, whereas various clinical trials are working on the efficient targeted delivery to the solid tumor by concentrating on their intricate mechanisms for the effective deliverance along with the cancer treatment. The significant advantages of contrast sensitivity, binding avidity, multivalency, specificity sensitivity of nanoparticles, and suitable nanoparticle fabrication procedures can enhance the prognosis and direct diagnosis with quantitative accuracy in solid tumors based on their severity. Although different nanoparticles exhibit variable in-vivo actions that demand the process of translation from lab bench to bedside, which necessitates further reformation (Petersen et al. 2012). Research findings in the article Duncan (2006) have focused on the encapsulation of doxorubicin within the PEGylated nanoparticle permits extended circulation half-life along with increased tumor concentration of drug. At present, several drug delivery methods using nanomedicine include doxorubicin-loaded liposome and paclitaxel bound albumin nanoparticles have been endorsed by the food and drug administration for clinical application. Clinical trial methods have shown better pharmacokinetics as well as decrease side effects and limelight towards the fabrication of an efficient nanocarrier for better penetration at the tumor site.

Key Highlights of the Chapter

1. Solid tumors classification based on their tissue of origin and also focussing on their tumor microenvironment for the eradication of cancer cells at that site.
2. Solid tumor is heterogeneous in nature comprising of multitude of cells that has to be overseen keenly to avoid the relapse of the tumor.
3. Nanomedicine aided nanoparticles pave the way towards a vast breach by studying their intricate cellular composition at the molecular level as well as fabrication of nanoparticles and penetration intrinsically at the intended site holds the main attribute towards the solid tumor treatment.

4. The physiological barriers, type of solid tumor, tumor microenvironment architecture, immune rejections, and other biological consequences have to be met by the nanomedicine-based nanoparticle designed accordingly and doped along with adjuvants and imaging agents to observe the distribution of drug at the site of the tumor. Nanomedicine method shows all the signs for enhanced control of photosensitizer bio-distribution by photodynamic therapy infused along with nanoparticles fabricated for tumor-specific deliverance in the solid tumor.

4.13 Future Perspective

Cancer usually evokes in wound-repair pathways, employing blood vessel cells, basal laminal cells as well as tumor assisting macrophages to aid in their growth and survival of tumor cells. Tumor cells usually desire anaerobic metabolic pathways and partial hypoxia of the tumor niche. While focusing on the pH gradients shifting from extracellular to intracellular space makes them to revert back to the tumor tissue while comparing the normal tissue. Different solid tumors over express surface proteins in comparison with the normal cells wherein the over the profusion of specific surface protein is not assured to selectivity using targeted therapy where finally, few drugs will end up out of the targeted site target affecting the non-cancerous cells. The selection of an accurate surface marker is the most significant feature for the targeted delivery to work efficiently. Thus, the emergence of nanomedicine corresponds to considerable advancement in drug delivery parameters that should be intricately fabricated to establish as an effective anticancer therapy and focusing on the administration methods for safety and efficacy parameters through the biocompatible nanocarrier precisely. Recent oncology drug development considerably utilizes biomarkers as well as imaging technologies such as MRI, US imaging, PET, and CT with functionalized nanoparticles to facilitate in diagnostics for patient stratification as well as for enhanced drug targeting in solid tumors. Conclusively, numerous clinical experimentations are required for validating the fabricated nanoparticle to emerge as an effective technique for targeted drug delivery to not only eradicate the solid tumor but also the tumor microenvironment effectively via various enzymes loaded in the nanocarrier to avoid the recurrence of the tumor at that site which is considered to be a non-invasive procedure to reduce the side effects and pain undergone by the patients undergoing chemotherapy significantly.

Acknowledgement The authors are thankful to Chettinad Academy of Research and Education (CARE) for providing the support to complete this piece of work.

Author Contribution Surajit Pathak conceived the idea of the article. Janani Gopi, Surajit Pathak, Madhumala Gopinath, Antara Banerjee, Secunda Rupert and Rossy Vanilla had written the manuscript. All the authors read and approved the final version of the manuscript.

References

Albini A, Sporn M (2007) The tumour microenvironment as a target for chemoprevention. Nat Rev Cancer 7(2):139e47

Banerjee D, Harfouche R, Sengupta S (2011) Nanotechnology-mediated targeting of tumor angiogenesis. Vasc Cell 3:3

Borowik A, Banasiuk R, Derewonko N, Rychlowski M, Krychowiak-Masnicka M, Wyrzykowski D, Ziabka M, Woziwodzka A, Krolicka A, Piosik J (2019) Interactions of newly synthesized platinum nanoparticles with ICR-191 and their potential application. Sci Rep 9(1):1–11

Chen F, Zhuang X, Lin L, Yu P, Wang Y, Shi Y et al (2015) New horizons in tumor microenvironment biology: challenges and opportunities. BMC Med 13:45

Duncan R (2006) Polymer conjugates as anticancer nanomedicines. Nat Rev Cancer 6(9):688–701

Ekdawi SN, Jaffray DA, Allen C (2016) Nanomedicine and tumor heterogeneity: concept and complex reality. Nano Today. https://doi.org/10.1016/j.nantod.2016.06.006

El-Readi MZ, Althubiti MA (2019) Cancer nanomedicine: a new era of successful targeted therapy. Hindawi J Nanomater 2019:13

Gao H (2016) Shaping tumor microenvironment for improving nanoparticles delivery. Curr Drug Metab 17:731–736

Gavhane YN, Shete AS, Bhagat AK, Shinde VR, Bhong KK, Khairnar GA, Yadav AV (2011) Solid tumors: facts, challenges and solutions. Int J Pharm Sci Res (IJPSR) 2(1):1–12

Guerrini L, Garcia-Rico E, Alvarez-Puebla R (2018) The role of nanoscience in cancer diagnosis. In: Handbook of nanomaterials for cancer theranostics. Elsevier, Amsterdam, pp 177–197

Klemm F, Joyce J (2015) Microenvironmental regulation of therapeutic response in cancer. Trends Cell Biol 25:198e213

Ma Y-Y, Jin K-T, Wang S-B, Wang H-J, Tong X-M, Huang D-S, Mou X-Z (2017) Molecular imaging of cancer with nanoparticle-based theranostic probes. Hindawi Contrast Media Mol Imaging:11

Master A, Livingston M, Gupta AS (2013) Photodynamic nanomedicine in the treatment of solid tumors: perspectives and challenges. J Control Release 168(1):88–102

Parodi A, Haddix SG, Taghipour N, Scaria S, Taraballi F, Cevenini A, Tasciotti E (2014) Bromelain surface modification increases the diffusion of silica nanoparticles in the tumor extracellular matrix. ACS Nano 8:9874–9883

Peer D, Karp JM, Hong S, Farokhzad OC, Margalit R, Langer R (2007) Nanocarriers as an emerging platform for cancer therapy. Nat Nanotechnol 2(12):751

Petersen AL, Hansen AE, Gabizon A, Andresen TL (2012) Liposome imaging agents in personalized medicine. Adv Drug Deliv Rev 64:1417–1435

Rizwanullah M, Amin S, Mir SR, Fakhri KU, Rizvi MM (2018) Phytochemical based nanomedicines against cancer: current status and future prospects. J Drug Target 26(9):731–752

Siegler EL, Jeong Kim Y, Wang P (2016) Nanomedicine targeting the tumor microenvironment: therapeutic strategies to inhibit angiogenesis, remodel matrix, and modulate immune responses. J Cell Immunother:1–10

Wang R, Billone PS, Mullett WM (2013) Nanomedicine in action: an overview of Cancer nanomedicine on the market and in clinical trials. J Nanomater. https://doi.org/10.1155/2013/629681

William M (2003) Grady. Genetic testing for high-risk colon cancer patients. Gastroenterology 124 (6):1574–1594

Xia D, Leon AJ, Cabanero M et al (2020) Minimalist approaches to cancer tissue-of-origin classification by DNA methylation. Mod Pathol. https://doi.org/10.1038/s41379-020-0547-7

Xu X, Ho W, Zhang X, Bertrand N, Farokhzad O (2015) Cancer nanomedicine: from targeted delivery to combination therapy. Trends Mol Med 21(4)

Zhang Y-R, Lin R, Li H-J, He W-l, Du J-Z, Wang J (2018) Strategies to improve tumor penetration of nanomedicines through nanoparticle design. WIREs Nanomed Nanobiotechnol:e1519

Nanomaterials for Early Cancer Diagnostics 5

Sumit Kumar, Pooja Kumari, Gaurav Rathee, and Brijesh Rathi

Abstract

Cancer is unquestionably a serious and potentially life-threatening illness. All over the world, cancer is the second leading cause of death, and early detection of cancer provides a golden opportunity of possibly saving a life. Biomarkers remain a key tool for the early diagnosis of cancer. Biomarkers like microRNAs have been reported for early detection of prostate, breast, ovarian, lung, and many different types of cancer. The current technical progression eyeing at the applications and advantages of nanomaterials makes them a good choice for targeting various biomarkers, which can help in screening, diagnosing, grading, monitoring or prognosticating different cancers. This chapter mainly focuses on the recent research in the field of utilizing nanomaterials as an early diagnostic tool for cancer disease.

Keywords

Cancer · Nanomaterials · Biomarkers · DNA · RNA

S. Kumar (✉) · P. Kumari
Department of Chemistry, Deenbandhu Chhotu Ram University of Science and Technology, Murthal, Sonepat, Haryana, India
e-mail: sumitmalik.chem@dcrustm.org

G. Rathee
Senior Resident, Department of General Medicine, N C Medical College and Hospital Israna, Panipat, India

B. Rathi
Laboratory For Translational Chemistry and Drug Discovery, Department of Chemistry, Hansraj College, University of Delhi, Delhi, India

A. Malik et al. (eds.), *Nanomedicine for Cancer Diagnosis and Therapy*,
https://doi.org/10.1007/978-981-15-7564-8_5

5.1 Introduction

Biomarkers are biological markers, which are helpful indicators for identifying the biological state of a disease. Recent research and advancements in the search for new biomarkers, especially with the utilization of nanoparticle techniques have given new hope for early diagnosis of various cancers. The "early diagnosis" is such a great help to oncologists in the treatment of cancer that it can make a difference of complete cure versus a death warrant. A patient diagnosed at an early-stage may get a complete cure by the various treatment modalities available, and on the other hand, if a patient is diagnosed in the late stage, when most of the treatment options are not effective or possible, the patient may end up with the only help of palliative care. In addition to the help in early diagnosis, some biomarkers can also be possibly used in determining the severity and grade of the disease, and thus can assist with treatment options and estimate the prognosis. Further, many biomarkers could also be useful in monitoring for recurrence of cancer during follow-up of the treated patients. Those new biomarkers with greater sensitivity may be used to design screening tests for mass population or for high-risk populations, and would prove helpful in making early diagnosis; on the other hand, those new biomarkers, which have high specificity, may prove utility in confirming the diagnosis in a suspected patient. This may help in avoiding invasive procedures, specially tissue sampling/biopsies, in many suspected patients. Similarly, the use of such biomarkers could also decrease the need for repetitive tissue sampling to confirm or refute the recurrence of cancer. By determining the receptors and/or antigens which are specifically expressed by the cancer cells, targeted therapy can be planned, providing significantly improved outcomes with a lesser number of drug related toxicities/adverse effects. In brief, with the new prospective nanoparticle biomarkers in line, we are looking forward to a new era of early diagnosis, non-invasive diagnostic approaches, and better determinant of severity and grade, better modalities of monitoring on follow up, better determinants of prognosis, and help for targeted therapy with better results and minimum drug toxicities. Biomarkers and nanotechnology are two prime factors recognized in the field of expanding diagnostic methods in screening and monitoring of early cancer.

Biomarkers can be protein, nucleic acids like DNA or RNA-based materials (Choi et al. 2010). Colossal studies have been conducted in the field of nanotechnology area and many nanomaterial-based techniques have been implemented in early-stage detection of cancer (Fig. 5.1). Nanomaterials like quantum dots, gold particles, biosensors, etc., have been utilized in detecting cancer biomarkers and cancer diagnostics (Zhang et al. 2019). While the scope of the application of micro/nanomotors-based delivery systems is limited at the cellular level (Wang et al. 2020a). Herein, we have discussed various types of cancer and their early detection techniques using nanomaterials.

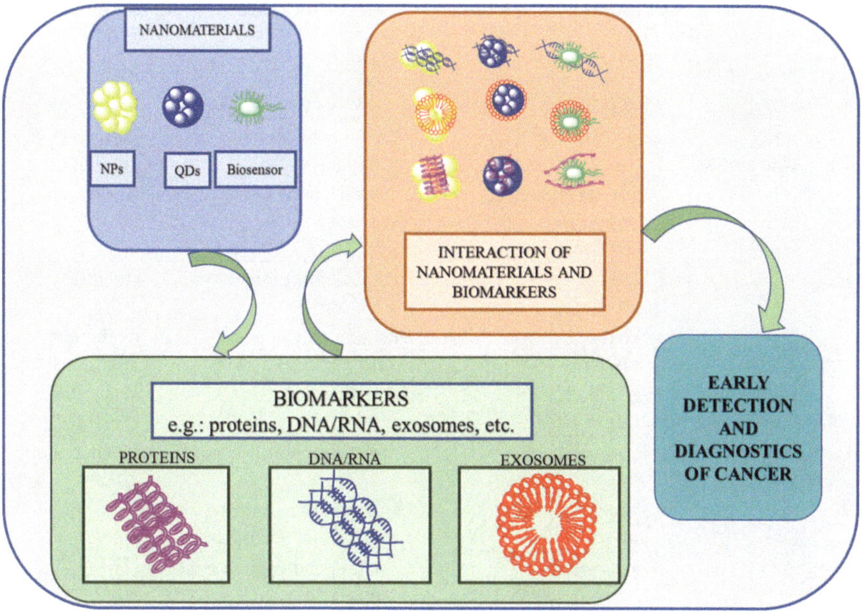

Fig. 5.1 Nanomaterials for detecting the cancer biomarkers and cancer diagnostics

5.2 Cancer and Biomarkers

Different biomarkers are identified for indicating specific type of cancer with the help of nanoparticle techniques (Table 5.1).

5.2.1 Early Detection of Prostate Cancer

Prostate cancer, one of the common cancers, has many types like acinar and ductal adenocarcinoma, squamous cell cancer, and transitional cell cancer, but acinar adenocarcinoma is the most prevalent type. Various biomarkers like miR-21, prostate-specific antigen (PSA), prostate-specific membrane antigen (PSMA), human interleukin-6, IgG proteins, DU145 and LNCaP cells biomarker, microRNAs (miR-107), etc., have been exploited for early detection of prostate cancer. Early detection and treatment will have an advantage, specially using nanomaterials. Various efforts have been made for different types of nanoparticles; an electrochemical biosensor built on single-walled carbon nanotubes (SWCNT) grafted dendritic Au nanostructures have been used for detecting miR-21 (Sabahi et al. 2020). Photoelectrochemical biosensor synthesized from TiO2 mesocrystals coupled with polyamidoamine dendrimers has shown promising results for detecting prostate-specific antigen and human interleukin-6 as biomarkers (Dai et al. 2016).

Table 5.1 A summary of nano techniques used for detection of various types of cancer with their respective biomarkers

Sl. no.	Type of cancer	Biomarker	Type of nanomaterial	Reference
1	Early detection of prostate cancer	miR-21 biomarker	Electrochemical nano-genosensor	(Sabahi et al. 2020)
		Prostate-specific antigen and human interleukin-6	Photoelectrochemical biosensor	(Dai et al. 2016)
		Prostate-specific membrane antigen	Electrochemiluminescence immunosensor	(Juzgado et al. 2017)
		Prostate-specific antigen (PSA)	Electrochemical immunosensor	(Rafique et al. 2015)
		Prostate-specific antigen (PSA)	Silicon nanowire	(Rani et al. 2018)
		Prostate-specific antigen	Silicon nanowire biosensor	(Huang et al. 2013)
		Prostate-specific antigen	Electrochemiluminescence immunoassay technique	(Wang et al. 2020b)
		IgG proteins	Citrate ligand capped gold nanoparticles	(Zheng et al. 2015)
		DU145 and LNCaP cells	GaDu-loaded mesoporous silica nanoparticles	(Gu et al. 2020)
		Prostate-specific membrane antigen	Manganese oxide-mesoporous silica nanoparticles	(Du et al. 2020)
		Prostate-specific antigen	Luminous nanorods	(Zhao et al. 2019)
		Prostate-specific antigen	Plasmonic and photothermal immunoassay	(Liu et al. 2019)
		Prostate-specific antigen	Surface-enhanced Raman scattering (SERS)-based immunoassay	(Zhou et al. 2018)
		MicroRNAs (miR-107)	Nanozyme-patterned hollowed nanocuboids	(Li et al. 2019)
		Testosterone	Polymerized nanocomposites	(Tang et al. 2015)
2	Early detection of breast cancer	Twist mRNA	MaBiDZ fluorescent sensor	(Bakshi et al. 2019)
		Cellular biomarkers	"Caged" carbon nanoparticles	(Mohammad et al. 2020)
		4 T1	Magnetic-fluorescent iron oxide-carbon hybrid nanomaterials	(Cuiping et al. 2019)
		MCF-7 cancer cells	Electrochemical aptamer cytosensor	(Dan et al. 2019)
		Biomarker anti-ErbB2	Immunosensor	(Md. Azahar et al. 2015)

(continued)

Table 5.1 (continued)

Sl. no.	Type of cancer	Biomarker	Type of nanomaterial	Reference
		Tissue plasminogen activator (tPA)	Immunosensor	(Nabiabad et al. 2018)
		miRNA-155	Field-effect transistor (FET) biosensor	(Mansouri et al. 2018)
		Human epidermal growth factor receptor-2 (HER-2)	Amine-functionalized MoO @RGO nanohybrid-based biosensor	(Shine et al. 2019)
		Plasma miRNA-155	Electrochemical nano-biosensor	(Azimzadeh et al. 2016)
		BRCA1	Biosensor	(Kazerooni and Nassernejad 2016)
		MUC1 and VEGF165 biomarker	Dual-aptamer probe	(Kun et al. 2015)
		C595	Nanoprobes; superparamagnetic iron oxide nanoparticles (SPIONs)	(Moradi et al. 2017)
		MDA-MB-231 and MCF-7	Surface-enhanced Raman spectroscopy	(Linhu et al. 2019)
		Human epidermal growth factor receptor 2 (HER2-ECD)	Electrochemical sensing platforms	(Maria et al. 2019)
3	Early detection of lung cancer	Telomerase	Hemin–graphene nanomaterial	(Xu et al. 2017)
		EGFR cells	Sulforaphane-conjugated carbon dots	(Lu et al. 2019)
		VOC (volatile organic compounds) biomarkers	Surface-enhanced Raman scattering (SERS)	(Xuezhi et al. 2018)
		VOC biomarkers	Monolayer-capped gold nanoparticles (MCNP)	(Fernandes et al. 2015)
		DNA methylation biomarker plasma	Nanoparticle-based DNA extn. (MOB) followed by qMSP	(Chen et al. 2020)
		MicroRNAs	Electrochemical nano-biosensors	(Roghayeh et al. 2020)
		Calpain 2 (CAPN2)	Peptide sensor	(Seung-Hae et al. 2020)
		Marker ProGRP	Biosensor	(Zheng et al. 2019)
		Carcinoembryonic antigen (CEA) and neuron-specific enolase (NSE)	Electrochemical aptasensor	(Yang et al. 2019)

(continued)

Table 5.1 (continued)

Sl. no.	Type of cancer	Biomarker	Type of nanomaterial	Reference
		VOC biomarkers	Nanocomposites based on carbon nanotubes	(Lisday et al. 2016)
		microRNA	Electrocatalysis-assisted biosensor	(Lin et al. 2019)
		EGFR	Electronic nose system	(Dekel et al. 2017)
		microRNAs	Nano-quantum dots microarray	(Lihong et al. 2016)
		miRNA	Semiconductor quantum dot	(Lihong et al. 2015)
		microRNA	Gold nanoshells probe	(Yi et al. 2019)
4	Early detection of liver cancer	SerpinB3 antigen	AuNP@PEG-PreS1 nanostructures	(Francesca et al. 2019)
		Serum microRNA and α-fetoprotein	DNA probes	(Cheng et al. 2018)
		Alpha fetoprotein	Nano optical sensor	(Attia et al. 2018)
		mRNA	Hybridization probe	(Yuli et al. 2012)
5	Early detection of oral cancer	FaDu and HaCaT cells	N-doped carbon nanospheres	(Das et al. 2019)
		Interleukin-8	DNA-templated quantum dots	(Jue et al. 2020)
		DAK cells	OCT by plasmonic gold clusters	(Soo et al. 2018)
		SCC-9 cells	pLGA-DTX nanoconjugate	(Parul et al. 2018)
		ORAOV1	Photoelectrochemical biosensor	(Fangjing et al. 2020)
6	Early detection of pancreatic cancer	Carbohydrate antigen (19-9) CA-19-9 marker	Biomolecular corona of graphene oxide nanoflakes	(Massimiliano et al. 2019)
		CD326	Gadolinium ion-doped upconversion nanoparticles (UCNPs)	(Yong et al. 2018)
		ESA marker	Co-SPIONs nanoparticles	(Vita et al. 2014)
		MUC4, CEACAM6, and CD44v6	Iron oxide nanoparticle composite	(Yinting et al. 2020)
		GPC1 biomarker	GPC1-targeted, gemcitabine (GEM)-loaded multifunctional gold nanocarrier	(Wenli et al. 2019)
		Exosomes (glypican-1 and CD63)	Electro-kinetic chips	(Lewis Jean et al. 2018)
		Glypican-1 (GPC-1)	Gd-Au-NC-GPC-1 nanocluster	(Xin et al. 2018)

(continued)

Table 5.1 (continued)

Sl. no.	Type of cancer	Biomarker	Type of nanomaterial	Reference
		PTR86 peptide	Multimodal imaging nanoprobes	(Yasaman et al. 2017)
		Claudin 4 and prostate stem cell antigen (PSCA)	Indium phosphide (core)-zinc sulfide (shell) quantum dots	(Ken-Tye et al. 2009)
		Biomarker CA199	Biosensors	(Anshu et al. 2017)
		Biomarker CA199	Impedance spectroscopy based biosensors	(Soares Andrey et al. 2015)
7	Early detection of ovarian cancer	microRNA biomarker	DNA–AuNP probes	(Wang and Xu 2015)
		siRNA	NIR-II fluorescent probes	(Xiangnan et al. 2016)
		ESA marker	Co-SPIONs nanoparticles	(Vita et al. 2014)
		CA125, Mucin 1, HE4, and prostasin biomarker	Nanomaterial-based biosensors	(Rinky and Sushmee 2020)
8	Early detection of human cervical cancer	HeLa cells	SERS and MEF nanoprobes	(Wu et al. 2018)
		MicroRNA	Silicon nanowire biosensors	(Guo-Jun et al. 2012)
		HPV-16 E6 oncogene	IDE-based nano-biosensor	(Thevendran et al. 2019)
		CEM/PTK7 aptamer	Photoelectrochemical cytosensors	(Robabeh et al. 2018)
		Human papillomavirus	Electrochemical biosensor	(Avelino Karen et al. 2020)
		HeLa and HEK-293T	ZnO quantum dots	(Yang et al. 2020)
9	Early detection of bladder cancer	Micro-RNA-181a	Nanophotonic biosensor	(Huertas et al. 2016)
		Galectin1 (Gal-1) protein	Immunosensor	(Cheng-Hsin et al. 2016)
10	Early detection of head and neck cancer	Human papillomavirus (HPV16)	Electrochemical genosensor	(Leila et al. 2020)
11	Early stage detection of colon cancer	p53 autoantibodies	Gold-loaded nanoporous iron oxide nanocubes	(Yadav et al. 2017)
		HT-29 cells	Optical cytosensor	(Jafar et al. 2020)

Electrochemiluminescence immunosensors with multi-walled carbon nanotubes and silicon nanoparticles and polymer brush [oligo (ethylene glycol) methacrylate-co-glycidyl methacrylate] have been reported for recognizing prostate-specific membrane antigen (PSMA) and prostate-specific antigen (Juzgado et al. 2017; Rafique et al. 2015). Silicon nanowire field-effect transistor (poly-Si NWFET) composed biosensors and quantum dot-based electrochemiluminescence immunoassay technique have been used for early detection of prostate-specific antigens (Rani et al. 2018; Huang et al. 2013; Wang et al. 2020b). Citrate ligand capped gold nanoparticles have been reported for detecting the IgG proteins as a biomarker (Zheng et al. 2015). While, GaDu-loaded mesoporous silica nanoparticles have been reported for the detection of DU145 and LNCaP cells for timely detection and early diagnostics of prostate cancer (Gu et al. 2020). Manganese oxide–mesoporous silica nanoparticles developed from PSA-Mn-Msn-Cy7 have been utilized for detecting the prostate-specific membrane antigen (Du et al. 2020). Luminous nanorods composed of Au@Ag@SiO nanoparticles for detecting the prostate-specific antigen and detection of prostate cancer and malignant cancer (Zhao et al. 2019). Plasmonic and photothermal immunoassay based on gold nanostars has been utilized for detecting prostate-specific antigen and premature detection of prostate cancer (Liu et al. 2019). SERS (Surface-enhanced Raman scattering)-based immunoassay composed of silver nanoparticles (AgNPs) as immune probes utilized for detecting the prostate-specific antigen (Zhou et al. 2018). A new class of nanomaterials based on nucleic acid sequences having controllable plasmonic functionalities for Surface Enhanced Raman Scattering (SERB)-based bioanalysis applications have been reported. Wherein the microRNAs (miRNAs) act as a biomarker as well as a self-assembly trigger. The mi-RNA triggered nanostructure approach has shown the potential of miR-107 in clinical patient samples as a non-invasive prostate cancer diagnostic biomarker. Polydopamine imprinting layer coated MWCNT (multi-walled carbon nanotube) has been utilized for determining the testosterone level in prostate cancer LNcap cells (Tang et al. 2015).

5.2.2 Early Detection of Breast Cancer

Breast cancer includes DCIS (ductal carcinoma in situ), metastatic breast cancer, inflammatory breast cancer, and IDC (invasive ductal carcinoma). While, its biomarkers include ER (estrogen receptor) Mib1/Ki-67 proliferation index, PR (progesterone receptor), HER2 (human epidermal growth factor receptor), and mRNA biomarkers. DNA-modified nanoparticles have been used for the detection of mRNA biomarkers cultured in MCF-7 cells and were also found to induce its downregulation (Bakshi et al. 2019). Polyethyleneimine (PEI) encapsulated bare-surface carbon nanoparticles (CNPs) have been developed and used for caging and de-caging to produce a unique emission PL for each type of cell leading to their identification and separation (Mohammad et al. 2020). Magnetic-fluorescent iron oxide–carbon hybrid nanoparticles (MCNPs) composed of FeCl, $FeCl{\cdot}4H_2O$, citric acid, and ethylenediamine in diethylene glycol when conjugated to CD44 (monoclonal antibody) exhibited specific effect in 4T1 breast cancer cells thus helps to distinguish them from normal cells (Cuiping et al. 2019). A sandwich-type cytosensor was designed to analyze MCF-7 cancer cells depending on metal organic framework PCN-224 and DNA tetrahedron associated with dual-aptamer and found to be an efficient strategy for detecting breast cancer cells (Dan et al. 2019). Highly sensitive and label-free immunosensor conjugated with mesoporous zinc oxide nanofibers fabricated for detection of a biomarker in early-stage detection of breast cancer (Md. Azahar et al. 2015). Immunosensors composed of single-walled carbon nanotubes has been reported for early detection of human tissue plasminogen activator (tPA) in myocardial infarction and breast cancer (Nabiabad et al. 2018). Molybdenum disulfide (MoS2) field-effect transistor (FET) biosensor developed for ultrasensitive detection of breast cancer biomarker miRNA-155, which is present in human serum and cell-line samples (Mansouri et al. 2018). A label-free amine-functionalized molybdenum trioxide anchored on reduced graphene oxide (MoO_3@RGO) Nanohybrid-Based Biosensor has been reported for detecting early breast cancer detection using human epidermal growth factor receptor-2 (HER-2) as an analyte with improved sensitivity. Electrochemical nano-biosensor based on graphene oxide and gold nanorod has been used for detecting the plasma miRNA-155 (Azimzadeh et al. 2016) and electrochemical biosensor synthesized from nitrogen-doped graphene aerogels (SIL-g-(N) GAs) has been used for detecting the BRCA1 gene and early diagnosis of the breast cancer (Kazerooni and Nassernejad 2016). Dual-aptamer probe composed of MUC1 and VEGF165 with PtAu nanoparticles was used for detection of MUC1 and VEGF165 biomarker (Kun et al. 2015) and the nanoprobes composed of superparamagnetic iron oxide nanoparticles have been reported for detecting the C595 biomarkers (Moradi et al. 2017). While surface-enhanced Raman spectroscopy-based nanoprobes have been utilized for detecting MDA-MB-231 and MCF-7 biomarkers and early detection of breast cancer (Linhu et al. 2019). Moreover, electrochemical sensing platforms composed of multi-walled carbon nanotubes combined with AuNPs have been reported for detecting HER2-ECD (human epidermal growth factor receptor 2) and early detection (Maria et al. 2019).

5.2.3 Early Detection of Lung Cancer

Lung cancer ranks among the top for the deaths related to cancer and it comprises several subtypes, but the most frequent are adenocarcinoma, large cell lung carcinoma, and squamous cell carcinoma. Early detection through biomarkers will considerably change oncologic therapy decisions. Hemin–graphene nanomaterials were used for quantification of human telomerase activity in urine, where telomerase is a cancer biomarker used in the early detection of cervical, breast, and lung cancer (Xu et al. 2017). Multifunctional nano-system from SFN-CDs (sulforaphane-conjugated carbon dots) having thiourea skeleton has been used to detect EGFR overexpressing cancer cells for lung cancer (Lu et al. 2019). SERS technique has been implemented for the detection of VOC (volatile organic compounds) biomarkers and lung cancer (Xuezhi et al. 2018). VOC biomarkers are also utilized by chemiresistors coated with gold nanoparticles for early detection of lung cancer (Fernandes et al. 2015). MOB-qMSP nanoparticle system has been developed by linking it to DNA methylated extension for detection of the DNA methylated biomarkers (Chen et al. 2020). Also, the electrochemical nano-biosensors have been reported for detecting the early-stage lung cancer related microRNAs biomarkers (Roghayeh et al. 2020). HSA-CAPN2 (human serum albumin Calpain 2) peptide sensor CAPN2 enzyme-activable near IR was developed to detect the Calpain-2 biomarker and early-stage detection of lung cancer (Seung-Hae et al. 2020). A biosensor composed of CPE/TiO2/(CS + AuNPs)/anti-ProGRP/BSA/ProGRP nanoparticles has been expended for detecting the marker Progastrin-releasing peptide (ProGRP) and early detection of lung cancer (Zheng et al. 2019). Electrochemical aptasensor composed of amine functionalized graphene-thionin-gold particles and PB-PEDOT (Prussian blue-poly (3,4-ethylenedioxythiophene)-AuNPs nanocomposites were used to detect the biomarkers CEA and NSE (Yang et al. 2019). Quantum resistive sensors composed of nanocomposites based on carbon nanotubes were utilized for the detection of VOC biomarkers and early-stage lung cancer (Lisday et al. 2016). Electrocatalysis-assisted biosensor composed of iron-embedded nitrogen-rich carbon nanotubes (Fe-CNTs) for detecting microRNA for lung cancer (Lin et al. 2019). A nanoarray sensors for exhaled VOC have been utilized to detect EGFR mutation and early detection of lung cancer (Dekel et al. 2017). Nano-quantum dots microarray is utilized for detecting the microRNAs and early detection of non-small cell in lung cancer (Lihong et al. 2016). Cd/Ge semiconductor quantum dot with 3–6 nm size used to prepare DNA probe for detecting circulating miRNA and early detection of lung cancer (Lihong et al. 2015). Gold nano shells probe composed of EMSNAs (Erythrocyte membrane-bio interfaced spherical nucleic acids) has been developed to detect microRNA for early detection of lung cancer (Yi et al. 2019).

5.2.4 Early Detection of Liver Cancer

Hepatocellular carcinoma (HCC) is the most common cancer type among various types of liver cancer. AFP (alpha fetoprotein) and DCP (des-γ-carboxy prothrombin) are the main biomarkers for HCC. SERRS (surface enhanced resonance Raman scattering) technique has been reported with active gold nanoparticles, which were engineered with PreS1-peptide for the detection of SerpinB3 antigens overexpressed in liver cancer (Francesca et al. 2019). DNA probes have been implemented for detecting the serum microRNA and alpha-fetoprotein biomarkers and the early diagnosing of liver cancer (Cheng et al. 2018). Nano optical sensor synthesized from binuclear Pt-2aminobenzimidazole-bipyridine reported for detection of alpha fetoprotein and for early diagnosis of liver cancer (Attia et al. 2018). The test kit comprising of hybridization probe was applied for detecting the marker mRNAs and early detection of liver cancer (Yuli et al. 2012).

5.2.5 Early Detection of Oral Cancer

Squamous cell carcinoma and verrucous carcinoma are the main cancers that occur in the oral cavity. The genomic biomarkers like Integrin α3 and β4, VEGF (vascular endothelial growth factor), receptor tyrosine kinase (RTK), and B-cell lymphoma-2, etc. have been used to predict oral squamous cell carcinoma. NCQD (N-doped carbon quantum dot)-deposited carbon capsules used for the detecting FaDu cells for early diagnostics of oral cancer (Das et al. 2019). DNA-templated quantum dots have been synthesized from CdTe/CdS QDs and employed for the detection of biomarker interleukin-8 and early detection of oral cancer (Jue et al. 2020). The stimuli-responsive plasmonic gold nanoclusters were used as a contrast agent for OCT in the detection of the early stages oral cancer (Soo et al. 2018). The PLGA-DTX conjugate (poly (lactic-co-glycolic acid) nanoparticles encapsulated with DTX drug) has been expended for detecting the SCC-9 cells and treatment of oral cancer (Parul et al. 2018). DNA rolling motor based photoelectrochemical biosensor with synergistic effect among DNA–Ag NCs (DNA-templated silver nanoclusters), GO (graphene oxide), and hemin have been used for detecting ORAOV1 biomarkers and early diagnosis of oral cancer (Fangjing et al. 2020).

5.2.6 Early Detection of Pancreatic Cancer

Adenocarcinoma is the most common pancreatic cancer with a most common biomarker, namely, CA 19-9 (carbohydrates antigens). Blood test based on the characterization of the BC (biomolecular corona) that forms around graphene oxide (GO) nanoflakes have shown great potential for early diagnosis of pancreatic cancer (Massimiliano et al. 2019). Gadolinium ion-doped up conversion nanoparticles (UCNPs) have been reported for detecting the CD326 cells and improved the diagnostic efficacy of early pancreatic cancer (Yong et al. 2018). While superparamagnetic cobalt ferrite nanoparticles have been reported for detecting the ESA biomarkers (Vita et al. 2014). Iron oxide nanoparticle composite comprises PEGylated iron oxide nanoparticle and three single-chain antibodies where these three single-chain antibodies anti-MU C4 single-chain antibody, anti-CEACAM6 single-chain antibody, and anti-CD44v6 single-chain antibody have been reported possessing applications for the treatment of pancreatic cancer (Yinting et al. 2020). GPC1, a biomarker targeted by GEM (gemcitabine)-loaded multifunctional gold nanocarrier shown good potential for early detection of pancreatic cancer (Wenli et al. 2019). Moreover, electro-kinetic chips have been reported for detecting the exosomes (glypican-1 and CD63); which are potential biomarkers for pancreatic cancer (Lewis Jean et al. 2018). Dual-modal imaging probe has been used by conjugating Glypican-1 (GPC-1) antibody with Gd–Au nanoclusters for early detection as Glypican-1 are overexpressed cells in pancreatic cancer (Xin et al. 2018). Multimodal imaging nanoprobes composed of magnetic iron oxide nanoworms have been reported with applications for detecting PTR86 peptide and early detection of pancreatic cancer (Yasaman et al. 2017). Indium phosphide–zinc sulfide QDs have been used for detecting the Claudin 4 and PSCA (prostate stem cell antigen) novel biomarkers for early detection of pancreatic cancer (Ken-Tye et al. 2009). Highly sensitive biosensors have been synthesized from carbon nanotube for detecting the biomarker CA19–9 (Anshu et al. 2017). An architecture based on a self-assembled monolayer (SAM) and layer-by-layer (LbL) films of polysaccharide chitosan and the protein Con A was implemented for detecting the biomarker CA19–9 of pancreatic cancer for early diagnosis (Soares Andrey et al. 2015).

5.2.7 Early Detection of Ovarian Cancer

Ovarian cancers have been demarcated by the type of cell from which it starts. The main types are surface epithelium tumours (starts from epithelial cells), stromal tumours (starts from structural tissue cells), and germ cells tumours (starts from the egg-producing cells). Wang et al. have compiled the work on microRNA biomarker for early detection of ovarian cancer, including the use of DNA probes and gold nanoparticles (Wang and Xu 2015). NIR-II fluorescent probes composed of down-conversion nanoparticles, quantum dots, SWCNTs, and organic dyes have been utilized for detecting siRNA biomarkers and diagnosing ovarian cancer (Xiangnan et al. 2016). Superparamagnetic cobalt ferrite nanoparticles have been reported for detecting the ESA biomarkers and early stage detection of pancreatic and ovarian cancer (Vita et al. 2014). Nanomaterial-based biosensors have been synthesized to detect CA125, Mucin 1, HE4, and prostasin and diagnosis of ovarian cancer (Rinky and Sushmee 2020).

5.2.8 Early Detection of Human Cervical Cancer

Squamous cell carcinoma is the main type of cervical cancer, followed by adenocarcinoma. SERS and MEF (metal-enhanced fluorescence) are ultrasensitive methods for the detection and identification of HeLa cells in human cervical cancer (Wu et al. 2018). PNA (peptide nucleic acid) functionalized silicon nanowires biosensors have been reported for detection of microRNA biomarkers which regulates gene expression in cancer initiation and progression, thus detecting the early-stage of cervical cancer (Guo-Jun et al. 2012). IDE-based nano-biosensors composed of gold-hybridized zinc oxide nanorods found effective for detecting virulent DNA signature of HPV-16 in cervical cancer (Thevendran et al. 2019). Photoelectrochemical cytosensors synthesized from g-C3N4AgI/ITO nanocomposites photoelectrode were able to detect the cervical cancer HeLa cells in early stages (Robabeh et al. 2018). Electrochemical biosensor composed of metal–polymer hybrid nanomaterial and gold nanoparticles has been applied for detecting Human papillomavirus and early detection of cervical cancers (Avelino Karen et al. 2020). ZnO quantum dots have been implemented for diagnostic applications, particularly the detection of HeLa cervical cancer cells and HEK-293 T human embryonic kidney cells (Yang et al. 2020).

5.2.9 Early Detection of Bladder Cancer

UCC (Urothelial carcinoma) is the main bladder cancer, along with squamous cell carcinoma and adenocarcinoma. Various biomarkers for bladder cancer are extracellular vesicles, CEA (carcinoembryogenic antigen), Ca19-9 (gastrointestinal cancer antigen), and TPA (tissue-polypeptide antigen). Nanophotonic biosensors like interferometric bimodal nano-waveguides (BiMW) have been utilized for detecting the early microRNA-181a biomarkers of bladder cancer (Huertas et al. 2016). Immunosensor composed of nanoprobes Gal-1 antibodies coupled with alumina nanoparticles has been reported for the detection of Galectin1 protein (Gal-1), which is used as a biomarker for the early detection (Cheng-Hsin et al. 2016).

5.2.10 Early Detection of Head and Neck Cancer

Squamous cell carcinoma is the most common type of head and neck cancer and its biomarkers include EGFR (epidermal growth factor receptor), VEGF, CCND1 (cyclin D1), and Bcl-2 (B-cell lymphoma 2). Electrochemical genosensor synthesized from amine-ionic liquid functionalized reduced graphene oxide immobilized on MWCNT has served as a tool for detecting human papillomavirus (HPV16) DNA limit to 1.3 nM (at 3σ) and early detection (Leila et al. 2020).

5.2.11 Early Detection of Colon Cancer

Major type of colon cancer is adenocarcinoma, while others are gastrointestinal carcinoid tumors, gastrointestinal stromal tumors, squamous cell carcinomas, and primary colorectal lymphomas. It has various biomarkers like methylated genes (MLH1, SEPT9, and VIM); however, due to poor prognosis, there is an urgent need for predictive biomarkers by using nanomaterials. Gold-loaded nanoporous iron oxide nanocubes synthesized and used for p53 autoantibodies detection and early diagnosing of colon cancer (Yadav et al. 2017). Detection of HT-29 cells and early-stage detection of colon cancer demonstrated by optical cytosensor synthesized from terbium-doped dendritic fibrous nano-silica (Jafar et al. 2020).

5.3 Conclusion

Nanoparticle-based techniques are the new era of technology that holds a promise of early-stage cancer detection. Complete understanding of the different type of biomarkers present in the tumor cell environment and their detection with nanoparticle techniques have paved the way for better and earlier cancer detection and its treatment.

In this chapter, we have discussed tumor-related biomarkers along with the techniques used for early diagnostics of cancer. Biomarkers such as a prostate-specific antigen, miRNA 21, IgG protein have been reported for early detection of prostate cancer. Twist mRNA, MCF-7 cancer cells MUC1 and VEGF165, anti-ErbB2, cellular biomarkers have been utilized for early stage detection of breast cancer. Telomerase, microRNAs, DNA methylated biomarkers, etc., have been reported for early detection of lung cancer. Similarly, different types of biomarkers have been summarized in this chapter for the early detection of various cancers by utilizing nanomaterials-based techniques.

References

Anshu T, Coatrini SA, Coatrini SJ, Taj AI, Diogo V, Eliseo MM, Guerreiro FJHT, Lopes CA, Oliveira Osvaldo N (2017) Carbon nanotube matrix for highly sensitive biosensors to detect pancreatic cancer biomarker CA199. ACS Appl Mater Interfaces 9(31):25878–25886

Attia MS, Youssef AO, Khan ZA, Abou-Omar MN (2018) Alpha fetoprotein assessment by using a nano optical sensor thin film binuclear Pt-2aminobenzimidazole-Bipyridine for early diagnosis of liver cancer. Talanta 186:36–43

Avelino Karen YPS, Oliveira Léony S, Norma L-S, Pinto d MC, Andrade César AS, Oliveira Maria DL (2020) Metal-polymer hybrid nanomaterial for impedimetric detection of human papillomavirus in cervical specimens. J Pharm Biomed Anal 185:113249

Azimzadeh M, Rahaie M, Nasirizadeh N, Ashtari K, Naderi-Manesh H (2016) An electrochemical nanobiosensor for plasma miRNA-155, based on graphene oxide and gold nanorod, for early detection of breast cancer. Biosens Bioelectron 77:99–106

Bakshi S, Zakharchenko A, Minko S, Kolpashchikov DM, Katz E (2019) Towards nanomaterials for cancer theranostics: a system of DNA-modified magnetic nanoparticles for detection and suppression of RNA marker in cancer cells. Magnetochemistry 5(2):24

Chen C, Xiaojie H, Wei Y, Muyun P, Wu F, Wu X, Jingqun T, Mingjiu C, Wang X, Alicia H et al (2020) Ultrasensitive DNA hypermethylation detection using plasma for early detection of NSCLC: a study in Chinese patients with very small nodules. Clin Epigenetics 12(1):39

Cheng L, Zhikun Z, Duo Z, Zhu W, Jie Z, Qingdao Z, Yang D, Min L, Yuliang Z (2018) Ultrasensitive detection of serum MicroRNA using branched DNA-based SERS platform combining simultaneous detection of α-fetoprotein for early diagnosis of liver cancer. ACS Appl Mater Interfaces 10(41):34869–34877

Cheng-Hsin C, Yi-Chun D, Wu T-F, Cheng-Ho C, Lee D-H, Shih-Min C, Chi HT, Wu H-P, Omar SM (2016) Immunosensor for the ultrasensitive and quantitative detection of bladder cancer in point of care testing. Biosens Bioelectron 84:126–132

Choi Y, Kwak J, Won Park JW (2010) Nanotechnology for early cancer detection. Sensors 10:428

Cuiping H, Aiwei Z, Ying K, Nana Y, Ting X, Binru D, Ke L, Yong W, Jingjing L, Kai X (2019) Multifunctional iron oxide-carbon hybrid nanoparticles for targeted fluorescent/MR dual-modal imaging and detection of breast cancer cells. Anal Chim Acta 1067:115–128

Dai H, Zhang S, Hong Z, Lin Y (2016) A potentiometric addressable photoelectrochemical biosensor for sensitive detection of two biomarkers. Anal Chem 88(19):9532–9538

Dan O, Duanping S, Liang Z, Bowen C, Lin X, Zuanguang C (2019) A novel cytosensor for capture, detection and release of breast cancer cells based on metal organic framework PCN-224 and DNA tetrahedron linked dual-aptamer. Sensors Actuators B Chem 285:398–404

Das RK, Snigdharani P, Sekhar BC, Bhutia SK, Sasmita M (2019) N-doped carbon quantum dot (NCQD)-deposited carbon capsules for synergistic fluorescence imaging and photothermal therapy of oral cancer. Langmuir 35(47):15320–15329

Dekel S, Manal A, Ori L, Jair B, Naomi G-M, Maya I, Amir O, Alon B-N, Hossam H, Nir P (2017) Nose detection of lung cancer and EGFR mutation by electronic system. J Thorac Oncol 12 (10):15441551

Du D, Fu H-J, Ren W-w, Li X-L, Guo L-H (2020) PSA targeted dual-modality manganese oxide-mesoporous silica nanoparticles for prostate cancer imaging. Biomed Pharmacother 121:109614
Fangjing M, Min C, Hui M, Wu J, Yingzi F (2020) A DNA rolling motor for photoelectrochemical biosensing of oral cancer overexpressed 1. Sensors Actuators B Chem 309:127824
Fernandes MP, Venkatesh S, Sudarshan BG (2015) Early detection of lung cancer using nano-nose - a review. Open Biomed Eng J 9:228–233
Francesca B, Santina Q, Gianmarco V, Cristian T, Alessandra B, Lucio L, Maria R, Moreno M, Patrizia P, Marina G (2019) PreS1 peptide-functionalized gold nanostructures with SERRS tags for efficient liver cancer cell targeting. Mater Sci Eng C Mater Biol Appl 103:109762
Gu C, Li C, Zhang J, Li X, Wang L, Ju Y, Liu Y, Xu Y (2020) Ultra-effective near-infrared photothermal therapy for the prostate cancer nursing care through novel intended and surface tailored photo-responsive Ga-Au@MPS nanovesicles. J Photochem Photobiol B 202:111685
Guo-Jun Z, Preedy VR, Patel VB (2012) Detection of miRNA with silicon nanowire biosensors. In: Biosensors and cancer. CRC Press, Boca Raton, FL, pp 248–267
Huang Y, Wu C, Chuang C-K, Pang S-T, Pan T-M, Yang Y-S, Ko F-H (2013) Real-time and label-free detection of the prostate-specific antigen in human serum by a polycrystalline silicon nanowire field-effect transistor biosensor. Anal Chem 85(16):7912–7918
Huertas CS, David F, Lechuga LM (2016) Direct and label-free quantification of micro-RNA-181a at attomolar level in complex media using a nanophotonic biosensor. ACS Sens 1(6):748–756
Jafar S, Mohammad H, Nasrin S, Hossein SM, Abolghasem J (2020) Spectrofluorimetric cytosensing of colorectal cancer cells using terbium-doped dendritic fibrous nanosilica functionalized by folic acid: a novel optical cytosensor for cancer detection. J Pharm Biomed Anal 180:113077
Jue X, Xiaomeng Y, Linshen X, Meiying S (2020) Facile incorporation of DNA-templated quantum dots for sensitive electrochemical detection of the oral cancer biomarker interleukin. Anal Bioanal Chem 412(11):2599–2606
Juzgado A, Solda A, Ostric A, Criado A, Valenti G, Rapino S, Conti G, Fracasso G, Paolucci F, Prato M (2017) Highly sensitive electrochemiluminescence detection of a prostate cancer biomarker. J Mater Chem B Mater Biol Med 5(32):6681–6687
Kazerooni H, Nassernejad B (2016) A novel biosensor nanomaterial for the ultraselective and ultrasensitive electrochemical diagnosis of the breast cancer-related BRCA1 gene. Anal Methods 8(15):3069–3074
Ken-Tye Y, Hong D, Indrajit R, Wing-Cheung L, Bergey EJ, Anirban M, Prasad PN (2009) Imaging pancreatic cancer using bioconjugated InP quantum dots. ACS Nano 3(3):502–510
Kun W, Daoqing F, Yaqing L, Erkang W (2015) Highly sensitive and specific colorimetric detection of cancer cells via dual-aptamer target binding strategy. Biosens Bioelectron 73:1–6
Leila F, Sodeh S, Mojtaba S, Shahab S (2020) Electrochemical genosensor based on carbon nanotube/amine-ionic liquid functionalized reduced graphene oxide nanoplatform for detection of human papillomavirus (HPV16)-related head and neck cancer. J Pharm Biomed Anal 179:112989
Lewis Jean M, Vyas Ankit D, Yuqi Q, Messer Karen S, Rebekah W, Heller Michael J (2018) Integrated analysis of Exosomal protein biomarkers on alternating current electrokinetic chips enables rapid detection of pancreatic cancer in patient blood. ACS Nano 12(4):3311–3320
Li J, Koo Kevin M, Wang Y, Trau M (2019) Native microRNA targets trigger self-assembly of nanozyme-patterned hollowed nanocuboids with optimal interparticle gaps for plasmonic-activated cancer detection. Matt Small 15(50):1904689
Lihong F, Bo S, Hao C (2015) Semiconductor quantum dot-based microchip for early diagnosis of lung cancer and method for preparing DNA probe thereof. Faming Zhuanli Shenqing, CN 105018591 A 20151104
Lihong F, Huiwei Q, Junliang T, Bo S, Hao C, Wang C, Qing X (2016) Identification of serum miRNAs by nano-quantum dots microarray as diagnostic biomarkers for early detection of non-small cell lung cancer. Tumor Biol 37(6):7777–7784

Lin C, Wang M, Bing S, Shiyun A, Wang S, Chun-yang Z (2019) Substrate-free and label-free electrocatalysis-assisted biosensor for sensitive detection of microRNA in lung cancer cells. Chem Commun 55(8):1172–1175

Linhu L, Liao M, Yingfan C, Beibei S, Ming L (2019) Surface-enhanced Raman spectroscopy (SERS) nanoprobes for ratiometric detection of cancer cells. J Mater Chem B Mater Biol Med 7 (5):815–822

Lisday D, Sananda S, Mickael C, Veronique B, Jean-Francois F, Philippe G (2016) Artificial noses from biopolymers or supramolecular assembly based on cyclodextrins for the detection of lung cancer VOC biomarkers. Abstracts of papers, 252nd ACS national meeting & exposition, Philadelphia, PA, United States, POLY-188

Liu Y, Pan M, Wang W, Jiang Q, Wang F, Pang D, Liu X (2019) Plasmonic and photothermal immunoassay via enzyme-triggered crystal growth on gold nanostars. Anal Chem 91 (3):2086–2092

Lu W, Fangfang D, Xuewei Z, Lihong S, Shaomin S, Tracy CX, Dong C (2019) Sulforaphane-conjugated carbon dots: a versatile nanosystem for targeted imaging and inhibition of EGFR overexpressing cancer cells. ACS Biomater Sci Eng 5(9):4692–4699

Mansouri MS, Abdollah S, Foad G (2018) An ultrasensitive detection of miRNA-155 in breast cancer via direct hybridization assay using two dimensional molybdenum disulfide field-effect transistor biosensor. Biosens Bioelectron 105:6–13

Maria F, Nouws HPA, Delerue-Matos C (2019) Electrochemical sensing platforms for HER2-ECD breast cancer biomarker detection. Cristina Electroanal 31(1):121–128

Massimiliano P, Valentina P, Luca D, Francesca G, Sara P, Gabriele C, Giordano P, Damiano C, Cristina CM, Chiara C et al (2019) Converting the personalized biomolecular corona of graphene oxide nanoflakes into a high-throughput diagnostic test for early cancer detection. Nanoscale 11(32):15339–15346

Md. Azahar A, Kunal M, Chandan S, Bansi DM, Ashutosh S (2015) Anti-epidermal growth factor receptor conjugated mesoporous zinc oxide nanofibers for breast cancer diagnostics. Nanoscale 7(16):7234–7245

Mohammad A, Indrajit S, Jairaj N, Dipanjan P (2020) Array-based on differential switchable photoluminescence of macromolecularly "caged" carbon nanoparticles for the discrimination of human cells. Abstracts of Papers, 259th ACS National Meeting & Exposition, Philadelphia, PA, United States, COLL-0767

Moradi KP, Majid AMSA, Asif M, Moradi KB, Shahbazi-Gahrouei D, Jaafar MS (2017) Breast cancer cell targeted MR molecular imaging probe: anti-MUC1 antibody-based magnetic nanoparticles. J Phys Conf Ser 851:012014

Nabiabad HS, Piri K, Kafrashi F, Afkhami A, Madrakian T (2018) Fabrication of an immunosensor for early and ultrasensitive determination of human tissue plasminogen activator (tPA) in myocardial infarction and breast cancer patients. Anal Bioanal Chem 410(16):3683–3691

Parul G, Manjri S, Rajiv K, Jodi B, Rishi S, Dwivedi Premendra D, Srinivas S, Singh Surinder P (2018) Synthesis and in vitro studies of PLGA-DTX nanoconjugate as potential drug delivery vehicle for oral cancer. Int J Nanomedicine 13:67–69

Rafique S, Bin W, Bhatti AS (2015) Electrochemical immunosensor for prostate-specific antigens using a label-free second antibody based on silica nanoparticles and polymer brush. Bioelectrochemistry 101:75–83

Rani D, Pachauri V, Madaboosi N, Jolly P, Vu X, Estrela P et al (2018) Top-down fabricated silicon nanowire arrays for field-effect detection of prostate-specific antigen. ACS Omega 3 (8):8471–8482

Rinky S, Sushmee B (2020) Recent advancements in fabrication of nanomaterial based biosensors for diagnosis of ovarian cancer: a comprehensive review. Microchim Acta 187(3):181

Robabeh MM, Liqin G, Hui J, Wang X (2018) A label-free aptamer-based cytosensor for specific cervical cancer HeLa cell recognition through a g-C3N4AgI/ITO photoelectrode. J Mater Chem B Mater Biol Med 6(31):5039–5049

Roghayeh S, Omolbanin S, Leili H, Milad S, Sahar M, Hajie L, Younes P-S, Zahra B, Sarraf ZS, Ziba N et al (2020) Electrochemical nano-biosensors as novel approach for the detection of lung cancer-related microRNAs. Curr Mol Med 20(1):13–35

Sabahi A, Salahandish R, Ghaffarinejad A, Omidinia E (2020) Electrochemical nano-genosensor for highly sensitive detection of miR-21 biomarker based on SWCNTgrafted dendritic Au nanostructure for early detection of prostate cancer. Talanta 209:120595

Seung-Hae K, Taemin W, Yong P, Woo KM, Lee G, Takumi H, Hoon CJ, Lee R (2020) Noninvasive early detection of calpain 2-enriched non-small cell lung cancer using a human serum albumin-bounded calpain 2 nanosensor. Bioconjug Chem 31(3):803–812

Shine A, Pragati K, Malhotra BD (2019) Amine-functionalized MoO @RGO nanohybrid-based biosensor for breast cancer detection. ACS Appl Bio Mater 2(12):5366–5378

Soares Andrey C, Soares Juliana C, Shimizu Flavio M, Melendez Matias E, Carvalho Andre L, Oliveira Osvaldo N (2015) Controlled film architectures to detect a biomarker for pancreatic cancer using impedance spectroscopy. J ACS Appl Mater Interfaces 7(46):25930–25937

Soo KC, Dominique I, Petra W-S, Zhongping C, Jik KY (2018) Stimuli-disassembling gold nanoclusters for diagnosis of early stage oral cancer by optical coherence tomography. Nano Converg 5(1):3/1–3/11

Tang X, Liu W, Chen J, Jia J, Ma Z, Shi Q, Gao Y, Wang X, Xu S, Wang K et al (2015) Preparation and evaluation of polydopamine imprinting layer coated multi-walled carbon nanotubes for the determination of testosterone in prostate cancer LNcap cells. Anal Methods 7(19):8326–8334

Thevendran R, Loong FK, Haarindraprasad R, Jeyachristy SA, Maheswaran S (2019) Gold-hybridized zinc oxide nanorods as real-time low-cost nanobiosensors for detection of virulent DNA signature of HPV-16 in cervical carcinoma. Sci Rep 9(1):1–17

Vita P, Agata M, Rasa P, Aleksander KJ, Marius S, Simona S, Vilius P, Vitalijus K, Urte S, Marija M et al (2014) Accumulation and biological effects of cobalt ferrite nanoparticles in human pancreatic and ovarian cancer cells. Medicina (Kaunas) 50(4):237–244

Wang Z-h, Xu C-j (2015) Research progress of microRNA in early detection of ovarian cancer. Chin Med J 128(24):3363–3370

Wang J, DongR WH, Cai Y, Ren B (2020a) A review on artificial micro/nanomotors for cancer-targeted delivery, diagnosis, and therapy. Nano-Micro Lett 12:11

Wang W, Liu Y, Shi T, Sun J, Mo F, Liu X (2020b) Biosynthesized quantum dot for facile and ultrasensitive electrochemical and electrochemiluminescence immunoassay. Anal Chem 92 (1):1598–1604

Wenli Q, Huifeng Z, Xiao C, Lina S, Wenjing C, Shuai R, Wang Y, Guo K, Donghui L, Rong C et al (2019) A GPC1-targeted and gemcitabine-loaded biocompatible nanoplatform for pancreatic cancer multimodal imaging and therapy. Nanomedicine (London) 14(17):2339–2353

Wu X, Yan P, Xiaomei D, Yang L, Jinze L, Wang F (2018) Homologous gold nanoparticles and nanoclusters composites with enhanced surface Raman scattering and metal fluorescence for cancer imaging. Nano 8(10):819/1–819/12

Xiangnan D, Li G, Jifa Q, Santiago C, Zhang G, Belcher AM, Hammond PT (2016) Layer-by-layer assembled fluorescent probes in the second near-infrared window for systemic delivery and detection of ovarian cancer. Proc Natl Acad Sci U S A 113(19):5179–5184

Xin H, Chengqi F, Huanhuan Z, Wenjun L, Shaobin C, Xin C, Wei L, Fulei Z, Yong H, Donglu S et al (2018) Glypican-1-antibody-conjugated Gd-Au nanoclusters for FI/MRI dual-modal targeted detection of pancreatic cancer. Int J Nanomedicine 13:2585–2599

Xu X, Wei M, Liu Y, Liu X, Wei W, Zhang Y, Liu S (2017) A simple, fast, label-free colorimetric method for detection of telomerase activity in urine by using hemingraphene conjugates. Biosens Bioelectron 87:600–606

Xuezhi Q, Bensheng S, Cong L, Qian S, Dan L, Mo G, Tie W (2018) Selective surface enhanced Raman scattering for quantitative detection of lung cancer biomarkers in superparticle@MOF structure. Adv Mater 30(5):1702275

Yadav S, Masud MK, Islam MN, Gopalan V, Lam A K-y, Tanaka S, Nguyen N-T, Al Hossain MS, Li C, Yamauchi MY, Shiddiky MJA (2017) Gold-loaded nanoporous iron oxide nanocubes: a novel dispersible capture agent for tumor-associated autoantibody analysis in serum. Nanoscale 9(25):8805–8814

Yang W, Jinping L, Juntao L, Shuai S, Ying X, Yuanyuan M, Shi Y, Yue Y, Huabing Y, Xinxia C (2019) Label-free microfluidic paper-based electrochemical aptasensor for ultrasensitive and simultaneous multiplexed detection of cancer biomarkers. Biosens Bioelectron 136:84–90

Yang Y, Zhenhua S, Wu W, Xu A, Shuangyu L, Shaoping J (2020) ZnO quantum dots induced oxidative stress and apoptosis in HeLa and HEK-293T cell lines. Front Pharmacol 11:131

Yasaman A, Genady K, Mor O-H, Wolfgang W, Markus M, Arie O, Siroos M, Peter K (2017) In vivo magnetic resonance imaging of pancreatic tumors using iron oxide nanoworms targeted with PTR86 peptide. Colloids Surf B Biointerfaces 158:423–430

Yi Y, Lan X, Ji Z, Chao L, Yue H, Yang X, Zhaoxia W, Genxi L (2019) Erythrocyte membrane-biointerfaced spherical nucleic acids: robust performance for microRNA quantification. Anal Chim Acta 1080:189–195

Yinting C, Kaihong H, Jinmao Z, Guoda L, Shaojie C, Shangxiang C, Yaqing L, Xuanna L, Ying T (2020) Iron oxide nanoparticle composite and preparation method and application thereof. China CN110841072 A 2020-02-28

Yong H, Yanli A, Gang J, Wang X, He C, Yinan D, Qiusha T (2018) Facile assembly of upconversion nanoparticle-based micelles for active targeted dual-mode imaging in pancreatic cancer. J Nanobiotechnol 16:7/1–7/13

Yuli Z, Lin Q, Yunfu Z, Jianying Q (2012) Detection of mRNA level of JAGGED1 gene at early stage of liver cancer metastasis by in situ hybridization. China, CN102605049 A 2012-07-25

Zhang Y, Li M, Gao X, Chen Y, Liu T (2019) Nanotechnology in cancer diagnosis: progress, challenges and opportunities. J Hematol Oncol 12(137):1

Zhao Y, Zheng F, Shi L, Liu H, Ke W (2019) Autoluminescence-free prostate-specific antigen detection by persistent luminous nanorods and Au@Ag@SiO nanoparticles. ACS Appl Mater Interfaces 11(43):40669–40676

Zheng T, Pierre-Pierre N, Yan X, Huo Q, Almodovar AJO, Valerio F et al (2015) Gold nanoparticle-enabled blood test for early stage cancer detection and risk assessment. ACS Appl Mater Interfaces 7(12):6819–6827

Zheng W, Xiaoping C, Junping Z, Junming F, Jiangyan X, Liran X (2019) High sensitive immunoelectrochemical measurement of lung cancer tumor marker ProGRP based on TiO2Au nanocomposite. Molecules 24(4):656

Zhou L, Liu Y, Wang F, Jia Z, Zhou J, Jiang T, Petti L, Chen Y, Xiong Q, Wang X (2018) Classification analyses for prostate cancer, benign prostate hyperplasia and healthy subjects by SERS based immunoassay of multiple tumour markers. Talanta 188:238–244

Role of Nanomedicine for Cancer Immunotherapy

6

Simran Nasra, Ramesh Chaudhari, and Ashutosh Kumar

Abstract

Cancer is the second leading cause of death worldwide and has become a global concern because of its inadequate effective treatment. Immunotherapy is one of the four key pillars in the treatment of cancer apart from surgery, radiotherapy, and chemotherapy. Cancer immunotherapy cures the initial tumor progression and also inhibits metastasis and the relapse of the tumor. Despite its high anti-tumor potential, there are some limitations that impede its frequent clinical use. Dose-limiting toxicity and low response rates of patients pertaining to cancer immunotherapy pose a major challenge in cancer. Cancer immunotherapy exhibits lower clinical advances as antigens associated with cancer are not successfully delivered to the cells of the immune system. Solid tumors have been reported to escape the anti-cancer immune response by creating an immune-suppressive and immune-deprived tumor microenvironment (TME).

Nanomedicine works as an excellent carrier, as its smaller size facilitates the effective delivery of the therapeutic agent in cancer cells and decreases the off-target transport. The present chapter focusses on the prospects of nanomedicine in cancer immunotherapy by its high efficacy to deliver the immunomodulatory agents at the location of the tumor and in draining lymph nodes, reorienting the immunosuppressive cells in the tumor microenvironment, modifying the interaction of therapeutics to immune cells, and recruiting myeloid cells in the tumor site. It is expected that cancer immunotherapy will not only conquer the challenges faced in existing immunotherapy but will also create a synergistic association between nanoparticles and immune cells.

S. Nasra · R. Chaudhari · A. Kumar (✉)
Biological and Life Sciences, School of Arts and Sciences, Ahmedabad University, Ahmedabad, Gujarat, India
e-mail: ashutosh.kumar@ahduni.edu.in

A. Malik et al. (eds.), *Nanomedicine for Cancer Diagnosis and Therapy*,
https://doi.org/10.1007/978-981-15-7564-8_6

Keywords

Cancer · Immunotherapy · Nanomedicine · Targeted delivery · Tumor microenvironment

6.1 Introduction

Cancer is the second principal cause of death globally and is expected to reach 27.1 million people by the year 2030 (Cabral et al. 2018). The growing prevalence and mortality due to cancer have become a global concern, and cancer treatments are nowadays the focus of extensive research. Available treatment modalities for cancer are surgery, chemotherapy, and radiotherapy, but all of them have inadequate effectiveness against progressive cancer. Cancer immunotherapy and immune checkpoint blockers can be useful to robustly eradicate tumors in a particular division of patients with higher metastatic disease leading to increased survival rate and limited side effects (Sharma and Allison 2015).

William B. Coley manipulated the patient's natural defense processes using *Streptococcus* in 1891, which helped in eliminating the malignancies (Mccarthy 2006). His attempts showed positive results, and this became one of the first paradigms of immunotherapy. The initial accomplishment of cancer immunotherapy had opened a new avenue in cancer treatment studies (Yan et al. 2019). There are various therapeutic advantages of cancer immunotherapy over traditional treatments in the context o f providing wider prospects. The purpose of cancer immunotherapy is to augment immune responses against the tumor and to achieve lesser off-target properties. Immuno-therapeutic agents are utilized to activate the immune system or improve the activation of the immune cells to tackle the cancer cells via natural immunity mechanisms, which are also escaped during the onset and advancement of the disease (Riley et al. 2019).

Cancer immunotherapy targets to instruct the immune cells of host, present in draining lymphoid tissues and anti-tumor immune cells available at the tumor microenvironment to look for the cancer cells and eliminate them. Immunotherapy can prime the immune responses that can stimulate systemic immune surveillance and destroy local and circulating metastatic cancer cells. Moreover, as the immune cells of the host are involved in fighting the disease, a long-lasting memory can be created by immune cells and that can further help in preventing the relapse of the tumor. Due to the clinical triumph of immune checkpoint blockade, immunotherapy has now been recognized as a new pillar of cancer treatment. The most important achievement that was emphasized in 2018 by the Nobel Prize in Physiology or Medicine, awarded to James Allison and Tasuku Honjo, who discovered the immune checkpoints in cancer (Guo 2018). There are various challenges that need to be conquered in cancer immunotherapy to achieve an effective clinical application. First major challenge is the inadequate rate of response to immune checkpoint blockers, as according to clinical data, only 10–30% response rates are achieved in patients, depending upon the type and stage of cancer (Sharma et al. 2017). Immune checkpoint blocking comprises of systemic administration of monoclonal antibodies that can lead to off-target effects by stimulating the activation of T-cells that are reactive to self-antigens. The combination therapy of numerous immune checkpoint blockers largely enhances the clinical responses, but few studies suggest that it can also lead to several immune system related adverse effects giving rise to clinical complications such as hepatitis, colitis and dermatitis (Postow et al. 2018).

The US Food and Drug Administration (FDA) has approved various therapies pertaining to successful clinical trials of checkpoint blockade and chimeric antigen receptor (CAR) T-cell therapy in some subsets of cancer. Such immunotherapy provides promising potential in inducing sustained complete remissions (Maude et al. 2014). Subsequently, in 2011, a monoclonal antibody (mAb) that targets cytotoxic T-lymphocyte antigen 4 (CTLA4), the revolutionary checkpoint inhibitor ipilimumab, was approved for progressive melanoma. Novel immunotherapies like other checkpoint inhibitor mAbs that target programmed cell death 1 (PD-1) present on T-cell or its ligand, PD-1 ligand 1 (PD-L1) present on the surface of cancer cells (Ribas and Wolchok 2018; June et al. 2018). The arrival of ipilimumab and CAR T-cell therapies were milestones in cancer immunotherapy, as stressed by Science as the breakthrough of the year 2013. There are numerous immunotherapies approved for the treatment of cancer and many are in clinical trials. Immunotherapies fall into major classes like immune checkpoint blockade, CAR T-cell therapy, lymphocyte triggering cytokines, and other additional cellular therapies, antibodies that are agonists to co-stimulatory response receptors, oncolytic viruses, cancer vaccines, and bispecific antibodies. Nanomedicine can enhance several steps in anti-tumor immune mechanism, described in (Fig. 6.1). In cold tumors, there are less number of T-cells or there is lower expression of PD-L1, as the tumors are non-immunogenic, resulting into a weak response to immune checkpoint inhibitors (Tumeh et al. 2014). Similarly, patients with hot tumors that are immunogenic containing a high number of tumor-infiltrating T-cells and expressing high PD-L1 gain from immune checkpoint blockers with durable clinical immune responses.

A promising solution to escape the traditional drug formulation is to design a system that delivers the immunotherapeutics at the site of action and artificially modulates the dose, location, and time of release. Nanomedicine approaches make the use of carriers less than 100 nm in size, which avoids the systemic contact of chemotherapeutic molecules and enhances its exposure at the site of the tumor. This improved the uptake of these agents by the immune cells residing in tumor and recruit more anti-tumor immune cells and alter the signaling processes taking place in the cells (Irvine and Dane 2020).

6.2 Improving Cellular-Mediated Immunotherapy

The efficacy of cancer immunotherapy is dependent on the specificity associated with T-cells towards antigens which can be improved by genetic manipulations and redirecting T-cells to the antigen of interest, which are highly expressed in tumor cells. Self T-cells of patients can be engineered for expression of modified TCRs or

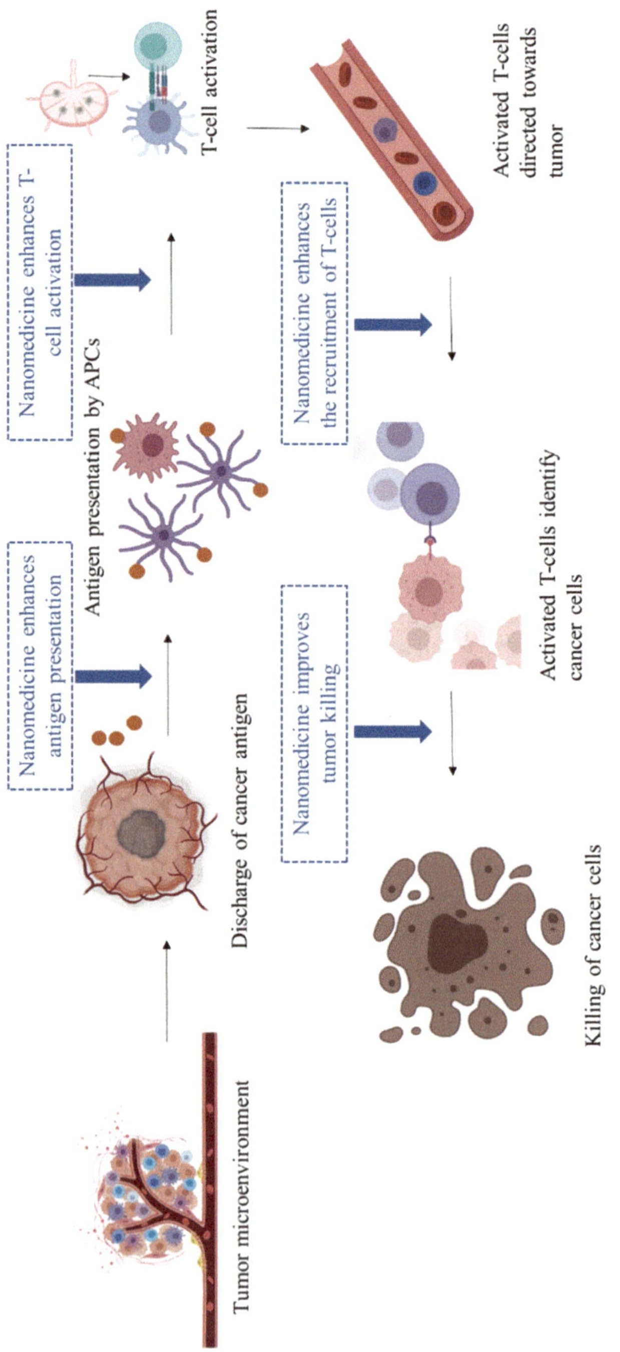

Fig. 6.1 Several roles of nanomedicine in enhancing the anti-tumor immunity

CARs which will increase the antigen specificity of T-cells and surmount the central and peripheral tolerance, eliminating the need for de-novo activation of T-cell and creating more target specific T-cells (Sharpe and Mount 2015).

For the treatment of acute lymphoblastic leukemia and refractory large B-cell lymphoma, CAR T-cell therapy is approved that includes virally transducing the autologous T-cells of patients with a synthetic antigen receptor directing CD19 (June and Sadelain 2018; Ruella et al. 2018). However, such adoptive cell therapy (ACT) has more modest accomplishments in epithelial cancers, thus providing the opportunity for encouraging trials to upgrade the potential of T-cells to overcome the hurdle of immunosuppressive nature of microenvironment in solid tumors (Miliotou and Papadopoulou 2018). A number of nanomedicine-based arenas are being exploited to improve the current ACT approach that can be long lasting and have enhanced functions in cell therapy (Qiu et al. 2017).

6.2.1 Combining Therapeutic Agents to Immune Cells

The immune system and many metabolic signaling pathways are extremely interactive and such signaling pathways can be helpful in deciding the fate and existence of T-cells. Manipulating these signaling pathways can help us to achieve higher survival and functional aspects. Several studies have demonstrated that immune suppression observed in cancer cells is due to dysregulation in the tumor microenvironment infiltrating T-lymphocyte (Kouidhi et al. 2017). Targeting such signaling pathways in T-cells can be useful in regulating the function, metabolism and, differentiation that works in favor of anti-tumor activity. Direct targeting of the specialized drugs to regulate the signaling pathways in lymphocytes seems as a difficult task as the systemic administration of drugs (the release of therapeutic agents in the circulatory system) leads to dose-limiting toxicity. This implies that the side effects of the therapeutic agents limit the possibility of an increase in dosage and level of that treatment. If lymphocytes are manipulated to express the helping factors like cytokines, then the therapeutic level can vary and it can result in either sustained release or show complete release. Such uncertain nature does not provide the opportunity to control the therapeutic levels in the cells.

New advent of emerging artificial nanocarriers and vehicles provides unconventional approaches for the engineering of cells leading to a robust increase in the efficacy of established cell-based treatments. Pertaining to the need for delivery of drugs in more targeted and controlled way to the site of the disease, isolated cells can be decorated with a ligand that defines more potent migration in the system, using artificial drug nanocarriers (Stephan and Irvine 2011). Conventional static drug targeting ligands like specific antibodies depend on passive transfer like enhanced permeation and retention for passing the vascular endothelium and accumulate at the target sites, primarily (Torchilin 2000). Modifying the cell-based therapy by attaching the nanoparticle to the immune cells significantly modifies the bio-distribution of the nanomedicine, as it gives the flexibility to use disease-relevant immune cells like tumor reactive T-cells and accumulate the particles at the site of cancer (Stephan et al. 2010). Similarly, other immune cells can be targeted, specific to a particular tumor microenvironment. Many chemotherapeutic drugs exhibit low solubility in water like Docetaxel, Camptothecin, and Paclitaxel, such drugs give enhanced aqueous solubility, protection from rapid degradation and lead to sustained delivery of the cargo (Narvekar et al. 2014).

In cell-based therapies, after the adoptive transfer, the cells migrate the endothelial and stromal cells and accumulate the surface displayed substance cargo at the pathological sites (Power and Bell 2008). The therapeutic drug can be encapsulated into the nanoparticles and then chemically attached to the plasma membrane of the adoptively transferred host immune cells. This leads to the controlled release of drug in a pre-estimated rate or in the relevant microenvironment, aiding uninterrupted pseudo-autocrine stimulation of transferred cells in vivo (Stephan et al. 2010). This limits the stimulation of other healthy tissue cells. Supporting cytokines like interleukin-2 (IL-2) and interleukin-15 (IL-15) are harmful if administered as a free drug that is distributed systemically. While, in preclinical trials the above discussed approach has shown delivery of a wider dosage range of cytokines and less toxicity (Xie et al. 2019; Singh and Bhaskar 2014).

Conjugation of nanocarriers with the surface protein of host cells triggers the nanoparticles to track the cell surface localization of the anchor proteins. Nanoparticles can be conjugated with CD45 (Freiberg et al. 2002), LFA1 (Li et al. 2009) and CD2 (Espagnolle et al. 2007) to move to the immune synapse at the initial phase of T-cell activation and subsequently in transport of such receptors in T-cell priming (Stephan et al. 2012; Huppa and Davis 2003). Immune cells interact by forming a receptor based adhesive zone of contact known as an immunological synapse (Dustin and Depoil 2011). T-cells remodel the membrane display receptors and downstream signaling molecules when antigen presenting cells (APCs) are encountered. These molecules are rearranged towards the T-cell and APC interaction zone for aiding in the interaction of stimulatory or inhibitory molecules to react with specific receptors. This will help in the expansion of T-cells and determine its destiny (Stephan et al. 2012). CD45 functions as a master regulator in T-cell activation, as it is expressed along with TCR into the central compartment of the initial immunological synapse (Freiberg et al. 2002). The time of cell activation can be regulated by controlling the release of encapsulated drug in particular environment. For instance, the release of drug conjugated with nanoparticle when the surface reduction potential is increased (Conlon et al., 2015, 2015), or in low oxygen levels (Zhang et al., 2020). However, associating the drug encapsulated nanoparticle with the host cell restricts the therapeutic intervention as the dosage of the drug is limited to the total time of cargo release from the nanoparticle (Fig. 6.2).

6.2.2 Directing Therapeutic Drugs to Immune Cells

Systematically administered nanoparticles are reported to be consumed more by non-tumor healthy cells than tumor cells. This provides a new prospect for nanomedicine mediated immunotherapy (Dai et al., 2018). Dendritic cells and

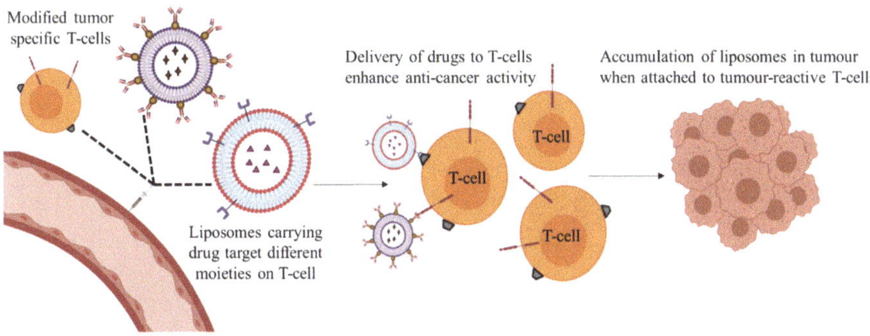

Fig. 6.2 The therapeutic agents are encapsulated into the nanoparticles and the donor T-cells are modified for relevant surface receptors. The nanoparticles carrying the drug attach to the modified tumor-specific T-cells in vivo and accumulate at the site of cancer

macrophages can engulf the nanoparticles within the tumor and enhance the recruitment of T-cells into the tumor. Phagocytic cells in the draining lymph nodes, spleen or in blood circulation can be a target of nanocarrier uptake. For example, in rodents, nanocarriers encapsulating immune checkpoint blockers are extensively delivered to phagocytic cells like dendritic cells and macrophages of spleen, facilitating dose for the highest benefit without much adverse effects (Ordikhani et al., 2018; Shi and Lammers, 2019).

Nanoparticles can effectively migrate from the site of administration into lymphatic vessels and then to lymph nodes. An emerging strategy is to target the lymph nodes by combining antigen peptides for CAR-T-cell to albumin-binding phospholipid polymers via a PEG spacer (Liu et al., 2014). CAR ligands could be transferred by albumin to lymph nodes, as peptide ligand for CAR is linked to the same lipid tail that subsequently inserts into the bilipid membrane of APCs displaying the peptide ligand from the surface of APCs (Liu et al., 2011; Ma et al., 2019). This decoration of peptide antigen on the surface of APCs can enhance the expansion and effector functions of CAR T-cells and lead to tumor rejection in mice model (Ma et al., 2019) (Fig. 6.3).

Another possibility is to use specific antibodies or other ligand or chemical moieties on the surface of nanoparticles and target the circulating endogenous lymphocytes in vivo or adoptively transferred lymphocytes. For targeting specific receptors, T-cell lineage markers like CD8 or functional markers as PD-1 are preferred markers. Immuno-modulators that aim for different inhibitory or co-stimulatory pathways efficiently lead to T-cell participation and encourage synergistic pro-activation signaling (Mi et al., 2019). Administration of anti-PD1 directed nanoparticles bearing small-molecule inhibitors of transforming growth factor-β (TGF- β) or a TLR-7/TLR-8 agonist led to prominent therapeutic efficacy that was not the case in nanoparticles without the target molecule or corresponding free drug doses (Schmid et al., 2017; Ahonen et al., 1999).

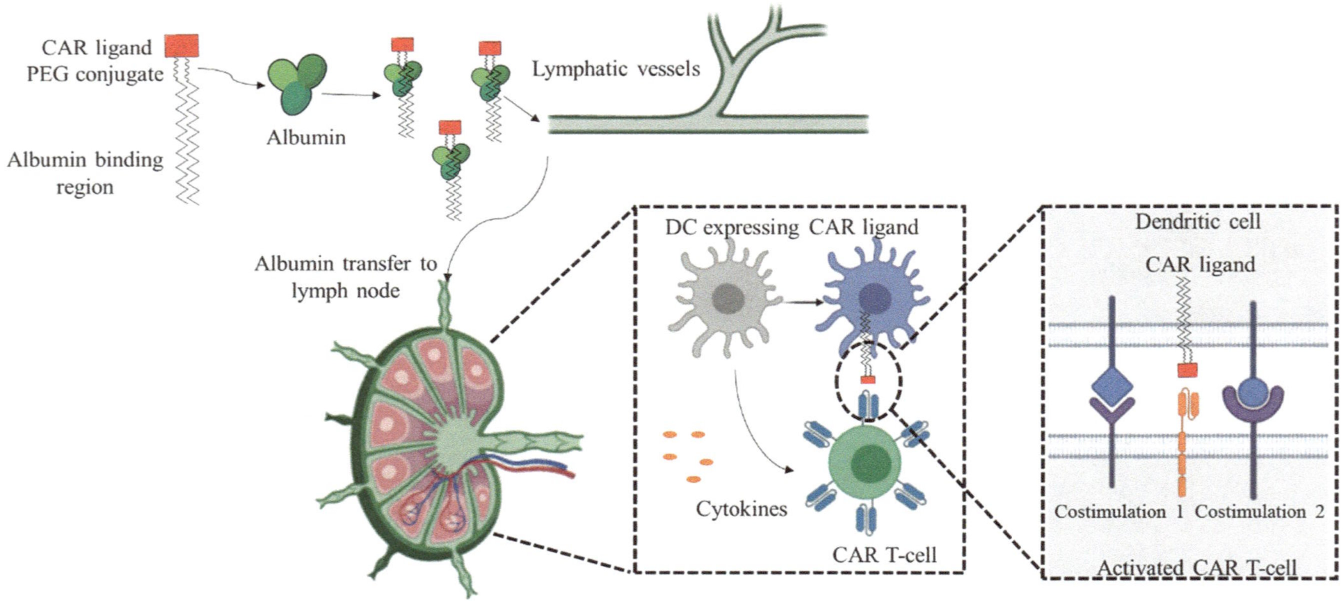

Fig. 6.3 Enhancing CAR T-cell activation and effector function. By conjugating the CAR specific ligand to albumin-binding region using a PEG spacer, efficiently delivers the ligand to lymph node draining dendritic cells via lymphatic vessels as albumin trafficking takes place in lymph node. The CAR ligand decorates on the surface of Dendritic cells (DCs) and improve the activity of CAR T-cells by as all the 3 stimulation is achieved in order to activate and produce effector CAR T-cells

6.2.3 Delivery of Gene in Lymphocytes

Viral vectors are widely used in transfection of cell with nucleic acid or to transform a cell with CARs or TCRs. But due to limitation in transgene insert size and lack of control over the cells that are transduced, it shows lower efficacy. Nanocarrier formulations with functionalized target ligand can exclusively transduce a target cell. Nanoparticles encapsulating the therapeutically appropriate transgenes can help in programming the cultured T-cells to express these transgenes. In-vitro, the nanoparticles are functionalized with appropriate ligands that target it to a particular cell, aiding them to release the mRNA cargo and result in the expression of such preferable proteins (Moffett et al., 2017).

In order to directly modify the cells in vivo, a polymeric nanoparticle is used to target transposon based DNA carrying a CAR to the circulating T-cells in lymphoma conditions. Here, transduction of a minor population of T-cells directed to T-cell expansion in 1–2 weeks and significant anti-tumor efficacy. Nanoparticles loaded with mRNA coding for a transcription factor (Foxo13A) promotes in guiding of CD62L+ T-cells towards a central memory, which is a long-lived memory and away from senescence. This can provide a robust platform to generate various immune responses (Mukalel et al., 2019; Kauffman et al., 2016).

6.3 Delivery Mechanism of Nanoparticle Therapeutics

6.3.1 Stimulating Immunogenic Cell Death (ICD)

Immunogenic cell death is characterized by the protracted exposure of DAMPs to the immune system and this leads to the generation of autoimmunity and elevated immune-mediated exclusion in the tumor microenvironment (TME). Nanoparticle encapsulation has been reported to enhance the action of chemotherapy drugs by limiting the dosage of drug accurately to subside the toxicity of constituents used in pharmacology (Zhou et al., 2019).

ICD provides the first hit by ICD inducers on perishing tumor cells and act as a vaccine for cancer that provokes anti-cancer immune reaction helping as a second hit for remaining cancer cells. This yields a sustainable gain and prevents initial drug cytotoxicity (Zitvogel et al., 2011; Galluzzi et al., 2012; Fang et al., 2011).

6.3.1.1 Nanosized Drug Carriers

For robust permeability and retention (EPR) effect of nanoparticles (Torchilin, 2011), a TME responsive nanocarrier was designed that carried two ICD inducers, mitoxantrone (MIT) and celastrol (CEL) (5:1) for melanoma model (Liu et al., 2018). The therapeutic dose delivered at the site of the tumor was more effective using nanocarrier than that of free drugs. Also, these inducers aid in improving $CD103^{+}$ DCs along with recruitment of anti-tumor memory $CD4^{+}$ and $CD8^{+}$ T-cells that uplifts the immune surveillance in the body. Similarly, a nanoparticle entrapping oxaliplatin generated more DAMPs release and improved the immune responses of DCs and T-lymphocytes more than oxaliplatin as a free drug (Zhao et al., 2016).

Doxil is a pegylated liposomal formulation of chemotherapeutic agent doxorubicin, along with a checkpoint inhibitor gives better anti-tumor activity than free drugs (Rios-Doria et al., 2015). Doxil stimulated higher CD8+ T-cell infiltration in the tumor site, higher co-stimulatory CD80 expression by DCs and macrophages and, the low fraction of regulatory T-cells (Kuai et al., 2018).

6.3.1.2 Nanopulse Stimulation

To induce ICD, nanopulse stimulation is a safer option as it uses ultrashort electrical pulses in nanosecond scale, which is much lesser invasive. These pulses infiltrate all the cells and cellular organelles in the cancer cells at elevated speed and large amplitude, which leads to calcium ion escape from the endoplasmic reticulum and trigger ER stress stimulating more release of ROS in ER (Nuccitelli et al., 2013).

Calreticulin (CRT) is one of the most powerful DAMPs signal. The translocation of ecto-CRT on the surface of cells functions as target signals for the antigen presenting cells and plays a crucial role in triggering anti-tumor immunity (Huang et al. 2019). NPS (Nanopulse stimulation) aids in ecto-CRT expression in cells along with HMGB1 (High mobility group box 1) and ATP which act as immunogenic cell death inducers, confirming its vital role in potent cancer immunotherapy (Kepp et al. 2014). Moreover, NPS is responsible for release in DAMPs with the help of ICD and stimulating antigen presentation by DCs. This shows the tendency to eradicate a high number of primary 4 T1 cancer by activating memory associated with the immune system (Guo et al. 2018).

6.3.2 Enhanced Presentation of Ligands to Immune Cells

Nanomedicine provides the capability to mimic the cell–cell junction boundary and shows a pivotal role in presenting ligands from the particle surface where various regulatory receptors and co-stimulatory interaction take place.

To activate a T-cell, a synchronization of different kinds of signaling molecules are involved including TCR and co-stimulatory signals. For more potent synchronization of receptors, paramagnetic nanoparticles are in use which can be gathered on the cell surface by the application of a magnetic field. Single signal nanoparticles can be introduced that can be combined systematically for more potent T-cell activation (Kosmides et al., 2018; Hashimoto-Tane and Saito, 2016). When a nanoparticle bearing peptide-MHC moieties and nanoparticles bearing anti-CD28 antibody is administered, it shows minimalistic T-cell activation. This is because crosslinking of the receptors does not take place and single signal is provided which is insufficient. Whereas, by applying a magnetic field helps in the coupling of the receptors and it triggers most robust T-cell activation and the effector functions (Kosmides et al., 2018; Walter et al., 2003). Nanoparticles that display both antibody against HER2 (Park et al., 2010) and calreticulin showed anti-HER2 efficacy in tumors along with a presentation of calreticulin as a DAMP to DCs to promote more uptake of tumor cells in the microenvironment. By activating more and more APC in tumor cells, higher T-cell recruitment in the cancer site takes place (Yuan et al., 2017).

6.3.3 Chronological Regulation of Immunostimulation

In order to prevent rapid clearance and obtain a sustained release of drug from nanoparticle, various nanomedicines have been created that co-operate with external energy like heat or light to release the drug from the nanoparticle in that controlled period of exposure to light or heat (Yan et al., 2011).

In order to achieve localized inflammation in TME and recruit tumor-specific immune cells in the location of cancer for enhanced survival rate in breast cancer positive rodents, NIR (near infrared light) sensitive nanoparticles are utilized. These nanoparticles carry a TLR9 agonist present on all the APCs and preferentially binds to the DNA of bacteria and viruses, activating the signaling that cause pro-inflammatory cytokine response (Chu et al., 2019). A potent agonist of TLR9 is CPG containing DNA. If such CPG containing DNA (Adamus and Kortylewski, 2018) is linked with light sensitive DNA fragment bound to photo-sensitive nanoparticles (Brieke et al., 2012; Zhou et al., 2015; Liu et al., 2016), then the splitting of the anchor DNA in the presence of NIR leads to localized inflammation because of the release of CPG containing DNA.

6.4 Modulation in Pharmacokinetics of Immunotherapy Agents

An antibody usually used as a free agent shows slow accumulation in tumor and high half-life in circulation. If a nanoparticle scaffold is used along with the antibody, then delivery of therapeutic agent in tumor site takes place in short duration. Also, it is cleared from the systemic circulation very rapidly and exhibits similar exposure of drug at tumor site but less exposure in other systems to eliminate off-target drug delivery. The target for delivery of nanoparticles carrying the drug can be cancer cells or the stromal cells like fibroblast or immune cells pertaining to tumor. Tumor-associated characteristics, like marginally acidic pH or the occurrence of higher concentrations of several enzymes, may operate as activators for the release of drugs from nanocarriers. Tumor-associated phagocytic cells can act as a depot for drugs or can themselves be the target of the treatment.

Activation of stimulator of interferon genes (STING) which is an intracellular receptor inhabiting in the endoplasmic reticulum, has proven to improve immunity against cancer by inducing pro-inflammatory cytokines (Su et al., 2019). Stimulation of STING activates an all-around IFN-I that helps in dendritic cell activation and cross-presentation of cancer antigens for the consequent activation of T-cells against tumor (Corrales et al., 2016). Nanomedicine provides an arena to administer such innate immunity activators like STING agonists, TLR agonists, and other DAMP signals. STING agonists are not effective when administered systemically but showed enhanced potential when nanocarrier is used and given intravenously in melanoma models. Such nanoparticle formulations improve the endosome escape to the cytoplasm where such receptors are present (Harlin et al., 2009).

6.5 Targeting Myeloid Cells

Tumor-associated macrophages (TAM) are recruited into tumor cells. They are derived from inflammatory monocytes and by targeting the circulating or lymphoid inhabitants monocytes, the production of TAM can be influenced (Movahedi et al., 2010). The first nanomedicine based inhibition in macrophages recruitment was reported in 2011. The approach involved the utilization of nanoparticles encapsulated with siRNA in order to inhibit chemokine receptor CCR2 that is essential in T-cell recruitment to the site of tumor. These designed nanoparticles collected in the spleen and bone marrow deliver the siRNA into the high Ly6C+ monocytes which usually gives rise to TAM (Leuschner et al., 2011; Movahedi et al., 2010). In order to destroy TAM, PLGA mannosylated nanoparticles are used to deliver doxorubicin to TAM and this lead to the depletion of TAM in melanoma model. This ultimately enhanced the efficacy of doxorubicin against the tumor (Niu et al., 2014).

By re-programming, the M2-like pro-tumor macrophages to M1-like anti-tumor macrophages, reorientation of TAM can be achieved (Sica and Mantovani, 2012; Mantovani et al., 2014; Torres Andon and Alonso, 2015). There are various reports of switching M2-like macrophages which is particularly immune-suppressive to M1-like macrophages that shows cytotoxicity in tumor (Vinogradov et al., 2014). IFN-γ has the tendency to activate M2 reorientation to M1 macrophages (Colombo et al., 1992). But due to adverse side effects, this does not hold any clinical application. This suggests the need for more efficient repolarization of M2 to M1 type.

Hydrazinocurcumin- packed legumain-targeted liposomes were in use to re-educate the TAM. Administration of this formulated nanoparticle suppresses the activity of STAT3 and exhibits a downfall in tumor proliferation, invasion, and migration in metastatic breast cancer models (Zhang et al., 2013; Wang et al., 2012). Similarly, legumain-targeted liposomes were used with another STAT3 inhibition, imidazole, which imparts protection from the relapse of tumor when used in a combination with HER-2 DNA vaccine (Liao et al., 2011).

6.6 Targeting Stromal Cell in TME

After extravasation of nanoparticles in the tumor, the delivery of the therapeutic agent to the immune-suppressed cells is difficult as it comprises malignant tumor cells, stromal cells, endothelial cells, immune cells, and fibroblast cells (Coussens et al., 2013; Mantovani et al., 2008; Hanahan and Weinberg, 2011). These cells together comprises of TME (Klemm and Joyce, 2015; Hanahan and Coussens, 2012;

Quail and Joyce, 2013). Apart from malignant cancer cells, all the other non-immune cells also contribute in TME resistance and critically regulate tumorigenesis (Egeblad et al., 2010). Fibroblasts associated with tumors proliferate uncontrollably and produce an extracellular matrix that induces hypoxic conditions and prevent the immune response by constricting blood vessels in tumor. To target the activity of these fibroblast cells, blockers of angiotensin receptors (Chauhan et al., 2019) were used but loses its clinical relevance due to systemic side effects. Formulated nanoparticles that released the angiotensin receptor blockers when the condition is acidic, particularly transport the inhibitor within the TME more effectively than the free drug. This was measured by accessing the concentration of active drugs in TME, when both the nanoparticle system and free drugs were used (Chauhan et al., 2019).

Fibroblast associated to the tumor, express fibroblast activation protein (FAP) on the surface of cells that can be targeted by using liposomes conjugated with FAP antibody Fv portions that aid in its internalization into endosome of cells that are FAP positive (Baum et al., 2007; Zhao and Rodriguez, 2013).

6.7 Limitations of Nanomedicines in Cancer Immunotherapy

For the formulation of effective cancer therapeutics, in-depth knowledge of tumor environment and obstacles relevant to cancer cells is very crucial (Navya et al., 2019). The development of the strategy and design of cancer nanomedicines is a huge challenge. The obstructions for drug delivery system to traffic to the location of cancer are broad-spectrum distribution, multifaceted tumor microenvironment, mononuclear phagocyte system, conflict with circulating blood cells, endosomal escape and multidrug resistance (Bhise et al., 2017). Very important attributes of nanoparticles are the size, stability, zeta potential, entrapment efficiency, release kinetics, and reaction to obligatory degradation. This is very difficult to achieve for large-scale production of nanoparticles. Clearance rate of highly negative nanoparticles is at higher pace and the charge of nanoparticles determine the adsorption associated with serum proteins which command the bio-distribution, pharmacokinetics, and pharmacodynamics of nanoparticles (Sau et al., 2018). The microenvironment associated with tumor is highly acidic and has poor drainage of the lymphatic system. The nanoparticles that are stable in such a harsh tumor environment are generally effective.

6.8 Conclusion and Future Perspectives

Several strategies are foreseen for the practise of nanomedicines to expand the efficacy of cancer immunotherapy. Noteworthy developments have been made in recent years at the preclinical stage and encouraging early trials has been accomplished in the clinic. For effective nano-immunotherapy in the future, biomarkers should be recognized to classify the immune-suppressive cells and immune-activating cells or signaling pathways that act as a target to safeguard the most favorable therapeutic results. Such comprehensions will monitor the formulation of nanomedicines that help in immune-modulation and provide a peak in clinical translation of nanomedicines that may impact the creation of more effective medications for cancer patients. Like reprograming the myeloid cells to live longer requires the exposure of innate immunity stimuli and this is being appreciated and learned from the molecular and genetic point of view. Inducing such trained immunity is a new arena for the development of anti-tumor agents and the ability of nanomedicine to effectively target the myeloid cells of primary lymphoid organs makes these immunotherapy strategies very promising. Such attempts not only involve the adaptive immune systems but also include the innate immune systems, increasing the overall immune surveillance.

Acknowledgements This work was supported by the Department of Biotechnology, Government of India [grant number BT/PR10414/PFN/20/961/2014] and DST SERB [grant number EMR/2016/005286]. Financial assistance by The Gujarat Institute for Chemical Technology (GICT) for the Establishment of a Facility for environmental risk assessment of chemicals and nanomaterials is also acknowledged.

Conflicts of Interest There are no conflicts to declare.

References

Adamus T, Kortylewski M (2018) The revival of CpG oligonucleotide-based cancer immunotherapies. Contemp Oncol 22:56

Ahonen CL, Gibson SJ, Smith RM, Pederson LK, Lindh JM, Tomai MA, Vasilakos JP (1999) Dendritic cell maturation and subsequent enhanced T-cell stimulation induced with the novel synthetic immune response modifier R-848. Cell Immunol 197:62–72

Baum P, Müller D, Rüger R, Kontermann RE (2007) Single-chain Fv immunoliposomes for the targeting of fibroblast activation protein-expressing tumor stromal cells. J Drug Target 15:399–406

Bhise K, Kashaw SK, Sau S, Iyer AK (2017) Nanostructured lipid carriers employing polyphenols as promising anticancer agents: quality by design (QbD) approach. Int J Pharm 526:506–515

Brieke C, Rohrbach F, Gottschalk A, Mayer G, Heckel A (2012) Light-controlled tools. Angew Chem Int Ed 51:8446–8476

Cabral BP, Fonseca MDGD, Mota FB (2018) The recent landscape of cancer research worldwide: a bibliometric and network analysis. Oncotarget 9:30474

Chauhan VP, Chen IX, Tong R, Ng MR, Martin JD, Naxerova K, Wu MW, Huang P, Boucher Y, Kohane DS (2019) Reprogramming the microenvironment with tumor-selective angiotensin blockers enhances cancer immunotherapy. Proc Natl Acad Sci 116:10674–10680

Chu H, Zhao J, Mi Y, Di Z, Li L (2019) NIR-light-mediated spatially selective triggering of anti-tumor immunity via upconversion nanoparticle-based immunodevices. Nat Commun 10:1–11

Colombo N, Peccatori F, Paganin C, Bini S, Brandely M, Mangioni C, Mantovani A, Allavena P (1992) Anti-tumor and immunomodulatory activity of intraperitoneal IFN-γ in ovarian carcinoma patients with minimal residual tumor after chemotherapy. Int J Cancer 51:42–46

Conlon KC, Lugli E, Welles HC, Rosenberg SA, Fojo AT, Morris JC, Fleisher TA, Dubois SP, Perera LP, Stewart DM (2015) Redistribution, hyperproliferation, activation of natural killer cells and CD8 T cells, and cytokine production during first-in-human clinical trial of recombinant human interleukin-15 in patients with cancer. J Clin Oncol 33:74

Corrales L, Mcwhirter SM, Dubensky TW, Gajewski TF (2016) The host STING pathway at the interface of cancer and immunity. J Clin Invest 126:2404–2411
Coussens LM, Zitvogel L, Palucka AK (2013) Neutralizing tumor-promoting chronic inflammation: a magic bullet? Science 339:286–291
Dai Q, Wilhelm S, Ding D, Syed AM, Sindhwani S, Zhang Y, Chen YY, Macmillan P, Chan WC (2018) Quantifying the ligand-coated nanoparticle delivery to cancer cells in solid tumors. ACS Nano 12:8423–8435
Dustin ML, Depoil D (2011) New insights into the T cell synapse from single molecule techniques. Nat Rev Immunol 11:672–684
Egeblad M, Nakasone ES, Werb Z (2010) Tumors as organs: complex tissues that interface with the entire organism. Dev Cell 18:884–901
Espagnolle N, Depoil D, Zaru R, Demeur C, Champagne E, Guiraud M, Valitutti S (2007) CD2 and TCR synergize for the activation of phospholipase Cγ1/calcium pathway at the immunological synapse. Int Immunol 19:239–248
Fang J, Nakamura H, Maeda H (2011) The EPR effect: unique features of tumor blood vessels for drug delivery, factors involved, and limitations and augmentation of the effect. Adv Drug Deliv Rev 63:136–151
Freiberg BA, Kupfer H, Maslanik W, Delli J, Kappler J, Zaller DM, Kupfer A (2002) Staging and resetting T cell activation in SMACs. Nat Immunol 3:911–917
Galluzzi L, Senovilla L, Zitvogel L, Kroemer G (2012) The secret ally: immunostimulation by anticancer drugs. Nat Rev Drug Discov 11:215–233
Guo ZS (2018) The 2018 Nobel Prize in medicine goes to cancer immunotherapy. Springer, Berlin
Guo S, Jing Y, Burcus NI, Lassiter BP, Tanaz R, Heller R, Beebe SJ (2018) Nano-pulse stimulation induces potent immune responses, eradicating local breast cancer while reducing distant metastases. Int J Cancer 142:629–640
Hanahan D, Coussens LM (2012) Accessories to the crime: functions of cells recruited to the tumor microenvironment. Cancer Cell 21:309–322
Hanahan D, Weinberg RA (2011) Hallmarks of cancer: the next generation. Cell 144:646–674
Harlin H, Meng Y, Peterson AC, Zha Y, Tretiakova M, Slingluff C, Mckee M, Gajewski TF (2009) Chemokine expression in melanoma metastases associated with CD8+ T-cell recruitment. Cancer Res 69:3077–3085
Hashimoto-Tane A, Saito T (2016) Dynamic regulation of TCR–microclusters and the microsynapse for T cell activation. Front Immunol 7:255
Huang Y, Kong L, Lu J (2019) Ecto-calreticulin expression after particle irradiation versus conventional photon irradiation in human Cancer cell lines. Int J Radiat Oncol Biol Phys 105: E643
Huppa JB, Davis MM (2003) T-cell-antigen recognition and the immunological synapse. Nat Rev Immunol 3:973–983
Irvine DJ, Dane EL (2020) Enhancing cancer immunotherapy with nanomedicine. Nat Rev Immunol:1–14
June CH, Sadelain M (2018) Chimeric antigen receptor therapy. N Engl J Med 379:64–73
June CH, O'connor RS, Kawalekar OU, Ghassemi S, Milone MC (2018) CAR T cell immunotherapy for human cancer. Science 359:1361–1365
Kauffman KJ, Webber MJ, Anderson DG (2016) Materials for non-viral intracellular delivery of messenger RNA therapeutics. J Control Release 240:227–234
Kepp O, Senovilla L, Vitale I, Vacchelli E, Adjemian S, Agostinis P, Apetoh L, Aranda F, Barnaba V, Bloy N (2014) Consensus guidelines for the detection of immunogenic cell death. Onco Targets Ther e955691:3
Klemm F, Joyce JA (2015) Microenvironmental regulation of therapeutic response in cancer. Trends Cell Biol 25:198–213
Kosmides AK, Necochea K, Hickey JW, Schneck JP (2018) Separating T cell targeting components onto magnetically clustered nanoparticles boosts activation. Nano Lett 18:1916–1924

Kouidhi S, Elgaaied AB, Chouaib S (2017) Impact of metabolism on T-cell differentiation and function and cross talk with tumor microenvironment. Front Immunol 8:270

Kuai R, Yuan W, Son S, Nam J, Xu Y, Fan Y, Schwendeman A, Moon JJ (2018) Elimination of established tumors with nanodisc-based combination chemoimmunotherapy. Sci Adv 4: eaao1736

Leuschner F, Dutta P, Gorbatov R, Novobrantseva TI, Donahoe JS, Courties G, Lee KM, Kim JI, Markmann JF, Marinelli B (2011) Therapeutic siRNA silencing in inflammatory monocytes in mice. Nat Biotechnol 29:1005

Li D, Molldrem JJ, Ma Q (2009) LFA-1 regulates CD8+ T cell activation via T cell receptor-mediated and LFA-1-mediated Erk1/2 signal pathways. J Biol Chem 284:21001–21010

Liao D, Liu Z, Wrasidlo WJ, Luo Y, Nguyen G, Chen T, Xiang R, Reisfeld RA (2011) Targeted therapeutic remodeling of the tumor microenvironment improves an HER-2 DNA vaccine and prevents recurrence in a murine breast cancer model. Cancer Res 71:5688–5696

Liu H, Kwong B, Irvine DJ (2011) Membrane anchored immunostimulatory oligonucleotides for in vivo cell modification and localized immunotherapy. Angew Chem Int Ed 50:7052–7055

Liu H, Moynihan KD, Zheng Y, Szeto GL, Li AV, Huang B, Van Egeren DS, Park C, Irvine DJ (2014) Structure-based programming of lymph-node targeting in molecular vaccines. Nature 507:519–522

Liu Z, Liu Y, Chang Y, Seyf HR, Henry A, Mattheyses AL, Yehl K, Zhang Y, Huang Z, Salaita K (2016) Nanoscale optomechanical actuators for controlling mechanotransduction in living cells. Nat Methods 13:143

Liu Q, Chen F, Hou L, Shen L, Zhang X, Wang D, Huang L (2018) Nanocarrier-mediated chemo-immunotherapy arrested cancer progression and induced tumor dormancy in desmoplastic melanoma. ACS Nano 12:7812–7825

Ma L, Dichwalkar T, Chang JY, Cossette B, Garafola D, Zhang AQ, Fichter M, Wang C, Liang S, Silva M (2019) Enhanced CAR–T cell activity against solid tumors by vaccine boosting through the chimeric receptor. Science 365:162–168

Mantovani A, Allavena P, Sica A, Balkwill F (2008) Cancer-related inflammation. Nature 454:436–444

Mantovani A, Vecchi A, Allavena P (2014) Pharmacological modulation of monocytes and macrophages. Curr Opin Pharmacol 17:38–44

Maude SL, Frey N, Shaw PA, Aplenc R, Barrett DM, Bunin NJ, Chew A, Gonzalez VE, Zheng Z, Lacey SF (2014) Chimeric antigen receptor T cells for sustained remissions in leukemia. N Engl J Med 371:1507–1517

Mccarthy EF (2006) The toxins of William B. Coley and the treatment of bone and soft-tissue sarcomas. Iowa Orthop J 26:154

Mi Y, Hagan Iv CT, Vincent BG, Wang AZ (2019) Emerging nano–/microapproaches for cancer immunotherapy. Adv Sci 6:1801847

Miliotou AN, Papadopoulou LC (2018) CAR T-cell therapy: a new era in cancer immunotherapy. Curr Pharm Biotechnol 19:5–18

Moffett H, Coon M, Radtke S, Stephan S, Mcknight L, Lambert A, Stoddard B, Kiem H, Stephan M (2017) Hit-and-run programming of therapeutic cytoreagents using mRNA nanocarriers. Nat Commun 8:389

Movahedi K, Laoui D, Gysemans C, Baeten M, Stangé G, van den Bossche J, Mack M, Pipeleers D, In't Veld P, de Baetselier P (2010) Different tumor microenvironments contain functionally distinct subsets of macrophages derived from Ly6C (high) monocytes. Cancer Res 70:5728–5739

Mukalel AJ, Riley RS, Zhang R, Mitchell MJ (2019) Nanoparticles for nucleic acid delivery: applications in cancer immunotherapy. Cancer Lett 458:102–112

Narvekar M, Xue HY, Eoh JY, Wong HL (2014) Nanocarrier for poorly water-soluble anticancer drugs—barriers of translation and solutions. AAPS PharmSciTech 15:822–833

Navya P, Kaphle A, Srinivas S, Bhargava SK, Rotello VM, Daima HK (2019) Current trends and challenges in cancer management and therapy using designer nanomaterials. Nano Converg 6:23

Niu M, Naguib YW, Aldayel AM, Shi Y-C, Hursting SD, Hersh MA, Cui Z (2014) Biodistribution and in vivo activities of tumor-associated macrophage-targeting nanoparticles incorporated with doxorubicin. Mol Pharm 11:4425–4436

Nuccitelli R, Lui K, Kreis M, Athos B, Nuccitelli P (2013) Nanosecond pulsed electric field stimulation of reactive oxygen species in human pancreatic cancer cells is Ca2+−dependent. Biochem Biophys Res Commun 435:580–585

Ordikhani F, Uehara M, Kasinath V, Dai L, Eskandari SK, Bahmani B, Yonar M, Azzi JR, Haik Y, Sage PT (2018) Targeting antigen-presenting cells by anti–PD-1 nanoparticles augments antitumor immunity. JCI Insight:3

Park S, Jiang Z, Mortenson ED, Deng L, Radkevich-Brown O, Yang X, Sattar H, Wang Y, Brown NK, Greene M (2010) The therapeutic effect of anti-HER2/neu antibody depends on both innate and adaptive immunity. Cancer Cell 18:160–170

Postow MA, Sidlow R, Hellmann MD (2018) Immune-related adverse events associated with immune checkpoint blockade. N Engl J Med 378:158–168

Power A, Bell J (2008) Taming the Trojan horse: optimizing dynamic carrier cell/oncolytic virus systems for cancer biotherapy. Gene Ther 15:772–779

Qiu H, Min Y, Rodgers Z, Zhang L, Wang AZ (2017) Nanomedicine approaches to improve cancer immunotherapy. Wiley Interdiscip Rev Nanomed Nanobiotechnol 9:e1456

Quail DF, Joyce JA (2013) Microenvironmental regulation of tumor progression and metastasis. Nat Med 19:1423

Ribas A, Wolchok JD (2018) Cancer immunotherapy using checkpoint blockade. Science 359:1350–1355

Riley RS, June CH, Langer R, Mitchell MJ (2019) Delivery technologies for cancer immunotherapy. Nat Rev Drug Discov 18:175–196

Rios-Doria J, Durham N, Wetzel L, Rothstein R, Chesebrough J, Holoweckyj N, Zhao W, Leow CC, Hollingsworth R (2015) Doxil synergizes with cancer immunotherapies to enhance antitumor responses in syngeneic mouse models. Neoplasia 17:661–670

Ruella M, Xu J, Barrett DM, Fraietta JA, Reich TJ, Ambrose DE, Klichinsky M, Shestova O, Patel PR, Kulikovskaya I (2018) Induction of resistance to chimeric antigen receptor T cell therapy by transduction of a single leukemic B cell. Nat Med 24:1499–1503

Sau S, Tatiparti K, Alsaab HO, Kashaw SK, Iyer AK (2018) A tumor multicomponent targeting chemoimmune drug delivery system for reprograming the tumor microenvironment and personalized cancer therapy. Drug Discovery Today 23:1344

Schmid D, Park CG, Hartl CA, Subedi N, Cartwright AN, Puerto RB, Zheng Y, Maiarana J, Freeman GJ, Wucherpfennig KW (2017) T cell-targeting nanoparticles focus delivery of immunotherapy to improve antitumor immunity. Nat Commun 8:1–12

Sharma P, Allison JP (2015) Immune checkpoint targeting in cancer therapy: toward combination strategies with curative potential. Cell 161:205–214

Sharma P, Hu-Lieskovan S, Wargo JA, Ribas A (2017) Primary, adaptive, and acquired resistance to cancer immunotherapy. *Cell* 168:707–723

Sharpe M, Mount N (2015) Genetically modified T cells in cancer therapy: opportunities and challenges. Dis Model Mech 8:337–350

Shi Y, Lammers T (2019) Combining nanomedicine and immunotherapy. Acc Chem Res 52:1543–1554

Sica A, Mantovani A (2012) Macrophage plasticity and polarization: in vivo veritas. J Clin Invest 122:787–795

Singh MS, Bhaskar S (2014) Nanocarrier-based immunotherapy in cancer management and research. ImmunoTargets Ther 3:121

Stephan MT, Irvine DJ (2011) Enhancing cell therapies from the outside in: cell surface engineering using synthetic nanomaterials. Nano Today 6:309–325

Stephan MT, Moon JJ, Um SH, Bershteyn A, Irvine DJ (2010) Therapeutic cell engineering with surface-conjugated synthetic nanoparticles. Nat Med 16:1035
Stephan MT, Stephan SB, Bak P, Chen J, Irvine DJ (2012) Synapse-directed delivery of immunomodulators using T-cell-conjugated nanoparticles. Biomaterials 33:5776–5787
Su T, Zhang Y, Valerie K, Wang X-Y, Lin S, Zhu G (2019) STING activation in cancer immunotherapy. Theranostics 9:7759
Torchilin VP (2000) Drug targeting. Eur J Pharm Sci 11:S81–S91
Torchilin V (2011) Tumor delivery of macromolecular drugs based on the EPR effect. Adv Drug Deliv Rev 63:131–135
Torres Andon F, Alonso MJ (2015) Nanomedicine and cancer immunotherapy–targeting immunosuppressive cells. J Drug Target 23:656–671
Tumeh PC, Harview CL, Yearley JH, Shintaku IP, Taylor EJ, Robert L, Chmielowski B, Spasic M, Henry G, Ciobanu V (2014) PD-1 blockade induces responses by inhibiting adaptive immune resistance. Nature 515:568–571
Vinogradov S, Warren G, Wei X (2014) Macrophages associated with tumors as potential targets and therapeutic intermediates. Nanomedicine 9:695–707
Walter S, Herrgen L, Schoor O, Jung G, Wernet D, Bühring H-J, Rammensee H-G, Stevanović S (2003) Cutting edge: predetermined avidity of human CD8 T cells expanded on calibrated MHC/anti-CD28-coated microspheres. J Immunol 171:4974–4978
Wang X, Zhang Y, Zhang X, Tian W, Feng W, Chen T (2012) The curcumin analogue hydrazinocurcumin exhibits potent suppressive activity on carcinogenicity of breast cancer cells via STAT3 inhibition. Int J Oncol 40:1189–1195
Xie Y-Q, Arik H, Wei L, Zheng Y, Suh H, Irvine DJ, Tang L (2019) Redox-responsive interleukin-2 nanogel specifically and safely promotes the proliferation and memory precursor differentiation of tumor-reactive T-cells. Biomater Sci 7:1345–1357
Yan B, Boyer J-C, Branda NR, Zhao Y (2011) Near-infrared light-triggered dissociation of block copolymer micelles using upconverting nanoparticles. J Am Chem Soc 133:19714–19717
Yan S, Zhao P, Yu T, Gu N (2019) Current applications and future prospects of nanotechnology in cancer immunotherapy. Cancer Biol Med 16:486
Yuan H, Jiang W, Von Roemeling CA, Qie Y, Liu X, Chen Y, Wang Y, Wharen RE, Yun K, Bu G (2017) Multivalent bi-specific nanobioconjugate engager for targeted cancer immunotherapy. Nat Nanotechnol 12:763–769
Zhang X, Tian W, Cai X, Wang X, Dang W, Tang H, Cao H, Wang L, Chen T (2013) Hydrazinocurcumin Encapsuled nanoparticles "re-educate" tumor-associated macrophages and exhibit anti-tumor effects on breast cancer following STAT3 suppression. PLoS One:8
Zhang P, Yang H, Shen W, Liu W, Chen L, Xiao C (2020) Hypoxia-responsive polypeptide nanoparticles loaded with doxorubicin for breast cancer therapy. ACS Biomater Sci Eng 6:2167–2174
Zhao G, Rodriguez BL (2013) Molecular targeting of liposomal nanoparticles to tumor microenvironment. Int J Nanomedicine 8:61
Zhao X, Yang K, Zhao R, Ji T, Wang X, Yang X, Zhang Y, Cheng K, Liu S, Hao J (2016) Inducing enhanced immunogenic cell death with nanocarrier-based drug delivery systems for pancreatic cancer therapy. Biomaterials 102:187–197
Zhou B, Shi B, Jin D, Liu X (2015) Controlling upconversion nanocrystals for emerging applications. Nat Nanotechnol 10:924
Zhou J, Wang G, Chen Y, Wang H, Hua Y, Cai Z (2019) Immunogenic cell death in cancer therapy: present and emerging inducers. J Cell Mol Med 23:4854–4865
Zitvogel L, Kepp O, Kroemer G (2011) Immune parameters affecting the efficacy of chemotherapeutic regimens. Nat Rev Clin Oncol 8:151

7 Targeting Tumor Microenvironment Through Nanotheranostics

Bhawna Deswal, Sonia Kapoor, and Adhiraj Roy

Abstract

Despite rigorous research endeavors and the discovery of novel therapeutic interventions such as immunotherapy and personalized medicine approaches, cancer tops the chart of global killers with an exceptionally high mortality rate along with deaths due to cardiac attack and stroke. Several factors including complex tumor heterogeneity, ineffective delivery of chemotherapeutic drugs to the tumor sites along with high cytotoxicity and acquisition of drug resistance by the cancer stem cells (CSC) make cancer a notorious pathology to treat and hence discovery of novel therapeutic interventions addressing these parameters are highly warranted. The tumor microenvironment (TME) consisting of the extracellular matrix (ECM), stromal cells, and immune cells plays a critical role in diseases progression by positively regulating several hallmarks of cancer including evasion of apoptosis, angiogenesis, and metastasis. Recently, cancer nanotheranostics, a nanotechnology-based diagnostic cum therapeutic approach utilizing the physicochemical and biological properties of nanoparticles has sparked global attention as novel intervention strategy for this deadly pathology. This chapter discusses the role of the TME in the development and progression of cancer and several nanotheranostic agents such as metallic, magnetic, and lipid nanoparticles that are currently utilized in targeted cancer therapeutics. Moreover, the *status quo* of applications of nanotheranostic agents in cancer biomarker detection, cancer imaging, and nano-formulations as improved drug delivery systems and novel therapeutic choices targeting the TME of several cancers are discussed.

B. Deswal · S. Kapoor · A. Roy (✉)
Amity Institute of Molecular Medicine and Stem Cell Research, Amity University, Noida, India
e-mail: bdeswal@amity.edu; skapoor4@amity.edu; aroy2@amity.edu

A. Malik et al. (eds.), *Nanomedicine for Cancer Diagnosis and Therapy*,
https://doi.org/10.1007/978-981-15-7564-8_7

Keywords

Tumor microenvironment · Nanotechnology · Cancer nanotheranostics · Nanoparticles · Cancer detection · Cancer therapeutics

7.1 Introduction

Despite decades of extensive research and the emergence of various prominent therapeutic strategies such as stem cell transplant therapy, immunotherapy, and targeted therapies, cancer remains as a global threat with more than 18 million cases and nine million deaths (Bray et al. 2018). The cellular and physiological properties of the tumor microenvironment (TME) play a pivotal role in disease development, progression and most importantly, acquisition of drug resistance (Gacche and Meshram 2013). Due to the heterogeneity of the tumor microenvironment (TME), cytotoxic effects of chemotherapy and radiotherapy such as infertility, immunosuppression, and heart disease, complex crosstalk between signaling pathways, and the TME-mediated drug resistance, researchers developed cancer nanotheranostics, a novel, nanotechnology-based diagnostic and therapeutic intervention which manipulates and exploits the unique properties of various nanoparticles (NPs) such as gold and magnetic NPs (Roy Chowdhury et al. 2016). Several key physical properties of the TME such as hypoxia, pH, and interstitial pressure are frequently targeted by nanotheranostic agents for effective therapeutic response (Sikkandhar et al. 2017). For example, the acidic pH environment of the TME due to high glycolytic activity (the Warburg effect) can be successfully targeted using several nanotheranostic probes and techniques such as gadolinium diethylenetriamine-penta-acetic acid bismethylamide (GdDTPA-BMA)-based MRI and functionalized gold nanostars (GNS)-based photoacoustic tomography. In this chapter, we have discussed the cellular and physiological properties of the TME and several novel nanotheranostic strategies that can be utilized to detect cancer biomarkers for early detection, cancer imaging and target the TME for improved drug delivery and therapy. Furthermore, we have also summarized the *status quo* of development of advanced nano-formulations that are currently used as therapeutic choices against several major human carcinomas.

7.2 The Tumor Microenvironment (TME) and its Components

Recent literature suggests that the tumor microenvironment (TME) is pivotal in tumorigenesis and acquisition of drug resistance, making it a novel therapeutic target (Gacche and Meshram 2013). In addition to the population of heterogeneous cancer cells, the tumor mass is also comprised of various infiltrated and resident immune cells, secreted growth factors, signaling proteins and Extracellular Matrix (ECM) which collectively form the Tumor Microenvironment (TME). The non-malignant cells of tumor microenvironment are believed to have dynamic and functional tumor

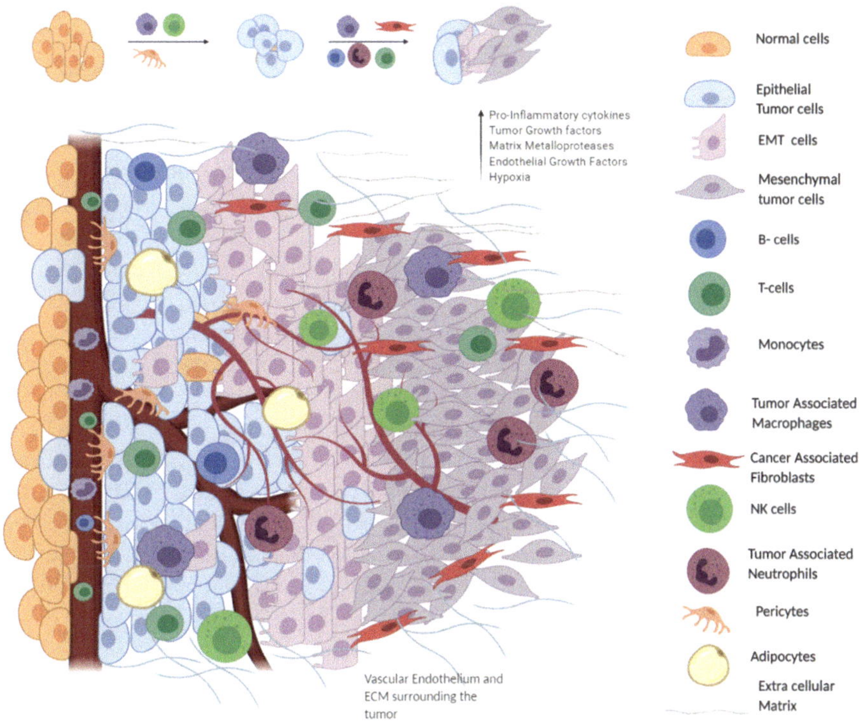

Fig. 7.1 The tumor microenvironment: The cells of innate and adaptive immune system such as B cells, T cells, Natural killer cells, Tumor associated Macrophages, Tumor associated Neutrophils, and Cancer associated fibroblasts enrich the tumor microenvironment with pro-inflammatory tumor promoting cytokines. Other components such as ECM, pericytes, adipocytes, proteases, and endothelial cells get altered and foster tumor growth, angiogenesis, and chemoresistance. As the complexity of tumor microenvironment increases, the cancer cells begin to attain more aggressive mesenchymal phenotype by undergoing Epithelial–Mesenchymal Transition (image prepared using Biorender)

promoting role during stages of tumor initiation as well as progression (Balkwill et al. 2012). The intercellular interaction between cancer cells and TME via secretion of various cytokines, chemokines, and growth factors drives the inflammatory and wound healing processes of tumor. Tumor vasculature, lymphatics, and other infiltrated cells such as pericytes and adipocytes are also key players along with altered immune cells such as macrophages, neutrophils, and Natural Killer cells (NK cells) (Hui and Chen 2015). Non-malignant cells of TME are also required to activate transcriptional programs in tumor cells which allow these cells to undergo changes like attaining mesenchymal phenotype, degrading ECM and to establish in distant organs and continuous crosstalk between microenvironment and cancer cells also boost up the resistance against anti-tumor therapies (Mbeunkui and Johann Jr. 2009). In this section, we summarize the components and physiological properties of the TME responsible for cancer progression (Fig. 7.1).

7.2.1 Cells of the Immune System

7.2.1.1 The T Cells

T cells are one of the cell types of adaptive immune system. The naive T cells ($CD44^{low}$, $CD67L^{hi}$) present in thymus get activated by foreign antigen and subsequently acquire the effector functions. These cells begin to proliferate, initiate secretion of effector cytokines, and subsequently the granzymes/perforin mediate cytotoxicity. Majority of the proliferated T cells die by apoptosis and the surviving ones remain in resting state as memory cells. These cells are responsible for inflammatory response, defense, and immunity against further infection (Jiang et al. 2015). The T cells target the foreign cells specifically; in contrast, tumor cells are self-molecules with weak immunogenicity. Therefore, T cells against tumor cells are of low T cell receptor (TCR) affinity as cells with increased affinity get deleted during thymic selection (Joyce and Fearon 2015).

The T cells can infiltrate the tumor are tumor infiltrating T cells/lymphocytes (TILs) and can be of $CD4^{+}$and $CD8^{+}$ subset. The failed effect of T cells against tumor is due to several reasons. Firstly, it has been suggested that the extravasation of T cells in tumor is regulated by tumor microenvironment itself. For example, the nitrated- C-C motif Chemokine Ligand 2 (N-CCL-2) secreted by tumor cells is essential for trapping the T cells in tumor surrounding in both prostate and colon cancer (Molon et al. 2011). Inhibition of N-CCL2 increases the infiltration of T cells (TILs) that are otherwise trapped in surrounding stroma. Inhibition of N–CCL2 also increases the success of Adaptive T cell therapy (ACT) which increases the immunity against tumor by increasing infiltration of TILs. Regulatory T cells, a subset of $CD4^{+}$ T cells regulate immune-suppression and are responsible for protecting the body against autoimmune diseases. It was found that tumor selectively increases the infiltration of Treg cells and other myeloid cells which boost up tumor's force against host immunity (Wang and Wang 2007). The secretions present in TME such as Vascular Endothelial Growth Factor (VEGF), Interleukin-10 (IL-10), and Prostaglandin E2 (PGE2) induce the expression of FasL apoptotic ligand in endothelial cells of tumor vasculature. Studies have found that there are fewer $CD8^{+}$ T cells in comparison with Treg cells in tumor with increased expression of FasL in their vasculature, Treg cells escape from this apoptotic mechanism due to increased expression of cFLIP (apoptotic inhibitor) on their surface (Motz 2014).

7.2.1.2 The B Cells

The role of T cells is well established in anti-tumor immunity and other innate and acquired responses. However, understanding the role of B cell generated antibodies and effector responses in tumorigenesis is the new emerging area. B cells can modulate immune cells of TME by presenting antigens, secreting cytokines, and by providing co-stimulatory signals. The role of B cells is still unclear as it evidently shows both anti- and pro-tumorous characteristics depending on population of different subtypes in the TME (Tsou et al. 2016). B cells in tumor microenvironment suppress the infiltration and activation of T cells along with the secretion of IL-10 and Immunoglobulin G (IgG). The B cell-driven antigen-IgG antibody complex can increase tumor progression by recruitment of immunosuppressive myeloid cells in TME, degradation of Extracellular Matrix (ECM), and enhanced angiogenesis in macrophage dependent manner (Sarvaria et al. 2017).

Like T cells, B cells also have different subsets, namely tumor infiltrating B-lymphocytes (B-TILs) and B regulatory cells (Bregs) and B-TILs derived lymphotoxins have been found to increase prostate cancer progression in NF-κB and STAT-3 dependent manner (Massimo Ammirante§ and Michael 2017). B regulatory cells show their immune modulatory functions by increasing the secretion of immunosuppressive factors such as Interleukin-10 (IL-10) and Tumor Growth Factor-β (TGF-β). Bregs evidently increase the production of Tregs from resting $CD4^+$ cells (Mizoguchi et al. 2002). Another important subset, i.e. $CD5^+$ B cells increases tumor progression by activating various signaling cascades by phosphorylating STAT-3 in IL-6 dependent manner in prostate, ovarian, and non-small lung cancer (Daniel and Shumer 2017). As mentioned earlier, B cells have several anti-tumoral roles as well. The anti-tumor effect is mainly mediated by increased cytotoxic T cells-dependent granzymes that affect tumor cells. The role of B cells as antigen presenting cells (APCs) is very essential to sustain the activation and proliferation of T cells in the TME. Most importantly, the secretion of autoantibodies by B cells associated with tumor is of prognostic value and their presence can predict onset of tumor along with the pattern of malignancies prior to months or years in some cases (Dowd and Barch 2017).

7.2.1.3 Tumor Associated Macrophages (TAMs)

Macrophages are essential cells of innate immune system that regulate the host immune response against pathogens, wound healing, and tissue homeostasis. During tumor initiation and progression, the circulating monocytes are recruited into the tumor to establish as macrophages which have been found to further accelerate the tumor development (Qian et al. 2015). Once entered the TME, the macrophages can potentially change their phenotype in response to microenvironmental signals from tumor and stromal cells. Based on these responses, macrophages can be broadly divided into anti-tumoral M1 and pro-tumoral M2 macrophages. The M1 phenotype is attained in response to Th1 cytokines such as interferon γ (INF-γ), toll-like receptors (TLRs), and lipopolysaccharides (LPS) which educate the macrophages in generating inflammatory response by secreting IL-6, IL-23, and Tumor Necrosis Factor-α (TNF-α). The M1 macrophages have a high expression of major histocompatibility complex type I and II (MHC I and MHC II) and help in antigen presentation. The Tumor Associated Macrophages (TAMs) closely resemble the M2 phenotype which is attained in response to Th2 cytokines, IL-4 and IL-13(Qiu et al. 2018).

The infiltration of monocytes in tumor is critically regulated by cytokines and growth factors secreted by tumor microenvironment. CCL-1 and Colony Stimulating Factor-1 (CSF-1) are two main cytokines which target the circulating monocytes and increase their infiltration in the TME (Paulus et al. 2006). Several evidences suggest that the hypoxia also drives infiltration of monocytes. Once activated, TAMs secrete immunosuppressive cytokines such as IL-10 and Tumor Growth Factor-β (TGF-β) which limit the infiltration of T cells into the tumor. Additionally, the M2 macrophages secrete proteolytic enzymes such as Matrix metalloproteases (MMPs), cathepsins, and plasminogens which have the potential to remodel the tumor surrounding ECM and increase tumor invasion and metastasis (Shree et al. 2011; Yang et al. 2015).

7.2.1.4 Tumor Associated Neutrophils (TANs)

Neutrophils are most abundant white blood cells in circulation and are first line of defense against a pathogen. Tumor Associated Neutrophils are cells of myeloid lineage with plasticity like that of TAMs as they exhibit pro-tumoral or anti-tumoral characteristics depending on surrounding microenvironment (Wu et al. 2019). The neutrophils are also classified as N1 (Anti-tumor neutrophils) and N2 (pro-tumor Neutrophils). The N1 Neutrophils are characterized by hypersegmented nucleus and increased cytotoxicity towards tumor due to secretion of cytokines such as TNF-α, Intercellular Adhesion Modecule-1 (ICAM-1), and FAS. Whereas N2 neutrophils show increased expression of Arginase, CCL2, CCL5, and cathepsin with increased tumor progression along with increased immunosuppression in TME. However, unlike macrophages no distinct markers are there to distinguish between N1 and N2 neutrophils (Kim et al. 2016). The recruitment of neutrophils into tumor is majorly regulated by three important players—CXCR-2, G-CSF, and IL-17. Tumor cells, immune cells, and cancer associated fibroblasts secrete CXCR-2-chemokine which attracts the $CXCR2^+$ neutrophils in a gradient dependent manner. Similarly, cells of TME secrete G-CSF, required for recruitment as well as maturation and proliferation of neutrophils (Martin et al. 2003). On the other hand, IL-17 stimulates secretion of factors such as IL-6, G-CSF, and CCL2 (MCP-1) which directly leads to neutrophil recruitment into tumor.

TANs have mostly been found to be significantly responsible for tumor progression upon modulation by tumor microenvironment. Neutrophils secrete myeloperoxide (MPO) and various other cytokines and chemokines which are responsible for recruitment of monocytes and their polarization to M2 phenotype in tumor microenvironment by (Ardi et al. 2007). Another mediatory role of neutrophils links inflammation and cancer. Studies have found that TANs show more anti-tumoral activity during early stages of tumor with increased secretion of TNF-α, Nitric Oxide (NO), and H_2O_2 (Hydrogen Peroxide). However, the cytotoxicity against tumor tends to get downregulated during later stages of tumor progression. One key feature of Neutrophils is release of Reactive Oxygen Species (ROS) from their phagolysosomes which cause DNA damage and mutations which is essential for tumor initiation, immune-suppression, and Epithelial–Mesenchymal transition (EMT). In breast cancer, production of Reactive Oxygen Species (ROS) can stabilize Hypoxia-Induced Factor-1 (HIF-1) which increases VEGF and hence increases tumor aggressiveness and resistance against chemotherapy. ROS such as hydrogen peroxide can activate various cancer progressive signaling such as MAPK/ERK2 pathway, PI3K/Akt pathway, and IKK/NFκB in various types of cancers. Other important factors secreted by neutrophils are TGF-β, Oncostatin M, and VEGF which can potentially increase tumor invasiveness (Kerfoot et al. 2001). In fact, study of over 25 cancer types in 500 cases has revealed that presence of polymorphonuclear (PMN cells including neutrophils) indicates lower survival rate. Similarly, higher Neutrophil to Lymphocyte Ratio (NLR) is related with worse prognosis (Gentles et al. 2015).

7.2.1.5 Natural Killer (NK) Cells

NK cells are important cells for host defense against tumor and metastasis, but their role is still unclear in tumor microenvironment. NK cells are found to be of prognostic significance in several types of cancers as their presence in tumor has been shown to be associated with increased survival rate of patients. It was found that tumor development was faster in that leukemia and prostate cancer models where NK infiltration was moderate as compared to those with higher NK infiltration (Stojanovic and Cerwenka 2011). Studies have found that in contrast to the adaptive NK cells activated by IL-2 (A-NK cell) cells, naïve NK cells have lesser tendency to infiltrate the tumor. The infiltration of A-NK cells was shown to be up to 20 folds higher than NK cells in lung cancer. Hence, lung cancer seems to show the potential effects of A-NK dependent tumor cytotoxicity. However, studies suggest that NK cells cannot exhibit their anti-tumor effect once the tumor extravasates in blood circulation (Paul and Lal 2017).

7.2.1.6 Cancer Associated Fibroblasts (CAFs)

Fibroblasts are spindle shaped cells that build up the ECM and hence provide mechanical strength to tissues. These cells are generally in their resting state and come into play during processes of tissue repair. Since tumor is a "wound that never heals," an increased activity of fibroblasts is observed i n tumor microenvironment as Cancer Associated Fibroblasts (CAFs). CAFs vary from normal fibroblasts in several aspects including their larger size, intense cytoplasmic network, and irregular nuclei (Wever et al. 2008). Fibroblasts lack metabolic and transcriptional activities, whereas CAFs are metabolically active and are also found to secrete tumor promoting growth factors such as TGF-β, VEGF, and IL-6. For instance, in Pancreatic Adenocarcinoma (PAAD), the expression of important CAF markers such as Fibroblast activation Protein (FAP), Platelet derive Growth Factor α/β (PDFG α/β), and ACTA2 was significantly up-regulated in comparison with normal tissue (Mace et al. 2013).

The conditions of normal tumor milieu such as oxidative stress, low glucose, and pH, and the presence of TGF-β, Epidermal Growth Factor (EFG), Fibroblast Growth Factor-2 (FGF-2), and PDGF lead to activation of and recruitment of CAFs in tumor microenvironment. Different subsets of CAFs are there depending on the presence of different markers on their surface such as α-SMA, FAP, S100A4, CD90, and PDFGR α/β. The α-SMA^{+} CAF (Smooth Muscle Actin) are pro-tumoral as they secrete MMP-2, TGF-β, and IL-6.In addition, they increase the proliferation of cancer stem cells through CXCL14-CXCR-4 axis (Kobayashi et al. 2019). Breast cancer harbors different phenotypes of CAFs depending on expression of CD146. CD146^{-} CAFs can decrease the responsiveness of breast cancer towards estrogen by suppressing the expression of estrogen receptor. Whereas the presence of CD146^{+}

CAFs can increase the sensitivity towards tamoxifen in luminal breast cancer (Brechbuhl et al. 2018). The original source for CAFs is very elusive and the heterogeneity of its subsets makes it very difficult but very important to understand and also a potential target for anti-cancer therapies (Sugimoto et al. 2006).

7.2.2 The Extracellular Matrix (ECM) and Surrounding Cells

7.2.2.1 The Adipocytes

Adipocytes are critical cellular components of our body. They are widely present in tumor stroma and a dynamic communication between adipocytes and cancer cells plays an important role in tumor progression (Bussard et al. 2016). The Cancer Associated Adipocytes (CAAs) are present in invasive front of tumor that is involved in inducing epithelial-to-mesenchymal transition (EMT), matrix remodeling, degradation of basement membrane, and survival of cancer cells (Choi et al. 2018). The CAAs show an increased expression of insulin like growth factor binding protein-2 (IGFBP-2) which is absent in normal adipocytes. In breast cancer, the increased expression of IGFBP-2 was correlated with increased metastasis in vitro in MCF-7 cells as well as in vivo conditions (Wang et al. 2015). Similar studies in breast cancer also showed that an increase in secretion of MMP-11, IL-6, and IL-1β from adipocytes has a significant contribution in breast cancer metastasis (Dirat et al. 2011). CAAs have been shown to increase tumor aggressiveness in ovarian cancer in IL-8 dependent manner. Co-culture studies have found that CAA increases β-oxidation in ovarian cancer suggesting that adipocytes can be an energy source for cancer cells (Nieman et al. 2011).

7.2.2.2 The Pericytes

Pericytes are slender and branched mural cells (vascular smooth muscle cells) of blood circulation that are essential for vasculature as they are present around the endothelial cells which form the capillaries and veins (Armulik et al. 2011). These cells are homing site for tumors and play essential role in tumor angiogenesis. Pericytes are critical for tumor progression as they stimulate the proliferation of endothelial cells (ECs) and secretion of proteases that pave the way for these ECs to migrate (Pietras and Östman 2010). The crosstalk between pericytes and ECs is regulated by paracrine signaling mediated by growth factors such as TGF-β for EC viability, angiopoietin 1/2 and Tie2 for mural cell differentiation, and PDGFβ/PDGFRβ for recruitment of pericytes (Geevarghese and Herman 2014). Recruitment of pericytes by PDGFβ is essential for angiogenesis and inhibition of PDGFβ can successfully inhibit the recruitment of pericytes in cancer and hence regression of tumor is observed (Lindblom et al. 2003).

7.2.2.3 Matrix Metalloproteases (MMPs) and Other Proteases

MMPs are a family of zinc dependent endopeptidases which helps in tissue remodeling, organ development, and regulation of inflammatory processes (Egeblad and Werb 2002). During early studies on cancer metastases, it was found that degradation of basement membrane (Collagen IV) was crucial for invasion which leads to discovery of Collagenase IV or MMP-2 to be responsible for its degradation. Till date, over 23 different types of MMPs have been identified which include MMP-1, 3, 7, 9, 12, and others which are secreted by tumor cells as well as from cells of the TME (Deryugina and Quigley 2006). In addition to degradation of basement membrane, overexpression of MMPs such as MMP-3 induces EMT by altering cell-cell adhesion due to cleavage of e-cadherin in breast cancer (Radisky et al. 2005). Many cells of tumor microenvironment secrete MMPs such as TAMs, TANs, and CAFs; and in turn, these MMPs can increase bioavailability of several growth factors such as TGF-b, VEGF, and FGF (Skrzydlewska et al. 2005). Overexpression of MMPs is found to be accompanied with increase in tissue inhibitors of metalloproteinases (TIMPs), as in case of lung carcinoma, in which elevated level of MMP-9 and TIMP-1 was found in serum of patients. Expression of TIMP-1 and TIMP-2 in TME was correlated with poor prognosis and increased tumor progression. Overexpression of TIMPs inhibits tumor growth in model system, however, no inhibition was observed in metastatic melanomas upon transfection with TIMP-2(Cho et al. 2003). Another prominent protease of tumor microenvironment is cysteine proteases, namely cathepsins which form a cascade of different proteases (Sloane et al. 2005). Pro-cathepsin B is activated to activate cathepsin B upon cleavage by Cathepsin D, Cathepsin D also activates Cathepsin L. One of the most important cathepsins is cathepsin B which is secreted by TAMs and is responsible for cleavage of ECM proteins and inhibitor or proteases (Skrzydlewska et al. 2005).

7.2.2.4 The Endothelial Cells

The progression of tumor is basically dependent on process of angiogenesis (formation of new blood vessels). These vessels are required for providing enough oxygen and nutrient supply to an aggressively growing tumor. A tumor with poorly developed vasculature will not be able to grow beyond a few millimeters and is likely to be relatively less harmful. Breast cancer patients with smaller tumor with poor angiogenesis were found to die because of other disease rather than cancer (Nielsen et al. 1987). The blood vessels and capillaries are made up of endothelial cells, whereas the blood vessels surrounding the tumor are made of Tumor Endothelial Cells (TECs) which show aberrant features (Hida et al. 2018). Vascular Endothelial Growth Factor (VEGF) is one of the key factors which is secreted by tumor cells that target the VEGF receptors (tyrosine kinase receptor) on endothelial cells and regulate tumor angiogenesis by stimulating formation of blood vessels. VEGFR-1, VEGFR-2, and VEGFR-3 are main receptors out of which VEGFR-1 and VEGFR-2 are found on blood Endothelial Cells and VEGFR-3 is found on lymphatic endothelial cells. Therapies against VEGF/VEGFR signaling are widely used in combination with other chemotherapeutic drugs to hamper growth of tumor (Shibuya and Claesson-Welsh 2006).

7.2.3 The TME, Inflammation, and Cancer

In 1863, Virchow hypothesized that most of the cancers originate from a site of chronic inflammation where a class of irritants and the injured tissues cause inflammation that leads to cell proliferation. The relationship between cancer and inflammation is well established now with tumor microenvironment being a critical player as it is the site for orchestration of most of altered immune cells and their pro-inflammatory secretions (Coussens et al. 2002). Epidemiological studies have shown a positive correlation between chronic inflammation and increased tumor progression in lung, breast, colon, pancreatic, and gastric cancer (Mantovani et al. 2008). Inflammatory immune cells such as leukocytes and phagocytic cells such as macrophages can increase tumor progression by increasing the secretion of reactive oxygen species (ROS) which increases DNA damage by forming peroxynitrite, a mutagenic agent that increases tumor initiation and proliferation (Maeda and Akaike 1998). In breast cancer, it has been found that altered adipocytes of tumor microenvironment stimulate pro-inflammatory surrounding that increases tumor (Iyengar et al. 2016). The mutation in p53, tumor suppressor gene can be observed in other inflammatory diseases such as rheumatoid arthritis is like that observed in cancer due to similar pattern of inflammatory conditions (Yamanishi et al. 2002).

7.2.4 Hypoxia in the TME

Oxygen deficiency is a key regulator of stress in tumor cells which develop a condition of hypoxia. Hypoxia induces the genes which regulate cell proliferation, matrix remodeling, and cell adhesion (Chan and Giaccia 2007). Hypoxic microenvironmental conditions control tumor cells in two ways; it limits growth of tumor cells on the one hand and induces cellular adaptations in malignant cells to increase their invasiveness. Adaptation to hypoxic environment induces the cells to undergo anaerobic glycolysis and increases genetic instability which ultimately leads to increased tumor invasiveness and angiogenesis (Pennacchietti et al. 2003). These modulations are achieved by activation of hypoxia related transcription factors, Hypoxia-Induced Factor (HIF) which include HIF-1, HIF-2, and HIF-3. In normal cells with optimum oxygen availability, hydroxylated HIF-1α is recognized by the tumor suppressor von Hippel–Lindau which acts as a ubiquitin ligase and modifies HIF-1α to undergo differentiation (Mole et al. 2001). Many chemotherapeutic approaches target rapidly proliferating cells; however, tumor cells of hypoxic environment grow with relatively slower rate which allows them to escape chemotherapy. Hence hyperbaric oxygen followed by administration of 100% oxygen after regular intervals is used during chemotherapies (Daruwalla and Christophi 2006).

7.3 The TME as an Attractive Therapeutic Target in Cancer

The components of the TME not only contribute to tumor progression but also cause a decreased efficacy against anti-tumor therapies. A regulated cross talk between tumor cells and cells of the TME increases secretion of cytokines, chemokines, and growth factors that play a pivotal role in protecting the tumor from chemo- and radiotherapies. However, the TME-mediated drug resistance is usually transient and requires cell–cell interaction, and these can often be reversed if the TME components get removed. These drug resistances include soluble factor-mediated drug resistance, cell adhesion-mediated drug resistance, and immune cells-mediated drug resistance (Wu and Dai 2017). For example, soluble factor-mediated drug resistance (SFM-DR) is mediated by cytokines and growth factors secreted by both tumor cells and stromal cells. One of such factors secreted by stromal cells is SDF-1 which interacts with CXCR4 on tumor cells and leads to tumor cell survival by activation of extracellular signal regulated kinase 1/2 (ERK 1/2) and Akt pathway, resistance to cytarabine and increased activation of MYC and anti-apoptotic BCL-XL in acute myeloid leukemia (AML)(Burger et al. 2005; Chen et al. 2013). Due to the failure of conventional drug delivery systems to release the cargo in the TME and extreme cytotoxic effects of the drugs, cancer nanotheranostics is emerging as an imperative approach as novel therapeutic intervention. In the next sections, we discuss several nanotheranostic agents, strategies, and their application in the early detection and successful treatment of this deadly pathology.

7.4 Cancer Nanotheranostic Agents that Target the TME

Nanotheranostics, one of the biggest scientific breakthroughs in personalized nanomedicine, utilizes both unique physiochemical and biological properties of nanoparticles (NPs) in detection of cancer biomarkers, cancer imaging, and treatment. Several properties of the TME such as acidic pH environment, immune cells, and hypoxia are exploited to target nanomedicines for improved diagnostic and therapeutic purposes and different nanotheranostic agents are used as personalized therapeutic interventions against certain cancer types (Roy Chowdhury et al. 2016; Roma-Rodrigues et al. 2019). In this section, we discuss recent advances in the TME modulation and therapeutic potential by different nanotheranostic agents.

7.4.1 Metallic Nanoparticles (NPs)

Metallic NPs are metals ranging between 10 and 100 nm size which can be used for molecular imaging, targeted delivery of ligands and small molecules to the TME (Kim et al. 2013). Out of numerous metallic NPs, gold NPs (AuNPs) are most widely used as nanotheranostic agent in cancer therapeutics followed by silver (AgNPs) and platinum NPs (PtNPs). AuNPs can be synthesized with a variety of diameters such as nanorods, nano shells, and nanocages by many methods including photochemical reduction of gold salts and reduction of plant extracts obtained from several species such as *Zingiber officinale* (Eustis et al. 2005). Functionally, effective localized surface plasmon resonance (LSPR), fluorescent-quenching ability, high atomic number, X-ray absorption coefficient combined with superior surface conjugation methods make AuNPs as excellent nanotheranostic choice in cancer management (Kim et al. 2013). Moreover, surface-enhanced Raman spectroscopy (SERS) nano-antenna synthesized by capping of AuNPs with Raman reporters entrapped in polymers is frequently used in cancer nanotheranostics including conjugation of several FDA-approved drugs such as cetuximab and cancer photoacoustic (Roy Chowdhury et al. 2016; Sonali et al. 2018). Other AuNPs such as gold nano-beacons (AuNBs), gold nanoclusters (AuNCs), and gold nanorods (AuNRs) are extensively implicated in treatment of various cancers including carcinomas of brain, head and neck, kidney, and lung due to their unique properties such as superior tissue specificity, enhanced cellular uptake, reduced cytotoxicity, low photobleaching, and enhanced Stokes-shifted emission (Roy Chowdhury et al. 2016). Apart from AUNPs, AgNPs and PtNPs have attracted great attention in cancer nanotheranostics due to unique physiochemical and biochemical properties such as superior nano-design architecture, enhanced Rayleigh scattering, enhanced SERS, resistance to photobleaching, limited cytotoxicity, and improved drug delivery kinetics (Porcel et al. 2010; Huy et al. 2020; Li et al. 2018). In summary, metallic NPs are superior nanotheranostic choice that can effectively target TME and exert superior patient management.

7.4.2 Magnetic Nanoparticles (MNPs)

MNPs, nanomagnetic particles fabricated from pure metals (such as iron, cobalt, and nickel), most frequently magnetite (Fe_3O_4), are frequently used in cancer diagnosis, drug delivery, and therapy (Wu and Huang 2017; Farzin et al. 2020). Recently, MNPs are utilized in hyperthermia cancer treatment, biosensing, magnetic resonance imaging (MRI), and controlled drug delivery to the TMC (Farzin et al. 2020). For cancer diagnostics, high special resolution and tomographic ability of MNPs along with surface modification such as induction of magnetic dipole interaction are exploited in MRI, one of the most practiced non-invasive tumor imaging techniques (Wu and Huang 2017). Besides MRI, magnetic particle imaging (MPI) and near infrared imaging (NIR) techniques using MNPs are frequently used for superior detection of many cancers such as carcinomas of the breast, lung, pancreatic, and prostate (Wu and Huang 2017). As potent drug carrier, MNPs are frequently coated with stabilizing polymer shells such as polyethylene glycol (PEG) and PLGA (Poly (DL-lactic-co-glycolic acid)), conjugated with several chemotherapeutic agents such as doxorubicin (DOX), cisplatin, and antibodies including anti-CD44 and anti-C595 and used to manage deadly pathologies such as ovarian cancer (Wu and Huang 2017). Recently, MNPs are utilized to treat cancers using several nanotheranostic methods such as magnetic hyperthermia (MHT), photodynamic therapy (PDT), and photothermal therapy (PTT) (Wu and Huang 2017). By carefully considering several factors such as magnetic field strength, MNP size, and concentration, MHT takes advantage of MNPs to convert electromagnetic energy into heat for the destruction of tumor cells (Farzin et al. 2020; Obaidat et al. 2015). In PDT, photosensitizing drugs (PD) conjugated with MNPs are localized to TME, photoexcited using appropriate wavelength in the presence of O_2 and cause cell death by producing reactive oxygen species (ROS)-leading to tumor tissue damage (Wu and Huang 2017). In PTT, MNPs such as Fe_3O_4 are often coated with a photothermal agent, delivered to the TME and exited with NIR irradiation inducing high temperature and cell death (Cheng et al. 2012). In summary, MNPs as novel nanotheranostic agents show exciting potential in improving early tumor detection, targeted drug delivery to the TME and increased success of cancer treatment.

7.4.3 Mesoporous Silica Nanoparticles (MSiNPs)

Several unique properties such as chemical stability, large surface area and pore volume, lower cytotoxicity and biocompatibility have made MSiNPs significant nanotheranostic agents (Iturrioz-Rodriguez et al. 2019). Superior porosity of MsiNPs allows them to be conjugated with a wide range of ligands such as antibody, peptide, and growth factors and delivered to various cancer cell types (Roy Chowdhury et al. 2016). For example, MsiNP conjugated with camptothecin, a human topoisomerase I inhibitor, DOX, and quantum dots has shown significant therapeutic promise against pancreatic cancer (Liu et al. 2000). Moreover, MiSPs exhibit superior biocompatibility, that is, they are readily degraded in physiological buffers, eliminated by renal clearance and display low cytotoxicity (Iturrioz-Rodriguez et al. 2019). Hence, MsiNPs are excellent cancer nanotheranostic agents and robust research is highly warranted to completely characterize these NPs for successful cancer therapy.

7.4.4 Nano-Graphenes (NGs)

Graphene, a 2D layer of sp2-hybridized carbon and graphene oxide (GO)-based nanotheranostic agents have great potential in targeted drug delivery to the TME and cancer chemotherapy (Pei et al. 2020). Large surface area, colloidal stability, improved aqueous solubility, easy surface functionalization by various functional groups such as hydroxyl, carbonyl, and epoxy groups have rendered NGs as excellent cancer nanotheranostic agents (Roy Chowdhury et al. 2016). Indeed, several therapeutic strategies such as image-guided tumor ablation by synergistic PTT, dendrimer-grafted nano-GO conjugated with gadolinium, GO conjugated with anti-cancer drug such as epirubicin and GO-AuNP composites have shown promising results in combating several pathologies such as ovarian cancer. In summary, NG-based theranostic approach shows immense possibility in targeting the TME and provides a novel therapeutic approach against cancer.

7.4.5 Polymeric-Based Nanotheranostic Particles (PNPs)

Polymeric-based NPs including nanospheres and nano-capsules are biodegradable polymer of various compounds such as poly(D,L-lactic-co-glycolic acid) (PLGA), PEG, and Poly(1-caprolactone) (PCL) that can serve as effective drug delivery systems to the tumor site (Sikkandhar et al. 2017; Parveen and Sahoo 2008). Due to the availability of various polymers and enhanced biocompatibility, a wide array of drugs can be conjugated with PNPs and effectively delivered to the TME. For example, poly-lactic acid-fabricated PNP encapsulating Endostar (recombinant human endostatin) conjugated with a targeted anti-angiogenic agent GX1 peptide and NIR dye 800CW has shown promise as a nanotheranostic agent against colorectal cancer (Du et al. 2015). Moreover, PNPs are frequently used in many tumor imaging techniques such as optical imaging (e.g., Indocyanine green encapsulated in PEG), MRI (e.g., paclitaxel-superparamagnetic iron oxide nanoparticle (SPION) loaded in PLGA-based micelle), and X-ray CT scan (Braeken et al. 2017). In summary, polymeric nanoassemblies demonstrated excellent potential in cancer nanotheranostics and could serve as a novel drug delivery system in personalized medicine platform fighting this deadly disease.

7.4.6 Lipid-Based Nanotheranostic Particles (LNPs)

LNPs such as liposome, nanostructured lipid carriers (NLCs), and solid lipid nanoparticles (SLNs) have proven to be effective theranostic agents in cancer therapy due to their ability to transport hydrophobic and hydrophilic drugs, negligible toxicity, prolonged half-life inside the TME, and easier in vivo customization such as PEGylation (Roy Chowdhury et al. 2016; Garcia-Pinel et al. 2019). Liposomes, composed primarily of phospholipids organized in a bilayer structure due to their amphipathic properties, are mostly studies LNPs and due to excellent biocompatibility and biodegradability, liposomes act as effective carrier of many chemotherapeutic drugs (Garcia-Pinel et al. 2019). SLNs are colloidal drug delivery systems which have improved site-specific targeting, controlled release of both hydrophilic and hydrophobic drugs and non-toxicity-making them important drug delivery candidates (Garcia-Pinel et al. 2019). NLCs developed from SLNs are often prepared from mixtures of liquid and solid fatty acids such as glyceryl dioleate and ethyl oleate and can also be used as an efficient delivery system for both hydrophilic and hydrophobic drugs (Garcia-Pinel et al. 2019). Due to their extensive use in cancer therapy, LNPs are used in several clinical trials and some of them, such as Doxil and Abraxane have been approved for cancer therapy (Garcia-Pinel et al. 2019). Hence, LNPs constitute a wide range of NPs with diverse physical and biological properties that are widely used as cancer nanotheranostic agents and present a great promise for effective management and therapeutic interventions for this deadly pathology.

7.4.7 Protein-Based Nanotheranostic Particles (PNPs)

Due to their natural availability and physiological camaraderie, PNPs such as engineered protein nanocage, nano-radio peptides, and fluorescent peptide nanoprobes have invoked high promise in cancer therapy (Roy Chowdhury et al. 2016; Madamsetty et al. 2019). Several proteins such as albumin, human serum albumin, ferritin, gelatine, and transferrin have been considered as promising drug delivery systems to the TME and many PNP-conjugated drug formulations such as Abraxane (albumin-bound paclitaxel) and ABI-009 (albumin-conjugated rapamycin) have successfully cleared stringent clinical trials for cancer therapy (Roy Chowdhury et al. 2016; Madamsetty et al. 2019). Further research on PNPs as novel cancer nanotheranostic agents will help the clinicians to better manage the pathology and improve patient life to a greater extend.

7.4.8 Viral-Based Nanotheranostic Particles (VLPs)

VLPs emerged as novel class of nano-delivery systems and due to their natural biocompatibility, excellent reproduction rate inside host cell and improved ability to contain both hydrophobic and hydrophilic chemotherapeutic drugs (Madamsetty et al. 2019). As naturally occurring scaffold or synthetically designed for tumor cell-specific drug delivery system, many VLPs such as filamentous bacteriophage M13, plant-based tobacco mosaic virus (TMV), cowpea mosaic virus (CPMV), and mammalian viruses including influenza A and hepatitis B have been used in cancer nanotheranostics (Beatty and Lewis 2019). VLPs are recently recognized as tools for non-invasive imaging applications involved in cancer diagnosis such as PET and MRI as photosensitive moieties including fluorescent dye, metals, and quantum dots can be incorporated into the viral particles (Madamsetty et al. 2019; Cho et al. 2014). For example, fluorescent CPMV sensors allowed researchers to visualize the blood flow in the vasculature of chicken embryo, a principle that has been further applied in tumor angiogenesis imaging (Suci et al. 2007; Lewis et al. 2006). Taken together, VLPs have emerged as valuable tools for early detection and novel therapeutic intervention against many deadly diseases such as cancer.

7.4.9 DNA-Based Cancer Nanotheranostic Platform

Deoxyribonucleic acid (DNA), the genetic material of a cell has drawn a lot of attention in DNA nanotechnology and cancer nanotheranostics due to its remarkable molecular recognition properties, predictable secondary structure, small size, mechanical rigidity, easy custom synthesis, and improved biocompatibility (Chen et al. 2018; Kumar et al. 2016). Moreover, efficient drug loading capacity and cellular internalization support DNA origami and DNA hydrogels as programmable "smart" building blocks for development of highly versatile, non-toxic drug delivery carriers (Kumar et al. 2016). Indeed, owing to its strong affinity toward DNA double helix, DOX can intercalate with self-assembled DNA origami and it is widely used in cancer nanotheranostics (Chen et al. 2018). More interestingly, drug-loaded DNA nanostructure called nanoflower, DNA nanorobots, DNA signal amplification-based cancer nanotheranostic approaches, DNA-integrated gold nanoparticle and gold nanorods have shown great potential for targeting the TME and efficient drug delivery (Chen et al. 2018). Therefore, despite some disadvantages such as induction of immune response, poor stability, and transport in the TME, DNA-based nanomaterials have shown considerable promise in cancer diagnosis and therapy and more research are highly warranted to improve their theranostic functions in cancer therapy.

7.5 Visualizing Cancer Through Nanotheranostics

Advanced biomedical imaging techniques are integral to cancer diagnosis and the use of NPs as contrast agents due to their ability to carry a high amount of contrast agents, increased in vivo half-life, and tumor-specific accumulation has revolutionized clinical oncology enabling accurate diagnosis and therapy of this lethal disease (Sivasubramanian et al. 2019). In this section, we summarize recent developments in the field of cancer imaging and therapeutic interventions using nanotheranostic approach such as MRI, CT scan, and PET.

7.5.1 Magnetic Resonance Imaging (MRI)

MRI is a non-invasive, non-ionizing imaging technique which is governed by the principle of excitation of protons by radio frequency in the presence of a magnetic field and relaxation of the high energy state to equilibrium by emitting MRI signal (Sivasubramanian et al. 2019). NP-based contrast agents can markedly improve the sensitivity of MRI by two distinct mechanisms: T1-weighted and T2-weighted, where T1 contrast agents produce bright MRI signal by longitudinal relaxation of water proton and T2 contrast agents produce dark images by transverse relaxation of water proton (Lin et al. 2009). Several nano-formulations such as gadolinium ion (Gd^{3+})-based Gd-chelates, MnO-based Mn-oleate complex and PEG shell loaded with Mn^{2+} and CaP (calcium phosphate) are used as T1-weighted contrast agents which are frequently applied for molecular imaging of several cancers such as glioma and breast cancer (Sivasubramanian et al. 2019). Whereas due to strong dipolar interaction between iron oxide magnetic movement and water proton, SPION NP-based contrast agents such as chlorotoxin-conjugated, PEGylated SPION serve as excellent T2-weighted contrast agents in MRI. Overall, NP-fabricated MRI emerged as an excellent diagnostic choice in cancer therapy and more research is underway to improve its imaging efficiency for improved management of this deadly pathology.

7.5.2 Photoacoustic Imaging (PAI)

PAI is a non-invasive technique which combines optical and ultrasound imaging and presents high tissue penetration and rich optical contrast due to high spatial and temporal resolution (Sivasubramanian et al. 2019). Due to high photostability, large absorption coefficient, and low cytotoxicity, several nanomaterials such as gold nanorod, gold nanocage, silver nanoplate are frequently used as contrast agents in PAI for detection of many cancers. For example, Homan et al. conjugated anti-EGFR (epidermal growth factor receptor) with silver nanoplate and utilized it as PAI contrast agent to detect pancreatic tumor (Homan et al. 2012). Indeed, this nano-formulation was rapidly taken up by pancreatic tumor cells overexpressing EGFR via receptor-mediated endocytosis and presented a high contrast image of the disease. Moreover, utilizing the principle of enzyme-activable probe, Wu et al. developed a PA (photoacoustic) probe that could image alkaline phosphatase in HeLa tumors with maximum contrast ratio of 2.3 folds after 4 h of in vivo administration (Wu et al. 2018).

7.5.3 Optical Imaging

Cancer nanotheranostics utilizes optical imaging as an extremely sensitive, non-invasive diagnostic technique due to physical interaction of light with tissues, leading to several physical events such as absorption, scattering, and emission-offering biochemical and morphological information of the tumor (Sivasubramanian et al. 2019). Several contrast agents such as quantum dot, AuNPs, protease activatable NIR-based nano-formulations, and fluorescent core shell NPs have been developed for precise detection and therapeutic intervention of tumors. For example, targeting the acidic, angiogenic TME with fluorescent nanoprobe, Wang et al. developed a sensitive imaging technique using various mouse cancer models (Wang et al. 2014). These non-toxic, ultra pH-sensitive fluorescent nano-reporters were strongly activated in response to acidic microenvironment of the tumor and nonlinearly amplified the TME signal, identified tumor tissues independent of histology and driver mutations and detected the treatment response much rapidly than conventional imaging techniques.

7.5.4 Nuclear Imaging

Nuclear imaging techniques such as PET and CT are overly sensitive diagnostic methods which use contrast agents that can be traced by radioactive decay or their ability to interact with high energy radiation (Sivasubramanian et al. 2019). [^{18}F]-fluoro-2-deoxy glucose (FDG) is primarily used as a contrast agent in PET to detect tumors with high glycolytic rate (van Straten et al. 2017). Due to large X-ray absorption coefficient and easy surface modification, AuNPs and bismuth (Bi)-based NPs are proven to be excellent nanotheranostic choice as contrast agents

(Kim et al. 2007). Moreover, superior imaging of the TME can also be achieved by CT scanning using several efficient NPs as contrast agents such as Bi subcarbonate nanotubes (BNT), metallic NPs (Au, Ag, Pt, and Fe), and PEGylated Fe_3O_4 (Sivasubramanian et al. 2019). Indeed, several nano-formulations using these contrast agents such as DOX-loaded BNT, hypoxia-sensitive AuNP, and ^{64}Cu-conjugated AuNP are shown to not only tumor-specific accumulation and enhanced tumor imaging but also exhibited excellently targeted delivery of the drugs to the TME (Sivasubramanian et al. 2019). In summary, NPs have advanced the field of cancer nanotheranostics by largely contributing to the development of efficient cancer imaging and diagnostic techniques and deeper understanding of tumor biology coupled with molecular nanomedicine will contribute to successful therapeutic intervention against cancer.

7.6 Nanotheranostics for the Detection of Cancer Biomarkers

Despite significant global research endeavors, cancer remains a major health challenge with high mortality rate and acute detection of this disease at early stage by identifying cancer biomarkers, molecules that produced by tumor cells as a consequence of disease progression might improve successful treatment and patient health (Zhang et al. 2019a). Despite development of several screening strategies such as prostate-specific antigen (PSA) test for prostate cancer, mammography for breast cancer, and Papanicolaou (Pap) smear test for cervical cancer and several imaging techniques such as MRI, PET, and endoscopy, inadequate specificity and sensitivity of biomarkers led the researchers to develop novel nanotheranostic approaches for early detection, diagnosis, and treatment of this deadly pathology. However, recently, nanotechnology has emerged as a promising tool for early detection of cancer owing to its high selectivity, sensitivity, and ability to offer simultaneous detections of multiple cellular targets (Zhang et al. 2019a). In this section, we summarize the recent development of novel nanotheranostic approaches towards early detection of cancer biomarkers.

7.6.1 Labeling Nanoparticles with Conjugates

For efficient detection of cancer biomarkers, NPs must be conjugated with several ligands by different surface modification techniques such as linker chemistry and hybridization. In this section, we summarize several ligand conjugation methods by which NPs are armed for cancer biomarker detection.

7.6.1.1 Chemical Crosslinking

In chemical crosslinking, molecules are couples by covalent bond and this method is often used in many techniques such as Western blotting. Using four major functional groups, primary amines, carboxyls, sulfhydryls and carbonyls, chemical crosslinking conjugates NPs with a wide array of ligands and natural occurrence of these functional groups in both NPs and ligands often enhance chemical coupling and reduce non-specific ligand activity (El-Sayed et al. 2013).

7.6.1.2 Biotin/Avidin Conjugation

The biotin-avidin conjugation system is one of the strongest, most stable, non-covalent biological interactions with dissociation constant (K_d) in the order of 4×10^{-14} M and hence, avidin and its analogues are successfully used in diagnostics and drug delivery strategies (Jain and Cheng 2017). Biotin-avidin and their analogues such as neutravidin, streptavidin, and strep-tag can be used to conjugate various ligands such as peptides (e.g. cell penetrating peptide and Tat peptide), monoclonal antibodies (e.g. anti-transferrin receptor antibody), and small molecule inhibitors (e.g. cisplatin, paclitaxel, and hyaluronic acid) and utilized in many imaging techniques required for early detection of cancers (Jain and Cheng 2017).

7.6.1.3 Click Chemistry

First conceptualized in 2001 by K. B. Sharpless et al., click chemistry, a group of chemical reactions with high stereospecificity, favorable reaction rate, orthogonality, and high yield, is proving to be a novel tool in nanotechnology and cancer theranostics (Yi et al. 2018). It is widely used to conjugate ligands such as antibodies and small molecule inhibitors to the surface of nanoparticles for targeted delivery to the TME. For example, Liu et al. developed an AuNP-based folate receptor (FR)-targeted SERS nanoprobe using click chemistry (Liu et al. 2017). Lee et al. used azide groups and bicyclo [6.1.0]nonyne (BCN) to enhance tumor-targeting by metabolic click chemistry and showed an efficient method for efficient drug delivery and tumor therapy (Lee et al. 2014).

7.6.2 Target Moieties for Identification of Cancer Biomarkers

A variety of cellular moieties, such as proteins, peptides, nucleic acids, and vitamins can be conjugated with the NPs to identify cancer biomarkers. For example, protein-based targeting of NPs includes antibodies and antibody fragments. For example, Ranzoni et al. developed a homogeneous assay to detect prostate cancer based on antibody-coated magnetic NPs which can detect serum PSA at picomole concentration (Ranzoni et al. 2012). Using peptide-based targeting strategy, Hong et al. showed that fluorescent zinc ZnO_2 nanowires coated with a peptide (RGD peptide) can selectively bind angiogenic and metastatic surface marker integrin $\alpha v\beta 3$ in human glioblastoma cell U87MG (Hong et al. 2011). Nucleic acid aptamers, small ligands (20–40 bps) with the ability to fold into novel 3D topology, are excellent tools that can bind targets with a high degree of specificity, and they are frequently used to identify cancer biomarkers. For example, quantum dots coated with aptamers against prostate-specific membrane antigen (PSMA) have been used for early detection of prostate cancer and delivery of DOX for cancer treatment (Chinen et al. 2015). Interestingly, small molecule-based targeting strategy has been successful in identifying cancer biomarkers owing to their cost-effective formulation. Several biologically active small molecules such as vitamins and folic acid-conjugated NPs are widely used for cancer detection. For example, due to high expression of folate receptor in tumor cells, folic acid-conjugated mesoporous silica NPs have been successfully used to treat cervical cancer (Rosenholm et al. 2009). In summary, novel nanoformulation-based theranostic approaches to detect cancer biomarkers show tremendous promise in early detection, management, and treatment of this deadly pathology and improvement of patient health.

7.7 Conclusion and Future Direction

As the development and effectiveness of cancer therapeutics often face several challenges, including precise tumor-specific delivery and efficacy of chemotherapeutic drugs, multidrug resistance, and tumor heterogeneity, the recent surge in cancer therapeutics research has been directed towards novel nanotheranostic approach, an emerging field which utilizes multimodal theranostic nanoprobes towards personalized therapy through early detection and effective treatment of this deadly pathology (Kundu et al. 2020). The major attraction of nano-chemotherapeutics in accurate tumor localization which is achieved due to enhanced permeability and retention rate (EPR) of the tumor or active targeting of nano-delivery vehicles (Fernandes et al. 2018). The basic protocol used for nano-chemotherapeutics is (1) priming of tumor for better uptake of nano-chemotherapeutic drugs and (2) targeting of tumor by drugs enclosed in nano-carriers such as metallic and viral-based NPs (Savla and Minko 2017). As illustrated in the earlier section, the TAMs have an important role in modulating the TME. The use of super paramagnetic iron oxide nano particles (SPIONs) has been found to shift anti-tumoral M2 macrophages towards pro-tumoral M1 phenotype with increased expression of CD86, TNF-α, and cathepsin L (Laskar et al. 2013). Ferumoxytol is an iron oxide-based NP, approved by FDA, whose interaction with macrophages increases ROS production, inhibits tumor growth and metastases and increases apoptosis as well (Zanganeh et al. 2016). Silica NPs have also been shown to inhibit macrophages in a concentration dependent manner. At high concentrations, they damage the macrophages by inducing double-membraned vacuoles in macrophages while at a lower concentrations, these NPs can reprogram the macrophages and change their phenotype to M1 macrophages (Marquardt et al. 2017). The CAFs can be inhibited by 20 nm gold AuNP and these NPs interfere with CAFs ability to promote tumor proliferation and invasion (Zhang et al. 2019b). Therefore, the TME has been proven to be effectively targeted by cancer nanotheranostic approach for improved therapeutic response.

Highlighting the *status quo,* recent literature suggests that cancer nanotheranostics has taken a significant leap with the development of several novel nano-formulations combined with improved diagnostics for the treatment of many lethal cancers such as carcinomas of the breast, prostate, and ovary by targeting the TME. Several nano-formulations such as lipid nano-capsules, liposomes, micelles, and AuNPs loaded with anti-cancer drugs including DOX, paclitaxel, and chitosan are successfully implicated in targeting the TME and treating melanoma (reviewed in (Pautu et al. 2017)). Tang et al. demonstrated that antiferromagnetic pyrite nanotubes could be successfully targeted to the TME and it could overexpress intratumoral peroxide leading to generation of hydroxyl radical and cell death (Tang et al. 2017). Moreover, higher valence state of the Fe in the surface of this nano-formulation enhanced MRI signals accompanied by chemodynamic therapy (CDT). In a proof-of-concept tumor microenvironment-induced ultra-small-nanodrug generation (TMIUSNG) strategy, Zhang et al. assembled photosensitizer sinoporphyrin sodium, DOX, and ferric ions which effectively targeted and released the drug to the TME (Zhang et al. 2018). Dou et al. demonstrated that S-nitrosothiol groups (SNO, a NO donor) and indocyanine green (ICG, a photosensitizer)-loaded mesoporous silica shells of Eu^{3+}-doped $NaGdF^4$ scintillating nanocrystals (NSC) were effective in targeting the TME and overcoming hypoxia-mediated radio-resistance (Dou et al. 2018). Using triple negative 4T1 breast cancer model system, Wang et al. loaded superparamagnetic iron oxide (SPIO) nanocrystals and NIFI dyes IR780 in an amphiphilic nanosystem and showed that this nano-formulation was effective in targeting acidic TME and showed anti-cancer activity owing to its nano-enzyme catalyzed phototherapy (Wang et al. 2020). Ling et al. developed a tumor microenvironment (TME)-activated NIR-II nanotheranostic system (FEAD1) loaded with the peptide Fmoc-His, mercaptopropionic-functionalized Ag2S quantum dots (MPA-Ag2S QDs), DOX, and NIR absorber A1094 into nanoparticles and demonstrated that this theranostic tool was effective in detecting and delivering the drug to the tumor site, hence, achieving precise tumor theranostics (Ling et al. 2020). Dai et al. developed a NIR light-activated, tumor cell-specific, hypoxia prodrug tirapazamine-loaded chlorin E6 liposome which could be efficiently targeted to the tumor and induce apoptosis (Dai et al. 2019). In another study, Feng et al. developed magnetic MnO_2 nanosphere with large nanopores for improved cancer theranostics (Feng et al. 2019). These nanoparticles loaded with DOX or chlorin E6 achieved TME-specific cargo release and enhanced therapeutic potential in human glioma cells U87MG. Therefore, several nanotheranostic strategies have been adopted to combat.

As we discussed herein, cancer nanotheranostics has significantly advanced early detection of the disease by identifying cancer biomarkers, cancer imaging, and broadening the therapeutic window, hence, significantly improving patient life conditions. Although several drawbacks of cancer nanotheranostics such as lack of commercially available nano-formulations approved by FDA and inadequate knowledge of dynamic physicochemical properties of the NPs in vivo render researcher and clinicians to dig deeper into this exciting field of cancer therapeutics, this novel diagnostic cum therapeutic approach has tremendous potential to revolutionize personalized medicine approach and overall quality of life of patients suffering from this fatal malady. Nonetheless, future research on cancer nanotheranostics must focus on clinical significance, translational feasibility, and commercialization of NPs and cancer imaging techniques to improve quality of life and patient survival.

Acknowledgement SK acknowledges funding from ECR, Department of Science and Technology, Govt. of India (ECR/2016/001173) and Department of Biotechnology, Govt. of India (BT/PR18562/BIC/101/424/2016). AR acknowledges RLSF, Department of Biotechnology, Govt. of India (BT/HRD/35/02/2006) for this work.

Declaration The authors declare that there is no conflict of interest.

References

Ardi VC, Kupriyanova TA, Deryugina EI, Quigley JP (2007) Human neutrophils uniquely release TIMP-free MMP-9 to provide a potent catalytic stimulator of angiogenesis. Proc Natl Acad Sci U S A 104(51):20262-7

Armulik A, Genové G, Betsholtz C (2011) Pericytes: developmental, physiological, and pathological perspectives, problems, and promises. Dev Cell 21(2):193–215

Balkwill FR, Capasso M, Hagemann T (2012) The tumor microenvironment at a glance. J Cell Sci 125(23):5591–5596

Beatty PH, Lewis JD (2019) Cowpea mosaic virus nanoparticles for cancer imaging and therapy. Adv Drug Deliv Rev 145:130–144

Braeken Y, Cheruku S, Ethirajan A, Maes W (2017) Conjugated polymer nanoparticles for bioimaging. Materials (Basel) 10(12):1420

Bray F, Ferlay J, Soerjomataram I, Siegel RL, Torre LA, Jemal A (2018) Global cancer statistics 2018: GLOBOCAN estimates of incidence and mortality worldwide for 36 cancers in 185 countries. CA Cancer J Clin 68(6):394–424

Brechbuhl HM, Finlay-schultz J, Yamamoto TM, Gillen AE, Cittelly DM, Tan AC, Sams S, Pillai MM, Elias AD, Robinson A et al (2018) Fibroblast subtypes regulate responsiveness of luminal breast cancer to estrogen. Clin Cancer Res 23(7):1710–1721

Burger M, Hartmann T, Krome M, Rawluk J, Tamamura H, Fujii N, Kipps TJ, Burger JA (2005) Small peptide inhibitors of the CXCR4 chemokine receptor (CD184) antagonize the activation, migration, and antiapoptotic responses of CXCL12 in chronic lymphocytic leukemia B cells. Blood 106(5):1824–1830

Bussard KM, Mutkus L, Stumpf K, Gomez-Manzano C, Marini FC (2016) Tumor-associated stromal cells as key contributors to the tumor microenvironment. Breast Cancer Res 18(1):1–11

Chan DA, Giaccia AJ (2007) Hypoxia, gene expression, and metastasis. Cancer Metastasis Rev 26 (2):333–339

Chen Y, Jacamo R, Konopleva M, Garzon R, Croce C, Andreeff M (2013) CXCR4 downregulation of let-7a drives chemoresistance in acute myeloid leukemia. J Clin Investig 123(6):2395–2407

Chen T, Ren L, Liu X, Zhou M, Li L, Xu J, Zhu X (2018) DNA nanotechnology for cancer diagnosis and therapy. Int J Mol Sci 19(6):1671

Cheng L, Yang K, Chen Q, Liu Z (2012) Organic stealth nanoparticles for highly effective in vivo near-infrared photothermal therapy of cancer. ACS Nano 6(6):5605–5613

Chinen AB, Guan CM, Ferrer JR, Barnaby SN, Merkel TJ, Mirkin CA (2015) Nanoparticle probes for the detection of cancer biomarkers, cells, and tissues by fluorescence. Chem Rev 115 (19):10530–10574

Cho NH, Shim HS, Rha SY, Kang SH, Hong SH, Choi YD, Hong SJ, Cho SH (2003) Increased expression of matrix metalloproteinase 9 correlates with poor prognostic variables in renal cell carcinoma. Eur Urol 44(5):560–566

Cho CF, Shukla S, Simpson EJ, Steinmetz NF, Luyt LG, Lewis JD (2014) Molecular targeted viral nanoparticles as tools for imaging cancer. Methods Mol Biol 1108:211–230

Choi J, Cha YJ, Koo JS (2018) Adipocyte biology in breast cancer: from silent bystander to active facilitator. Prog Lipid Res 69(November 2017):11–20

Coussens LM, Werb Z, Coussens LM, Werb Z (2002) Inflammation and cancer. Pharm Biotechnol 420(6917):860. Nature 2002;420(6917):860–867

Dai Y, Wang B, Sun Z, Cheng J, Zhao H, Wu K, Sun P, Shen Q, Li M, Fan Q (2019) Multifunctional theranostic liposomes loaded with a hypoxia-activated prodrug for cascade-activated tumor selective combination therapy. ACS Appl Mater Interfaces 11(43):39410–39423

Daniel E, Shumer NJNNPS (2017) CD5 binds to Interleukin-6 and induces a feed-forward loop with the transcription factor STAT3 in B cells to promote cancer. Physiol Behav 176 (12):139–148

Daruwalla J, Christophi C (2006) Hyperbaric oxygen therapy for malignancy: a review. World J Surg 30(12):2112–2131

Deryugina EI, Quigley JP (2006) Matrix metalloproteinases and tumor metastasis. Cancer Metastasis Rev 25(1):9–34

Dirat B, Bochet L, Dabek M, Daviaud D, Dauvillier S, Majed B, Wang YY, Meulle A, Salles B, Le Gonidec S et al (2011) Cancer-associated adipocytes exhibit an activated phenotype and contribute to breast cancer invasion. Cancer Res 71(7):2455–2465

Dou Y, Liu Y, Zhao F, Guo Y, Li X, Wu M, Chang J, Yu C (2018) Radiation-responsive scintillating nanotheranostics for reduced hypoxic radioresistance under ROS/NO-mediated tumor microenvironment regulation. Theranostics 8(21):5870–5889

Dowd EC, Barch DM (2017) CD11c-expressing B cells are located at the T cell B cell border in spleen and are potent antigen presenting cells. Physiol Behav 176(12):139–148

Du Y, Zhang Q, Jing L, Liang X, Chi C, Li Y, Yang X, Dai Z, Tian J (2015) GX1-conjugated poly (lactic acid) nanoparticles encapsulating Endostar for improved in vivo anticolorectal cancer treatment. Int J Nanomedicine 10:3791–3802

Egeblad M, Werb Z (2002) New functions for the matrix metalloproteinases in cancer progression. Nat Rev Cancer 2(3):161–174

El-Sayed R, Eita M, Barrefelt A, Ye F, Jain H, Fares M, Lundin A, Crona M, Abu-Salah K, Muhammed M et al (2013) Thermostable luciferase from Luciola cruciate for imaging of carbon nanotubes and carbon nanotubes carrying doxorubicin using in vivo imaging system. Nano Lett 13(4):1393–1398

Eustis S, Hsu HY, El-Sayed MA (2005) Gold nanoparticle formation from photochemical reduction of Au3+ by continuous excitation in colloidal solutions. A proposed molecular mechanism. J Phys Chem B 109(11):4811–4815

Farzin A, Etesami SA, Quint J, Memic A, Tamayol A (2020) Magnetic nanoparticles in cancer therapy and diagnosis. Adv Healthc Mater 9(9):e1901058

Feng Y, Ding D, Sun W, Qiu Y, Luo L, Shi T, Meng S, Chen X, Chen H (2019) Magnetic manganese oxide sweetgum-ball nanospheres with large mesopores regulate tumor microenvironments for enhanced tumor nanotheranostics. ACS Appl Mater Interfaces 11 (41):37461–37470

Fernandes C, Suares D, Yergeri MC (2018) Tumor microenvironment targeted nanotherapy. Front Pharmacol 9(October):1–25

Gacche RN, Meshram RJ (2013) Targeting tumor micro-environment for design and development of novel anti-angiogenic agents arresting tumor growth. Prog Biophys Mol Biol 113 (2):333–354

Garcia-Pinel B, Porras-Alcala C, Ortega-Rodriguez A, Sarabia F, Prados J, Melguizo C, Lopez-Romero JM (2019) Lipid-based nanoparticles: application and recent advances in cancer treatment. Nanomaterials (Basel) 9(4):638

Geevarghese A, Herman IM (2014) Pericyte-endothelial crosstalk: implications and opportunities for advanced cellular therapies. Transl Res 163(4):296–306

Gentles AJ, Newman AM, Liu CL, Bratman SV, Feng W, Kim D, Nair VS, Xu Y, Khuong A, Hoang CD et al (2015) The prognostic landscape of genes and infiltrating immune cells across human cancers. Nat Med 21(8):938–945

Hida K, Maishi N, Annan DA, Hida Y (2018) Contribution of tumor endothelial cells in cancer progression. Int J Mol Sci 19(5):1–12

Homan KA, Souza M, Truby R, Luke GP, Green C, Vreeland E, Emelianov S (2012) Silver nanoplate contrast agents for in vivo molecular photoacoustic imaging. ACS Nano 6 (1):641–650

Hong H, Shi J, Yang Y, Zhang Y, Engle JW, Nickles RJ, Wang X, Cai W (2011) Cancer-targeted optical imaging with fluorescent zinc oxide nanowires. Nano Lett 11(9):3744–3750

Hui L, Chen Y (2015) Tumor microenvironment: sanctuary of the devil. Cancer Lett 368(1):7–13

Huy TQ, Huyen PTM, Le AT, Tonezzer M (2020) Recent advances of silver nanoparticles in cancer diagnosis and treatment. Anti Cancer Agents Med Chem 20(11):1276–1287

Iturrioz-Rodriguez N, Correa-Duarte MA, Fanarraga ML (2019) Controlled drug delivery systems for cancer based on mesoporous silica nanoparticles. Int J Nanomedicine 14:3389–3401

Iyengar NM, Gucalp A, Dannenberg AJ, Hudis CA (2016) Obesity and cancer mechanisms: tumor microenvironment and inflammation. J Clin Oncol 34(35):4270–4276

Jain A, Cheng K (2017) The principles and applications of avidin-based nanoparticles in drug delivery and diagnosis. J Control Release 245:27–40

Jiang Y, Li Y, Zhu B (2015) T-cell exhaustion in the tumor microenvironment. Cell Death Dis 6 (6):1–9

Joyce JA, Fearon DT (2015) T cell exclusion, immune privilege and the TME. Sci Mag 348 (6230):74–80

Kerfoot SM, Raharjo E, Ho M, McCafferty D-M, Burns AR, Patel KD, Kubes P (2001) Exclusive neutrophil recruitment with oncostatin M in a human system. Am J Pathol 159(4):1531–1539

Kim D, Park S, Lee JH, Jeong YY, Jon S (2007) Antibiofouling polymer-coated gold nanoparticles as a contrast agent for in vivo X-ray computed tomography imaging. J Am Chem Soc 129 (24):7661–7665

Kim TH, Lee S, Chen X (2013) Nanotheranostics for personalized medicine. Expert Rev Mol Diagn 13(3):257–269

Kim J, Bae J-S, Tam ML (2016) Tumor-associated macrophages and neutrophils in tumor microenvironment. Mediat Inflamm 2016:6058147

Kobayashi H, Enomoto A, Woods SL, Burt AD, Takahashi M, Worthley DL (2019) Cancer-associated fibroblasts in gastrointestinal cancer. Nat Rev Gastroenterol Hepatol 16(5):282–295

Kumar V, Palazzolo S, Bayda S, Corona G, Toffoli G, Rizzolio F (2016) DNA nanotechnology for cancer therapy. Theranostics 6(5):710–725

Kundu P, Singh D, Singh A, Sahoo SK (2020) Cancer nanotheranostics: a nanomedicinal approach for cancer therapy and diagnosis. Anti Cancer Agents Med Chem 20(11):1288–1299

Laskar A, Eilertsen J, Li W, Yuan XM (2013) SPION primes THP1 derived M2 macrophages towards M1-like macrophages. Biochem Biophys Res Commun 441(4):737–742

Lee S, Koo H, Na JH, Han SJ, Min HS, Lee SJ, Kim SH, Yun SH, Jeong SY, Kwon IC et al (2014) Chemical tumor-targeting of nanoparticles based on metabolic glycoengineering and click chemistry. ACS Nano 8(3):2048–2063

Lewis JD, Destito G, Zijlstra A, Gonzalez MJ, Quigley JP, Manchester M, Stuhlmann H (2006) Viral nanoparticles as tools for intravital vascular imaging. Nat Med 12(3):354–360

Li Y, Chang Y, Lian X, Zhou L, Yu Z, Wang H, An F (2018) Silver nanoparticles for enhanced cancer theranostics: in vitro and In vivo perspectives. J Biomed Nanotechnol 14(9):1515–1542

Lin W, Hyeon T, Lanza GM, Zhang M, Meade TJ (2009) Magnetic nanoparticles for early detection of cancer by magnetic resonance imaging. MRS Bull 34(6):441–448

Lindblom P, Gerhardt H, Liebner S, Abramsson A, Enge M, Hellström M, Bäckström G, Fredriksson S, Landegren U, Nyström HC et al (2003) Endothelial PDGF-B retention is required for proper investment of pericytes in the microvessel wall. Genes Dev 17 (15):1835–1840

Ling S, Yang X, Li C, Zhang Y, Yang H, Chen G, Wang Q (2020) Tumor microenvironment-activated NIR-II nanotheranostic system for precise diagnosis and treatment of peritoneal metastasis. Angew Chem Int Ed Engl 59(18):7219–7223

Liu LF, Desai SD, Li TK, Mao Y, Sun M, Sim SP (2000) Mechanism of action of camptothecin. Ann N Y Acad Sci 922:1–10

Liu R, Zhao J, Han G, Zhao T, Zhang R, Liu B, Liu Z, Zhang C, Yang L, Zhang Z (2017) Click-functionalized SERS nanoprobes with improved labeling efficiency and capability for cancer cell imaging. ACS Appl Mater Interfaces 9(44):38222–38229

Mace TA, Ameen Z, Collins A, Wojcik S, Mair M, Young GS, Fuchs JR, Eubank TD, Frankel WL, Bekaii-saab T et al (2013) Pancreatic cancer-associated stellate cells promote differentiation of myeloid-derived suppressor cells in a STAT3-dependent manner. Cancer Res 73 (10):3007–3018

Madamsetty VS, Mukherjee A, Mukherjee S (2019) Recent trends of the bio-inspired nanoparticles in cancer theranostics. Front Pharmacol 10:1264

Maeda H, Akaike T (1998) Nitric oxide and oxygen radicals in infection, inflammation, and cancer. Biochemistry (Mosc) 63(7):854–865

Mantovani A, Allavena P, Sica A, Balkwill F (2008) Cancer-related inflammation. Nature 454 (7203):436–444

Marquardt C, Fritsch-Decker S, Al-Rawi M, Diabaté S, Weiss C (2017) Autophagy induced by silica nanoparticles protects RAW264.7 macrophages from cell death. Toxicology 379:40–47

Martin C, Burdon PCE, Bridger G, Williams TJ, Rankin SM, In VY (2003) Chemokines acting via CXCR2 and CXCR4 control the release of neutrophils from the bone marrow and their return following senescence. Immunity 19:583–593

Massimo Ammirante§ J-LLSGSN, Michael K (2017) B cell–derived lymphotoxin promotes castration-resistant prostate cancer Massimo. Am Cancer Soc 464(7286):302–305

Mbeunkui F, Johann DJ Jr (2009) Cancer and the tumor microenvironment: a review of an essential relationship. Cancer Chemother Pharmacol 63(4):571–582

Mizoguchi A, Mizoguchi E, Takedatsu H, Blumberg RS, Bhan AK (2002) Chronic intestinal inflammatory condition generates IL-10-producing regulatory B cell subset characterized by CD1d upregulation. Immunity 16(2):219–230

Mole DR, Maxwell PH, Pugh CW, Ratcliffe PJ (2001) Regulation of HIF by the von Hippel-Lindau tumour suppressor: implications for cellular oxygen sensing. IUBMB Life 52(1–2):43–47

Molon B, Ugel S, Del Pozzo F, Soldani C, Zilio S, Avella D, De Palma A, Mauri PL, Monegal A, Rescigno M et al (2011) Chemokine nitration prevents intratumoral infiltration of antigen-specific T cells. J Exp Med 208(10):1949–1962

Motz GT (2014) Tumor endothelium FasL establishes a selective immune barrier promoting tolerance in tumors gregory. Nat Med 20(6):607–615

Nielsen M, Thomsen JL, Primdahl S, Dyreborg U, Andersen JA (1987) Breast cancer and atypia among young and middle-aged women: a study of 110 medicolegal autopsies. Br J Cancer 56 (6):814–819

Nieman KM, Kenny HA, Penicka CV, Ladanyi A, Buell-Gutbrod R, Zillhardt MR, Romero IL, Carey MS, Mills GB, Hotamisligil GS et al (2011) Adipocytes promote ovarian cancer metastasis and provide energy for rapid tumor growth. Nat Med 17(11):1498–1503

Obaidat IM, Issa B, Haik Y (2015) Magnetic properties of magnetic nanoparticles for efficient hyperthermia. Nanomaterials (Basel) 5(1):63–89

Parveen S, Sahoo SK (2008) Polymeric nanoparticles for cancer therapy. J Drug Target 16 (2):108–123

Paul S, Lal G (2017) The molecular mechanism of natural killer cells function and its importance in cancer immunotherapy. Front Immunol 8:1124

Paulus P, Stanley ER, Schäfer R, Abraham D, Aharinejad S (2006) Colony-stimulating factor-1 antibody reverses chemoresistance in human MCF-7 breast cancer xenografts. Cancer Res 66 (8):4349–4356

Pautu V, Leonetti D, Lepeltier E, Clere N, Passirani C (2017) Nanomedicine as a potent strategy in melanoma tumor microenvironment. Pharmacol Res 126:31–53

Pei X, Zhu Z, Gan Z, Chen J, Zhang X, Cheng X, Wan Q, Wang J (2020) PEGylated nano-graphene oxide as a nanocarrier for delivering mixed anticancer drugs to improve anticancer activity. Sci Rep 10(1):2717

Pennacchietti S, Michieli P, Galluzzo M, Mazzone M, Giordano S, Comoglio PM (2003) Hypoxia promotes invasive growth by transcriptional activation of the met protooncogene. Cancer Cell 3 (4):347–361

Pietras K, Östman A (2010) Hallmarks of cancer: interactions with the tumor stroma. Exp Cell Res 316(8):1324–1331

Porcel E, Liehn S, Remita H, Usami N, Kobayashi K, Furusawa Y, Le Sech C, Lacombe S (2010) Platinum nanoparticles: a promising material for future cancer therapy? Nanotechnology 21 (8):85103

Qian B-Z, Zhang H, Li J, He T, Yeo E-J, Soong DYH, Carragher NO, Munro A, Chang A, Bresnick AR et al (2015) FLT1 signaling in metastasis-associated macrophages activates an inflammatory signature that promotes breast cancer metastasis. J Exp Med 212(9):1433–1448

Qiu SQ, Waaijer SJH, Zwager MC, de Vries EGE, van der Vegt B, Schroder CP (2018) Tumor-associated macrophages in breast cancer: innocent bystander or important player? Cancer Treat Rev 70:178–189

Radisky DC, Levy DD, Littlepage LE, Liu H, Nelson CM, Fata JE, Leake D, Godden EL, Albertson DG, Nieto MA et al (2005) Rac1b and reactive oxygen species mediate MMP-3-induced EMT and genomic instability. Nature 436(7047):123–127

Ranzoni A, Sabatte G, van Ijzendoorn LJ, Prins MW (2012) One-step homogeneous magnetic nanoparticle immunoassay for biomarker detection directly in blood plasma. ACS Nano 6 (4):3134–3141

Roma-Rodrigues C, Pombo I, Raposo L, Pedrosa P, Fernandes AR, Baptista PV (2019) Nanotheranostics targeting the tumor microenvironment. Front Bioeng Biotechnol 7:197

Rosenholm JM, Meinander A, Peuhu E, Niemi R, Eriksson JE, Sahlgren C, Linden M (2009) Targeting of porous hybrid silica nanoparticles to cancer cells. ACS Nano 3(1):197–206

Roy Chowdhury M, Schumann C, Bhakta-Guha D, Guha G (2016) Cancer nanotheranostics: strategies, promises and impediments. Biomed Pharmacother 84:291–304

Sarvaria A, Madrigal JA, Saudemont A (2017) B cell regulation in cancer and anti-tumor immunity. Cell Mol Immunol 14(8):662–674

Savla R, Minko T (2017) Nanoparticle design considerations for molecular imaging of apoptosis: diagnostic, prognostic, and therapeutic value. Adv Drug Deliv Rev 113:122–140

Shibuya M, Claesson-Welsh L (2006) Signal transduction by VEGF receptors in regulation of angiogenesis and lymphangiogenesis. Exp Cell Res 312(5):549–560

Shree T, Olson OC, Elie BT, Kester JC, Garfall AL, Simpson K, Bell-McGuinn KM, Zabor EC, Brogi E, Joyce JA (2011) Macrophages and cathepsin proteases blunt chemotherapeutic response in breast cancer. Genes Dev 25(23):2465–2479

Sikkandhar MG, Nedumaran AM, Ravichandar R, Singh S, Santhakumar I, Goh ZC, Mishra S, Archunan G, Gulyas B, Padmanabhan P (2017) Theranostic probes for targeting tumor micro-environment: an overview. Int J Mol Sci 18(5):1036

Sivasubramanian M, Chuang YC, Chen NT, Lo LW (2019) Seeing better and going deeper in cancer nanotheranostics. Int J Mol Sci 20(14):3490

Skrzydlewska E, Sulkowska M, Koda M, Sulkowski S (2005) Proteolytic-antiproteolytic balance and its regulation in carcinogenesis. World J Gastroenterol 11(9):1251–1266

Sloane BF, Yan S, Podgorski I, Linebaugh BE, Cher ML, Mai J, Cavallo-Medved D, Sameni M, Dosescu J, Moin K (2005) Cathepsin B and tumor proteolysis: contribution of the tumor microenvironment. Semin Cancer Biol 15(2):149–157

Sonali, Viswanadh MK, Singh RP, Agrawal P, Mehata AK, Pawde DM, Narendra, Sonkar R, Muthu MS (2018) Nanotheranostics: emerging strategies for early diagnosis and therapy of brain cancer. Nano 2(1):70–86

Stojanovic A, Cerwenka A (2011) Natural killer cells and solid tumors. J Innate Immun 3 (4):355–364

Suci PA, Varpness Z, Gillitzer E, Douglas T, Young M (2007) Targeting and photodynamic killing of a microbial pathogen using protein cage architectures functionalized with a photosensitizer. Langmuir 23(24):12280–12286

Tang Z, Zhang H, Liu Y, Ni D, Zhang J, Yao Z, He M, Shi J, Bu W (2017) Antiferromagnetic pyrite as the tumor microenvironment-mediated nanoplatform for self-enhanced tumor imaging and therapy. Adv Mater 29(47):1701683

Sugimoto H, Mundel TM, Kieran MW, Kalluri R (Dec 2006) Identification of fibroblast heterogeneity in the tumor microenvironment. Cancer Biology & Therapy. 5(12):1640–1646

Tsou P, Katayama H, Ostrin EJ, Hanash SM (2016) The emerging role of b cells in tumor immunity. Cancer Res 76(19):5591–5601

van Straten D, Mashayekhi V, de Bruijn HS, Oliveira S, Robinson DJ (2017) Oncologic photodynamic therapy: basic principles, current clinical status and future directions. Cancers 9(2):19

Wang HY, Wang RF (2007) Regulatory T cells and cancer. Curr Opin Immunol 19(2):217–223

Wang Y, Zhou K, Huang G, Hensley C, Huang X, Ma X, Zhao T, Sumer BD, DeBerardinis RJ, Gao J (2014) A nanoparticle-based strategy for the imaging of a broad range of tumours by nonlinear amplification of microenvironment signals. Nat Mater 13(2):204–212

Wang C, Gao C, Meng K, Qiao H, Wang Y (2015) Human adipocytes stimulate invasion of breast cancer MCF-7 cells by secreting IGFBP-2. PLoS One 10(3):1–17

Wang S, Mao J, Liu H, Huang S, Cai J, Gui W, Wu J, Xu J, Shen J, Wang Z (2020) pH-sensitive nanotheranostics for dual-modality imaging guided nanoenzyme catalysis therapy and phototherapy. J Mater Chem B 8(22):4859–4869

Wever OD, Demetter P, Mareel M, Bracke M (2008) Stromal myofibroblasts are drivers of invasive cancer growth. Int J Cancer 2238:2229–2238

Wu T, Dai Y (2017) Tumor microenvironment and therapeutic response. Cancer Lett 387:61–68

Wu M, Huang S (2017) Magnetic nanoparticles in cancer diagnosis, drug delivery and treatment. Mol Clin Oncol 7(5):738–746

Wu C, Zhang R, Du W, Cheng L, Liang G (2018) Alkaline phosphatase-triggered self-assembly of near-infrared nanoparticles for the enhanced photoacoustic imaging of tumors. Nano Lett 18 (12):7749–7754

Wu L, Saxena S, Awaji M, Singh RK (2019) Tumor-associated neutrophils in cancer: going pro. Cancers 11(4):564

Yamanishi Y, Boyle DL, Rosengren S, Green DR, Zvaifler NJ, Firestein GS (2002) Regional analysis of p53 mutations in rheumatoid arthritis synovium. Proc Natl Acad Sci U S A 99 (15):10025–10030

Yang C, He L, He P, Liu Y, Wang W, He Y, Du Y, Gao F (2015) Increased drug resistance in breast cancer by tumor-associated macrophages through IL-10/STAT3/bcl-2 signaling pathway. Med Oncol 32(2):352

Yi G, Son J, Yoo J, Park C, Koo H (2018) Application of click chemistry in nanoparticle modification and its targeted delivery. Biomater Res 22:13

Zanganeh S, Hutter G, Spitler R, Lenkov O, Mahmoudi M, Shaw A, Pajarinen JS, Nejadnik H, Goodman S, Coussens LM et al (2016) Iron oxide nanoparticles inhibit tumour growth by inducing proinflammatory macrophage polarization in tumour tissues. Nat Nanotechnol 11 (11):986–994

Zhang P, Wang J, Chen H, Zhao L, Chen B, Chu C, Liu H, Qin Z, Liu J, Tan Y et al (2018) Tumor microenvironment-responsive ultrasmall nanodrug generators with enhanced tumor delivery and penetration. J Am Chem Soc 140(44):14980–14989

Zhang Y, Li M, Gao X, Chen Y, Liu T (2019a) Nanotechnology in cancer diagnosis: progress, challenges and opportunities. J Hematol Oncol 12(1):137

Zhang Y, Xiong X, Huai Y, Dey A, Roy V, Elechalawar CK, Rao G, Bhattacharya R, Mukherjee P, City O et al (2019b) Gold nanoparticles disrupt tumor microenvironment - endothelial cell crosstalk to inhibit angiogenic phenotypes in vitro. Bioconjug Chem 30(6):1724–1733

Therapeutic Applications of Noble Metal (Au, Ag, Pt)-Based Nanomedicines for Melanoma

8

Arpita Roy, Papia Basuthakur, and Chitta Ranjan Patra

Abstract

Melanoma is considered to be the most aggressive form of skin cancer. It mostly occurs as a result of exposure to the ultra violet (UV) radiation from the sun or due to genetic predisposition. Recent reports suggested that melanoma causes around 60,000 deaths worldwide. Conventional therapeutic approaches that are being applied for the treatment of melanoma include chemotherapy, surgery, immunotherapy, and radiation. However, the adverse side effects and drug resistance associated with the above strategies are the major causes of low patient outcomes and threaten to pose serious clinical challenges. Currently, nanomedicines, including inorganic noble metal nanoparticles, especially gold, silver, and platinum, which are known to have versatile biomedical applications, are being considered as a potential therapeutic alternative for the treatment of melanoma. These nanoparticles are mostly used as therapeutic agents, as contrast agents for diagnosis, or as nanovehicles for carrying anti-cancer drugs, nucleic acids, antibodies, and peptides to target cells, to selectively curtail cancer tissues in the body. Although numerous studies have reported promising results of noble metals nanoparticles in the treatment of melanoma, a single review article or book chapter that offers a comprehensive demonstration of applications of these nanomedicines in melanoma therapy is hard to find. Therefore, in this book chapter, we compile and discuss the recent advancements in nanomedicinal

Arpita Roy and Papia Basuthakur contributed equally with all other contributors.

A. Roy · P. Basuthakur · C. R. Patra (✉)
Department of Applied Biology, CSIR-Indian Institute of Chemical Technology, Hyderabad, Telangana, India

Academy of Scientific and Innovative Research (AcSIR), Ghaziabad, India
e-mail: crpatra@iict.res.in

A. Malik et al. (eds.), *Nanomedicine for Cancer Diagnosis and Therapy*,
https://doi.org/10.1007/978-981-15-7564-8_8

approaches using these noble metal nanoparticles in treatment of melanoma. Finally, we address the major challenges that are still to be overcome in the path to the meritorious future of these nanomedicinal approaches.

Keywords

Melanoma · Skin cancer · Noble metal nanoparticles · Chemotherapy · Targeted drug delivery · Photothermal therapy

Abbreviations

A375	Human melanoma cells
AgNP	Silver nanoparticle
AuNP	Gold nanoparticles
B16F10	Murine skin melanoma cells
BRAF	A proto-oncogene B-Raf
C57BL/6	C57 black 6 mice strain
CD44	Cluster of differentiation 44
CMC	Carboxymethylcellulose
CTAB	Cetyltrimethylammonium bromide
DMBA	7,12-Dimethylbenz(a) anthracene
DNA	Deoxyribonucleic acid
DOX	Doxorubicin
EdU	5-ethynyl-2′-deoxyuridine
EPR	Enhanced permeability and retention
FDA	Food and drug administration
FLIM	Fluorescence lifetime imaging microscopy
FU	Fluorouracil
γ-GT	Gamma-glutamyl transferase
GNP	Gold nanoparticle
GOT	Glutamic oxaloacetic transaminase
GPT	Glutamic pyruvic transaminase
HA	Hyaluronic acid
HaCaT	Human keratinocytes
HDF	Human dermal fibroblast
HIV	Human immunodeficiency virus
ICG	Indocyanine green
ICR-191	Acridine mutagen
IGF-1	Insulin-like growth factor-1
IL-1β	Interleukin-1 beta
IL6	Interleukin 6
IL8	Interleukin 8
MART1	Melanoma antigen
MelJuSo	Human melanoma cell line

miRNA	Micro ribonucleic acid
MSH	Melanoma stimulating hormone
NIR	Near infra-red
PAMAM	Poly amido-amine
PAT	Photo acoustic tomography
PD-L1	Programmed death-ligand 1
PDT	Photodynamic therapy
PEG	Polyethylene glycol
PpIX	Protoporphyrin IX
PtNP	Platinum nanoparticle
PTT	Photothermal therapy
PVP	Polyvinylpyrrolidone
ROS	Reactive oxygen species
siRNA	Small interfering ribonucleic acid
SOX2	Transcription factor
SPBANP	Silver Prussian blue analogs nanoparticles
SPR	Surface plasmon resonance
STAT3	Signal transducer and activator of transcription 3
TAG	Titanium-dioxide-nanoparticle–gold-nanocluster–graphene
TAT	Twin-arginine translocation
TEM	Transmission electron microscope
TiO_2	Titanium dioxide
TNFα	Tumor necrosis factor alpha
TUNEL	TdT-mediated dUTP nick-end labeling
UV	Ultra violet
ZnO	Zinc oxide

8.1 Introduction

8.1.1 Melanoma

Melanoma is one of the types of skin cancer which occurs as a result of malignant transformation of melanocytes into tumor. These melanocytes are pigment producing cells that reside, among other places, in the skin epidermis, inner ears, eyes, and hair follicles in the body. Although melanoma can arise from mucosal surfaces, uveal tract, gastrointestinal tract, or brain, cutaneous form of melanoma is the most prevalent and deadliest (Domingues et al. 2018). Combination of a variety of factors like genetic mutations, environmental exposure, hereditary susceptibility, high intensity exposure to UV (UVA and UVB) radiations from the sun, history of blistering sunburns in childhood or adulthood, immunodeficiency, geographical influence like latitude, etc., contributes to the higher risk of the disease (Leonardi et al. 2018; D'Orazio et al. 2011). Besides, scientists have also found that individuals with Parkinson's disease, inflammatory bowel disease, xeroderma pigmentosum (inherited genetic syndrome), some phenotypic traits like fair skin, light or red hair, light eye color, freckles, a large number of moles, age, heavy metal exposure, etc., pose increased risk of causing melanoma (D'Orazio et al. 2011; Pan et al. 2011; Kimmel et al. 2016; Cozzi et al. 2019; Takebe et al. 1989; Sturm 2002).

Since melanin produced by melanocytes acts as a protective barrier to environmental UV radiation, fair-skinned Caucasians with decreased photo-protection due to reduced melanin pigment are more vulnerable to developing this form of cancer. Melanoma can be of different types that include: (1) Superficial spreading melanoma (SSM), which grows slowly and appears as peripherally spreading surface lesions at sun-exposed sites; (Busam 2018); (2) Nodular melanoma (NM), which appears as rapidly growing, crumble smooth vertical nodule that is either pigmented (dark-blue) or non-pigmented (colorless); (Watson et al. 2018); (3) Lentigo maligna (LM) melanoma, which grows inside the epidermal layers and appears as lesions around the sun-exposed regions like head and neck; (Marks and Miller 2017; Lee and Jeffrey 2010) (4) Acral lentiginous melanoma (ALM), which appears as dark spots such as those seen in case of fungal infections, bruises, or steaks on the palms, soles, under the toenails or finger nails, etc. They mostly occur as a result of a all the skin cancer cases genetic predisposition; (Marks and Miller 2017); (5) Amelanotic and desmoplastic melanomas occur as non-pigmented lesions in elderly people; (6) Ocular melanoma, which occurs in the uvea of eye or in conjunctiva and produced by the pigment producing cells in the eye (Liu and Sheikh 2014). Generally, melanoma accounts for 1% of all the skin cancer cases and is accountable for majority of deaths caused due to skin cancer. Although it mostly affects older generation, people below 30 are also prone to the disease (Siegel et al. 2019). In the last three decades, incidences of melanoma have increased considerably.

8.1.1.1 Global Statistics and Market

Melanoma is the 19th most common cancers worldwide. If left untreated, it is the most lethal (60% deaths) form of skin cancer. Around 287,723 cases reported along with 60,712 deaths worldwide in 2018. There has been a trending rise in the incidence rate worldwide over the past few decades and is prevalent in Australia, New Zealand, Asia, Africa, and Latin America. Among these geographically distant continents, Australia accounts for highest incidence rate in the world. Statistical estimation predicts that more than 100 thousand people are likely to be diagnosed with melanoma cancer by 2020. Almost 95,710 cases and close to 10,000 will succumb to the deadly disease in the USA itself in 2020 (Khazaei et al. 2019; Siegel et al. 2019). Compared to the western world, incidence of melanoma is relatively low in India with around 3048 cases reported recently and is also the least common among other forms of skin cancer (Globocan 2019).

Steady rise of chronic disease such as melanoma is an important driver of pharmaceutical market. Increase in the number of FDA approvals for novel therapeutics complemented by the constant endeavor of R&D companies for development of innovative molecules and drugs for melanoma therapy promises lucrative growth opportunities in global market. Reports (Grand view research) estimate that by 2025, melanoma therapeutics market value may touch 12 billion USD approximately (GVR 2017). Such a huge market value indicates high cost of treatment, which is often beyond the reach of people of developing countries. To this end, an economically viable alternative therapeutic approach is urgently required, that can be easily afforded by the majority of population of the world.

8.1.1.2 Treatment Strategies

With no end to the continuous and steady rise of incidences of melanoma, there has been rampant improvement in the understanding of key signaling molecules and oncogenes involved in the pathogenesis and progression of melanoma, thanks to the endeavors of scientists. Presently, for the mitigation of cancer, doctors rely on different standard therapies like surgery, radiation therapy, immunotherapy, and chemotherapy (Kirkwood et al. 2008; Wilson and Schuchter 2016; Christopherson et al. 2015).

Initially, surgical resection of tumor tissue was the sole remedial measure for melanoma. Although considered effective, such surgical or other invasive measures not only pose a risk of adverse histopathological outcomes in resected tissues but also fail to eliminate tumor completely from the body when the tumor has metastasized to other tissues (Strojan 2010). Further, discovery of crucial links between tumor cells, tumor microenvironment, and body's immune system gave the impetus to researchers to look for possible therapies targeting the immune system cells. This gave rise to immune therapies. Since cancer cells including melanoma tend to circumvent the immune surveillance of body's immune system, these immunotherapies mostly rely on reactivation of function of immune cells to destroy cancerous cells by stimulating inflammatory response of the body (Van Elsas et al. 1999). However, the numerous studies unveiling the cellular events that lead to rapid progress of cancer have led to the procreation of chemical drugs that offer therapeutic options by targeting the cellular events to curtail the advancement of fast-growing cancer cells. Among the above mentioned therapies, chemotherapy is the most common and widely recommended therapy for cancer treatment as it is non-invasive in nature, less costly compared to other treatment measures, and has shown promising results (Wilson and Schuchter 2016). Hence, these chemotherapeutic drugs have flourished the market. Majority of them function by inhibiting the growth of tumor tissue either by inducing apoptosis or necrosis of tumor cells or by arresting the cell cycle progress of tumor cells. Another therapeutic option includes targeted therapy where drugs are made to selectively target cancer cells and modulate paradox in signaling pathways that lead to progression of the disease (Janetka and Benson 2018). For instance, the BRAF inhibitor vemurafenib (Zelboraf), which inhibits uncontrolled proliferation of malignant melanoma cells by down-regulating the constitutive expression of mutated BRAF gene that directs cell growth (Davies et al. 2002; Long et al. 2015). Many chemotherapeutic drugs have been approved by Food and Drug Administration (FDA) such as doxorubicin, paclitaxel, gemcitabine, cisplatin, and many more (El-Readi and Althubiti 2019). Additionally, keeping in mind the involvement of epigenetic events in many disease progressions, cancer biologists have started to consider epigenetic modulations for reversing cancer progression. For example, up-regulation of MiR-15b is associated with melanoma progression, while its down-regulation enhances apoptosis of melanoma cells. miRNAs can be used to restore or abrogate the post-transcriptional regulation of certain cancer specific genes (Satzger et al. 2010). Another epigenetic target for cancer therapy involves modulating genetic methylation or histone acetylation status. For instance, one of the apoptotic pathways in melanoma is diminished by methylation and subsequent silencing of two tumor suppressor genes $p16^{INK4A}$ and $p14^{ARF}$. In this case, use of pharmacological methylation inhibitors like 5-Aza-deoxycytidine (5-AZA-dC) can restore normal pathway functions by re-establishing the functions of aberrantly silenced genes in melanoma cells (Freedberg et al. 2008).

Despite wide expansions in the versatility of clinical treatment measures, cancer still remains a challenging health problem. The overall response rate to these therapies is not so impressive. The chemotherapeutic drugs or radiations used to regress the tumor often affect the healthy cells and disrupt the normal body physiology, thus imparting a lot of side effects that may continue to deteriorate the quality of life even after recovery. Besides, several shortcomings like drug resistance of tumors cells (Gottesman 2002), ineffective drug delivery, increased risk of destruction of normal cells and tissues, abnormal pathological behavior of tumor microenvironment with their associated blood vasculature, failure for early detection are among the many barriers for successful eradication of the disease by conventional treatment measures (El-Readi and Althubiti 2019). Moreover, after metastasis of tumor cells to different parts of the body, malignant melanoma cannot be resected by surgical interventions. Finally, the complications due to drug resistance and generation of unwanted inflammatory reactions depreciate treatment eligibilities. Considering the limitations possessed by the conventional treatment strategies, there is an urgent and critical need to look for alternative treatment strategies that can improve patient outcomes (Tang et al. 2017).

In this context, nanotechnology is one of the emerging technologies to be widely used for various biological applications can be promising candidate for treatment of melanoma. To this end, we demonstrate the benefit of nanotechnology in the treatment of cancer especially melanoma.

8.1.2 Nanotechnology in Melanoma

Application of nanotechnology in biomedicine has brought about significant changes in the course of treatment and diagnosis of several types of life threatening cancers including melanoma. Various forms of nanoparticles such as liposomes, nanocapsules, dendrimers, nanorods, micelles, nanoshells, polymeric nanoparticles, nanotubes, inorganic nanomaterials, etc., have been developed over the years for the treatment of various cancers (Li et al. 2015). These nanoparticles act as carriers or vehicles to carry drugs (Fan et al. 2015), nucleic acids (Ni et al. 2018), antibodies

(Day et al. 2010); target ligands to tumor tissue actively or passively to improve treatment specificity (Bertrand et al. 2014), minimize off-target side effects (Samarasinghe et al. 2012), and overcome biological barriers (Kim et al. 2017; Blanco et al. 2015) and biocompatibility issues. Such nanomedicines take advantage of leaky tumor vasculature to enhance their penetration and retention in tumor tissues, by a mechanism called "enhanced permeability and retention effect" (EPR effect) (Golombek et al. 2018; Zhang et al. 2017). These nanovehicles protect the drugs from proteolytic degradation and also facilitate intracellular trafficking of drugs inside tumor cells. Over the years, nanomedicine have gained interest in cancer treatment due to their non-invasive therapeutic procedures (Kalluru et al. 2016).

As a step towards the implementation of nanomedicine for clinical translation, comprehensive in vitro cellular models have been developed to evaluate physico-chemical properties, dose response, and molecular mechanism of action of these nanomedicines. On the other hand, in vivo data assess the tissue/organ distribution, plausible side effects, rate of metabolism, and route of clearance of these nanodrugs from the whole body (El-Kenawy et al. 2017).

8.1.2.1 Nanoparticles for Melanoma

Till date, different types of nanomaterials have been developed for exploration of their applications in mitigating melanoma. Nanoparticles have always gained interest from researchers because they offer several advantages like high surface to volume ratio, easy modification of the surface area, protection of the therapeutic agent from the biological environment, bio-availability of the therapeutic agent, and many more which upgrade their functions in the cellular and molecular level (Ahmad et al. 2010). Owing to these features, metal nanoparticles find versatile biomedical applications like bio-imaging (Guo et al. 2017), bio-sensing (Devi et al. 2015), anti-inflammatory (Agarwal et al. 2019), antimicrobial (Oves et al. 2015), tissue engineering (Yan et al. 2018), etc. Scientists have developed or formulated various types of nanoparticles that can be tailored to manipulate biological events to produce desirable outcomes. Some of which are discussed below.

8.1.2.2 PAMAM

Scientists have developed various types of polymer based nanoparticles for application in multiple areas of biomedicine. Especially, for specific targeting of cancer cells, polymeric nanoparticles are optimized to deliver chemotherapeutic drugs. Such studies are briefly discussed below.

Tang and his colleagues developed a nanocarrier composed of carboxylated poly (amido-amine) (PAMAM) for loading chemotherapeutic drug temozolomide for delivery into the melanoma tumor tissues (Tang et al. 2018). For selective elimination of cancer cells, the nanocarrier was decorated with hyaluronic acid (HA) that targets CD44 receptors overexpressed in melanoma cells. Conjugation of organic fluorescent dye indocyanine green (ICG) to the HA decorated nanocarrier led to photothermal killing of melanoma cells. Irradiation of the ICG-loaded nanocarrier under near infra-red light (NIR) led to the generation of heat and singlet oxygen molecules that drastically reduced the viability of cancer cells. This method of receptor targeted anti-tumor therapy selectively killed the melanoma cells facilitated by binding of HA to the CD-44 expressed on the melanoma cells, thereby protected surrounding cells from degradation (Tang et al. 2018).

8.1.2.3 Zinc Oxide Nanoparticle

Zinc oxide nanoparticles have versatile applications in biology and medicine (Barui et al. 2020; Augustine et al. 2014; Jiang et al. 2018). Scientists have been harnessing the anti-cancer activity of zinc oxide nanoparticles over the years. In one study, Fakhar et al. demonstrated the synthesis of multilayer zinc oxide (ZnO) nanomaterial, conjugated with protoporphyrin IX (PpIX) for intracellular delivery into melanoma cells (FM55P), using femtotip silver capillary probe. UV irradiation of PpIX-conjugated ZnO nanomaterials inside the cells induce ROS generation, disruption in mitochondrial membrane and ultimately causing necrosis of the cells (Fakhar-e-Alam et al. 2017).

8.1.2.4 Titanium Dioxide Nanoparticle

Although few, but there are promising reports about cytotoxic effect of titanium dioxide nanoparticles against melanoma. One study demonstrated that polyethylene glycol encapsulated titanium dioxide nanoparticles effectively reduced the size of melanoma in experimental animal model (Behnam et al. 2018). Cheng et al. reported heterogenous nanocomposite composed of titanium-dioxide-nanoparticle–gold-nanocluster–graphene (TAG) can be made to efficiently utilize sunlight for inducing photodynamic therapy (PDT) in melanoma cells (B16F1) (Cheng et al. 2017). The TAG nanocomposite under stimulated sunlight irradiation induces several toxicological effects inside the cell that ultimately lead to cell death such as over-production of ROS, depletion of glutathione, stimulation of heme oxygenase-1 expression as well as dysfunction of mitochondria. Studies in B16F1 tumor xenograft bearing mice indicated that the nanocomposite can effectively reduce tumor growth when irradiated by stimulated sunlight (Cheng et al. 2017).

8.1.2.5 Vanadium Pentoxide Nanoparticle

Vanadium is a transition metal that is beneficial and required for the various biological activities. However, there are very few reports on vanadium nanoparticles as anti-cancer agent (Ivanković et al. 2006; Kostova 2009).

Very recently, our group established anti-tumor properties of cytocompatible and non-toxic vanadium pentoxide nanoparticles via extensive in vitro and in vivo studies (Das et al. 2020). The study demonstrated that the nanoparticles exert anti-tumor effect on melanoma cells (B16F10) by generation of ROS, inducing DNA damage and inhibiting cell cycle progression thus leading to apoptosis. On the other hand, the nanoparticles also exerted anti-angiogenic effect by inhibiting endothelial cells of blood vessels that nourish the tumor. This causes considerable regression of the tumor as it becomes deprived of blood, oxygen, and nutrient supply. In vivo studies using B16F10 xenograft mice also revealed that the newly established nanoparticle reduced tumor growth and also improved their survival rate (Das et al. 2020).

8.1.2.6 Copper Prussian Blue Nanoparticle

There are numerous applications of copper in biology (Din and Rehan 2017; Santhoshkumar et al. 2019). However, effective anti-cancer nanoparticle to be therapeutic molecule should be biocompatible. Therefore, our group designed and synthesized a complex with copper and Prussian blue which is approved by FDA (Adams and Casagrande 2019) to form biocompatible nanocomplex for delivery of anti-cancer drugs.

We established that doxorubicin conjugated copper Prussian blue nanoparticle showed anti-tumor effect on melanoma cells (B16F10). The nanoconjugate drastically reduced melanoma cell viability through promoted apoptosis by stimulating the expression of pro-apoptotic genes (Mukherjee et al. 2015).

Table 8.1 indicates such various other metal nanoparticles in the treatment of melanoma.

8.2 Importance of Noble Metal Nanoparticles in Biomedicine

Application of noble metal nanoparticles (gold, silver, platinum, rhenium, ruthenium, palladium, iridium, etc.) in the treatment of various other diseases proves its importance in the field of biomedicine. For instance, very recently Miao et al. reported the use of polyethylene glycol (PEG) encapsulated rhenium nanoclusters for photothermal ablation of tumor (Miao et al. 2019). On the other hand, Vankayala et al. revealed that the optical properties of Iridium nanoclusters can be used for in vitro imaging purposes. Again, considering the plausible toxicological impacts of chemically synthesized nanoparticles, some researchers have synthesized noble metal nanoparticles using biological elements like cells, microbes, or even plant products (Vankayala et al. 2013). These biological substances not only imparted some medicinal properties to the nanoparticles but also rendered them non-toxic. For example, Tahir et al. followed a biological approach for the synthesis of palladium nanoparticles from *Phoenix dactylifera* leaves extract. These nanoparticles were found to possess excellent anti-oxidant and antibacterial activities (Tahir et al. 2016). Such biomedical applications of biosynthesized noble nanoparticles and many other chemically synthesized nanoparticles have been mentioned in a tabulated form in Table 8.2. However, among these noble metal nanoparticles, Au, Ag, Pt have been widely used for treatment of various diseases such as gold nanoparticles conjugated with doxorubicin (Mukherjee et al. 2012) have been used for curing breast cancer, platinum nanoparticles (Subramaniyan et al. 2018) have been used for treating antibacterial infection and many more. In Table 8.3, a comprehensive list of clinical applications of gold, silver, and platinum nanoparticles has been provided.

Table 8.1 Metal nanoparticles in melanoma treatment other than noble metals

Sl. No.	Nanoparticle	Mechanism of action	References
1.	Cerium oxide nanoparticles (CeO_2)	Oxidative stress and genotoxicity	Ali et al. (2015)
2.	Palladium nanoparticles	Reactive oxygen species (ROS) mediated apoptosis and genotoxicity	Alarifi et al. (2017)
3.	Ferric oxide (Fe_2O_3)	Apoptosis by ROS production, mitochondrial membrane potential disruption, release of pro-apoptotic cytochrome c	Naserzadeh et al. (2018)
4.	Biosynthesized copper nanoparticles using *Quisqualis indica* extract	Oxidative stress induced apoptosis	Mukhopadhyay et al. (2018)
5.	Cuprous oxide nanoparticles (CONP)	Apoptosis of melanoma stem cells	Yu et al. (2017)
6.	Single walled carbon nanotube	Apoptosis by ROS production, mitochondrial membrane potential disruption, release of pro-apoptotic cytochrome c	Naserzadeh et al. (2018)
7.	siRNA conjugated hyaluronic acid-calcium phosphate hybrid nanoparticle	siRNA mediated silencing of anti-apoptotic Bcl2	Zhou et al. (2017)
8.	Polydopamine-coated Aluminum oxide (Al_2O_3) nanoparticles	Photothermal therapy (NIR light) and immunotherapy (cell mediated immune response)	Chen et al. (2018)
9.	Dacarbazine conjugate-folic acid grafted silica nanoparticles	Controlled and targeted release of chemotherapeutic drug dacarbazine	Liu et al. (2017)
10.	Sulfur nanoparticles	Inhibition of cell proliferation by detention of copper from cancer cells.	Liu et al. (2016)
11.	Biosynthesized zinc oxide nanoparticles from *Cardiospermum halicacabum*	Induction of ROS production and overexpression of pro-apoptotic genes	Duan et al. (2020)
12.	Drug conjugated cell membrane coated copper sulfide nanoparticles	Synergistic photothermal and chemotherapy	Wang et al. (2018)
13.	PEG conjugated titanium dioxide (PEG-TiO_2)	Photothermal therapy	Behnam et al. (2018)
14.	Doxorubicin conjugated and PVP coated Gadolinium oxide nanoparticle	Combination of chemotherapy and radiation therapy	Mahdavi et al. (2019)
15.	Superparamagnetic iron oxide nanoparticles (SPIONs)	Magnetic hyperthermia and radiotherapy	Rybka (2019)
16.	Gemcitabine conjugated lipid-coated calcium phosphate (LCP) nanoparticle	Reduced immunosuppression in tumor microenvironment and induced apoptosis	Zhang et al. (2019)

Table 8.2 Biomedical application of noble metals other than Au, Ag, Pt

Sl. No.	Nanoparticle	Biomedical application	References
1.	Rhenium nanoparticle immobilized DNA scaffolds	Spectroscopic analysis, catalysis	Anantharaj et al. (2016)
2.	Rhenium bipyridine decorated iron oxide nanoparticles	Radiation therapy and optical imaging	Carron et al. (2015)
3.	PEGylated rhenium nanoclusters	Photothermal ablation of tumor	Miao et al. (2019)
4.	Ruthenium nanoparticles modified with transferrin	Photothermal therapy of tumor	Zhao et al. (2018)
5.	Biosynthesized ruthenium nanoparticles from *Gloriosa superba* L.	Antibacterial activity	Gopinath et al. (2014)
6.	Glycolic poly(DL-lactic-co-glycolic acid) stabilized ruthenium nanoparticles	Cancer therapy (promyelocytic leukemia)	Nandakumar et al. (2014)
7.	Rhodium nanoparticles	Sensing of glucose and hydrogen peroxide	Choleva et al. (2018)
8.	Rhodium nanoparticles	Cancer therapy	Kang et al. (2018)
9.	Biosynthesized palladium nanoparticles from *Phoenix dactylifera* leaves extract	Anti-oxidant and antibacterial activity	Tahir et al. (2016)
10.	Palladium nanoparticles stabilized with chitosan grape polyphenols	Antibacterial activity	Amarnath et al. (2012)
11.	Chitosan oligosaccharide-coated palladium nanoparticles	Multi-modal imaging of tumor	Bharathiraja et al. (2018)
12.	PVP capped iridium nanoparticles	Cyto-protection by anti-oxidant activity	Su et al. (2015)
13.	Iridium nanoclusters	In vitro imaging	Vankayala et al. (2013)
14.	Iridium nanoparticles	Bio-sensing of hydrogen peroxide and xanthine	Cui et al. (2017)

8.3 Role of Noble Metals (Au, Ag, Pt) in Treatment of Melanoma

8.3.1 Gold (Au) Nanoparticles

Gold nanoparticles (AuNPs) are having versatile application in the field of biomedicine owing to their biocompatible nature, the high surface ratio for the ease of functionalization, and tagging of various biological agents or molecules and also surface plasmon resonance properties for photothermal or photodynamic applications. In recent years, given its high value in targeted drug delivery, therapy, and diagnosis, AuNPs are modified extensively to treat various cancers including melanoma. Herein, this study details the reports of recent studies of AuNPs as a novel theranostic agent in treating melanoma.

Table 8.3 Importance of noble metals in biomedicine

Sl. No.	Nanomedicine	Biomedical application	References
1	Bleomycin and doxorubicin conjugated gold nanoparticles	Anti-cancer therapy (cervical cancer)	Farooq et al. (2018)
2	Doxorubicin conjugated gold nanoparticles	Anti-cancer therapy (breast cancer)	Mukherjee et al. (2012)
3	Targeted delivery of gold nanoparticle conjugated p53 gene	Anti-cancer therapy (ovarian cancer)	Kotcherlakota et al. (2019b)
4	Gold nanoparticles biosynthesized from *Olax scandens*	Theranostic applications for cancer	Mukherjee et al. (2013)
5	Quercetin conjugated gold nanoparticles	Anti-cancer therapy (breast cancer)	Balakrishnan et al. (2017)
6	Gold nanoshell conjugated with VCAM-1 antibody	Photoacoustic imaging of atherosclerotic plaque	Rouleau et al. (2013)
7	Gold nanospheres	Photoacoustic imaging of mouse brain vasculature	Lu et al. (2010)
8	Gold nanorods	Photoacoustic imaging of cardiovascular system	Taruttis et al. (2010)
9	Platinum nanoparticles conjugated with scFv antibodies	Detection of prostate specific antigen in prostate cancer	Spain et al. (2016)
10	Platinum nanoparticles encapsulated with hyaluronic acid	Photothermal therapy of breast cancer	Zhu et al. (2017)
11	Biosynthesized platinum nanoparticles from fresh green spinach leaves	Antibacterial activity against *Salmonella typhi*	Subramaniyan et al. (2018)
12	Platinum nanoparticles	In vivo antibacterial activity (*Aeromonas hydrophila and E. coli) in zebra fish*	Ahmed et al. (2016)
13	Platinum nanoparticles functionalized tea polyphenol (TPP@Pt)	Anti-cancer therapy (Cervical cancer)	Alshatwi et al. (2015)
14	Platinum nanoparticles conjugated Schiff based ligands	Anti-cancer therapy (breast cancer) and antibacterial therapy	Gupta et al. (2020)
15	Platinum nanoparticle biosynthesized from *Boswellia serrata*	Sensing of mercuric ions in water	Kora and Rastogi (2018)
16	Platinum nanoparticles biosynthesized from fungus *Fusarium oxysporum*	Antimicrobial therapy	Gupta and Chundawat (2019)
17	Silver nanoparticles	Antifungal therapy	Bocate et al. (2019)
18	Silver nanoparticles biosynthesized from *Bacillus brevis*	Antibacterial activity	Saravanan et al. (2018)

(continued)

Table 8.3 (continued)

Sl. No.	Nanomedicine	Biomedical application	References
19	Silver nanoparticles biosynthesized from medicinal plants	Antiviral activity (Chikungunya virus)	Sharma et al. (2019)
20	Silver nanoparticles biosynthesized from *Klebsiella oxytoca*	Anti-cancer activity	Buttacavoli et al. (2018)

8.3.1.1 Drug Delivery

Delivery of pharmaceutical or chemotherapeutic agents for the effective therapy of various diseases is being established recently in order to mitigate the non-specificity and side effects of pristine drugs. In such an attempt, noble metal nanoparticles serve as the appropriate delivery vehicle of the drugs and among them gold nanoparticles are highly considered for studying the same. Herein, delivery of chemotherapeutic drugs using gold nanoparticles for the therapy of melanoma is being discussed briefly.

In one study, Zhang et al. described the effective treatment approach for melanoma using ultra-small gold nanoparticles (AuNPs) conjugated with doxorubicin (Au-Dox). The combination therapy considerably accelerated the reduction in tumor size than doxorubicin alone in BL16 xenograft mice. The nano-conjugate induced significant necrosis and apoptosis of tumor tissues, as observed by histopathological analysis of tumor tissues (Fig. 8.1) (Zhang et al. 2015). As we know that anti-cancer drugs are toxic to the non-target organs especially to the cardiomyocytes, in order to decrease the toxic effect, doxorubicin conjugated with gold nanoparticles (Au-Dox) was studied in both melanoma B16 cells and cardiomyocytes using real-time cell growth and fluorescence lifetime imaging microscopy (FLIM). The authors' demonstrated that the uptake pattern of both the cells was different where Au-Dox was accumulated more in the nuclei of B16 cells, whereas in the cardiomyocytes it persisted in the endosome. Thereby, using gold nanoparticle as carrier for the delivery of chemotherapeutic drugs might help in reducing the toxicity of healthy tissues (Tawagi et al. 2015).

Similarly, 5-fluorouracil (5-FU) was delivered topically by loading onto CTAB capped gold nanoparticles (GNPs) for anti-skin cancer therapy (Safwat et al. 2018). The nanoconjugate of 5-FU/CTAB-GNPs amalgamated into gel or cream base for topical application on skin. The permeability efficiency of the nanoconjugate showed twofold higher permeability than free 5-FU drug in ex vivo C57BL/6 mice dorsal skin. When the same formulation was applied on A431 tumor-bearing C57BL/6 mice, the 5-FU/CTAB-GNPs lowered tumor volume by 6.8- and 18.4-fold as well as tumor weight by maintaining the healthy mice body weight than the untreated control (Fig. 8.2). This showed enhanced efficacy of 5-FU when delivered using gold nanoparticles than the free drug (Safwat et al. 2018).

In another approach, betulin, a pentacyclic triterpene was conjugated through polyethylene glycol (PEG) with sodium citrate reduced gold nanoparticles (AuNP

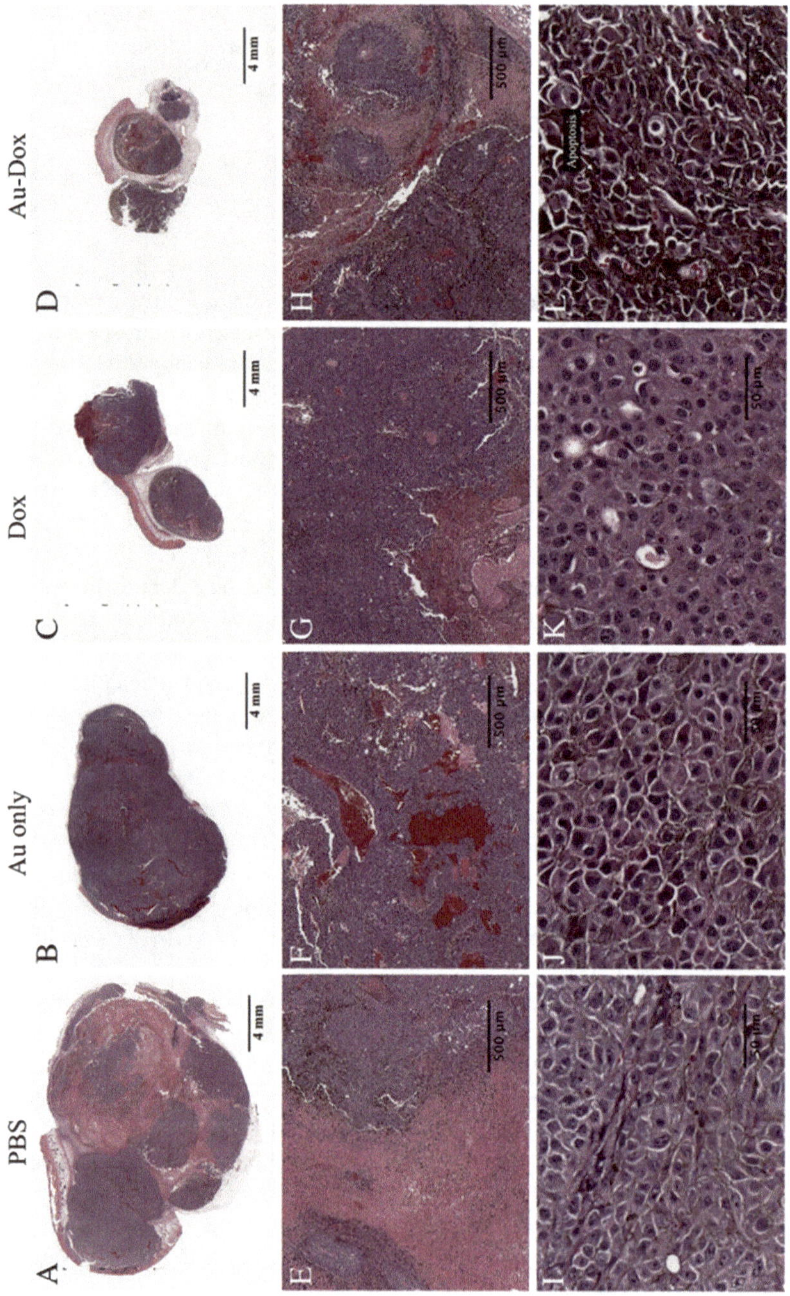

Fig. 8.1 Images of hematoxylin/eosin (H.E.) stained sections of B16 tumors at different magnifications after injection of (**a**, **e**, **i**) PBS, (**e**, **f**, **j**) unconjugated gold nanoparticles, (**c**, **g**, **k**) doxorubicin, and (**d**, **h**, **l**) Au–doxorubicin conjugates. The pink areas indicate necrosis, with individual apoptotic cells appearing black (arrow). Reproduced with permission from Zhang et al. (2015). Copyright © 2015 Elsevier Inc

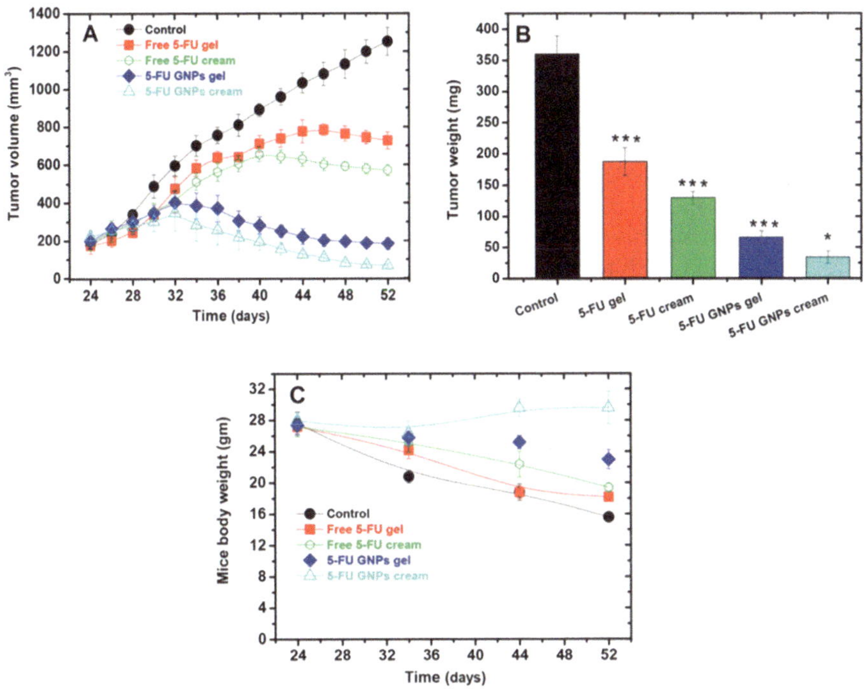

Fig. 8.2 (**a**) Growth curves of A431 tumors in C57BL/6 mice. (**b**) Weights of tumors at the end of the study. (**c**) Changes in the body weight of A431 tumor-bearing mice. Statistically significant differences were calculated using GraphPad Prism software. $^{***}p < 0.001$ compared with untreated control; $^{*}p < 0.05$ compared with 5-FU GNPs gel. Reproduced with permission from Safwat et al. (2018). Copyright © 2018 American Chemical Society

Peg + Bet) to inhibit melanoma cells. The in vitro assessment with the conjugated AuNP showed dose-dependent cytotoxicity and apoptosis in human melanoma cells (A375) and murine melanoma cells (B164A5), indicating potent anti-melanoma activity. Further, in vivo melanoma studies are required for the application of betulin conjugated gold nanoparticles to be deliberated as a therapeutic approach for patients with melanoma (Mioc et al. 2018).

8.3.1.2 Gene Delivery and Immunotherapy

Any mutation or anomaly in the expression of certain genes or proteins triggers a disease condition. Therefore, delivery of such identified gene for up-regulating or down-regulating the expression in order to maintain the healthy physiological condition in a diseased cells is necessary. Moreover, especially in the treatment of cancers, our immune system possesses the required potential to fight against it. In this regard, immunotherapy plays a pivotal role in diminishing the life threatening diseases like cancer. Gold nanoparticles are extensively studied for the delivery of gene as well as cancer immunization. Hence, various studies on the genetic material delivery and immunotherapy for the treatment of melanoma are discussed below.

Melanoma is mostly caused on the cutaneous layer of the skin and topical application of chemotherapeutic agent is ideal to avoid any complication of surgery, scar, etc. However, to penetrate the stratum corneum barrier by any drug is highly challenging. Therefore, Niu and group have developed a cationic gold nanoparticles based delivery platform to deliver miRNA221 inhibitor gene along with HIV-1 twinarginine translocation (TAT) cell-penetrating peptide (AuPT/pDNA-Mi221) for topical delivery of pDNA (Niu et al. 2017). The study was done using both in vitro (B16F10 cells) and in vivo (nude mice) models where the AuPT/pDNA-Mi221 significantly inhibited the melanoma progression and metastasis by inducing apoptosis detected by H&E staining, Tunel and EdU assay (Fig. 8.3) and up-regulating c-Kit and p27 gene expression (Niu et al. 2017).

In another approach for gene delivery, gold nanoparticles (AuNP) coated with chitosan (CS) was assembled layer-by-layer for iontophoretic delivery of STAT3 siRNA (AuNP-CS/siRNA/CS) for the treatment of melanoma (Labala et al. 2016). The formed nanocomplex inhibited the growth of B16F10 melanoma cells. Uptake mechanism showed time dependent cell uptake through clathrin mediated endocytosis of the nanocomplex. As expected, the nanoconjugate downregulated the STAT3 expression and induced late apoptosis of the B16F10 cells demonstrated with annexin V-FITC staining (Fig. 8.4). The skin penetration efficacy was also enhanced due to iontophoresis of the LbL-AuNP (Labala et al. 2016). In continuation to that, the same group utilized the LbL-AuNP for co-delivery of STAT3 siRNA and chemotherapeutic drug imatinib mesylate (IM) to treat melanoma. Along with the in vitro study, iontophoretic co-delivery of STAT3 siRNA and IM reduced the tumor volume and mass with the suppression of STAT3 protein expression as indicated by lower FITC signal in the immunohistochemical study as well as diminished density of tumorous cells visible in the H&E stained tumor sections showing apoptosis in melanoma tumor-bearing mice model as compared to only STAT3 siRNA or IM delivery using LbL-AuNP (Fig. 8.5). Thus, gold nanoparticles could be useful for the iontophoretic delivery of both gene and chemotherapeutic drug to treat melanoma (Labala et al. 2017).

Similarly, our group delivered STAT3 siRNA along with the immune check point protein PD-L1 siRNA to the melanoma bearing mice with the help of gold nanoparticles coupled with tumor vasculature targeting peptide CGKRK (Au-CGKRK) (Gulla et al. 2018). The gold nanocomplex with STAT3 siRNA and PD-L1 siRNA was further conjugated with NIR dye to track the biodistribution of the nanocomplex in the live animal as well as the tumor specific targeting. The authors showed that the intraperitoneal (i.p.) injection of the Au-CGKRK nanoconjugate in the melanoma bearing C57BL6/J mice specifically targeted the tumor resulting in higher accumulation in the tumor tissues. The Au-CGKRK +STAT3siRNA+PD-L1siRNA nanoconjugate significantly inhibited the tumor growth and increased the overall survivability of the tumor-bearing mice as compared to the untreated mice. Investigating of the molecular mechanism also supported that the tumor inhibition was the synergistic effect of STAT3 and PD-L1 pathway inhibition via T-cell driven process. This study could be a future approach for melanoma immunotherapy using gold nanoparticles (Gulla et al. 2018).

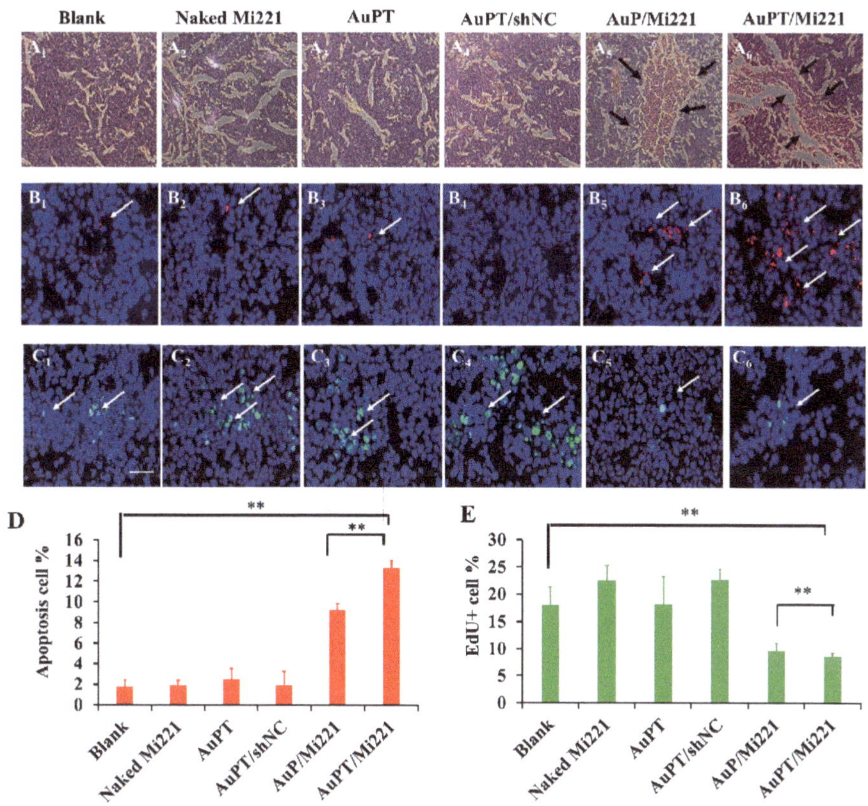

Fig. 8.3 H&E staining images of the tumor tissues harvested from mice treated with (A1) blank, (A2) Naked Mi221, (A3) AuPT, (A4) AuPT/shNC, (A5) AuP/Mi221, and (A6) AuPT/Mi221, on day 8. Scale bar represents 100μm. TUNEL staining (red fluorescence) images of the tumor tissues harvested from mice treated with (B1) blank, (B2) naked Mi221, (B3) AuP, (B4) AuPT/shNC, (B5) AuP/Mi221, and (B6) AuPT/Mi221. EdU staining (green fluorescence) images of the tumor tissues harvested from mice treated with (C1) blank, (C2) naked Mi221, (C3) AuP, (C4) AuPT/shNC, (C5) AuP/Mi221, and (C6) AuPT/Mi221. Scale bar represents 50μm. (D) Quantification of the number of melanoma cells with positive stain in TUNEL assay. (E) Quantification of the number of melanoma cells with positive stain in EdU assay. H&E stain was observed by a light microscope. TUNEL and EdU stains were observed. Reproduced with permission from Niu et al. (2017). Copyright © 2017 American Chemical Society

Likewise, our group also established genetic immunization against melanoma using gold nanoparticles. In this work, gold nanoparticle was functionalized and conjugated with mannose mimicking shikimoyl and transfection enhancer guanidyl functionalities along with melanoma antigen MART1 (Au-SGSH-pCMV-MART1) for delivery of DNA vaccine to dendritic cells (DCs) (Gulla et al. 2019). In vivo sub cutaneous immunization with Au-SGSH-MART1 nanoplex elicited immune response against mouse melanoma for around 180 days while considerably inhibiting the melanoma tumor growth. Studying the immunological markers IFN-γ

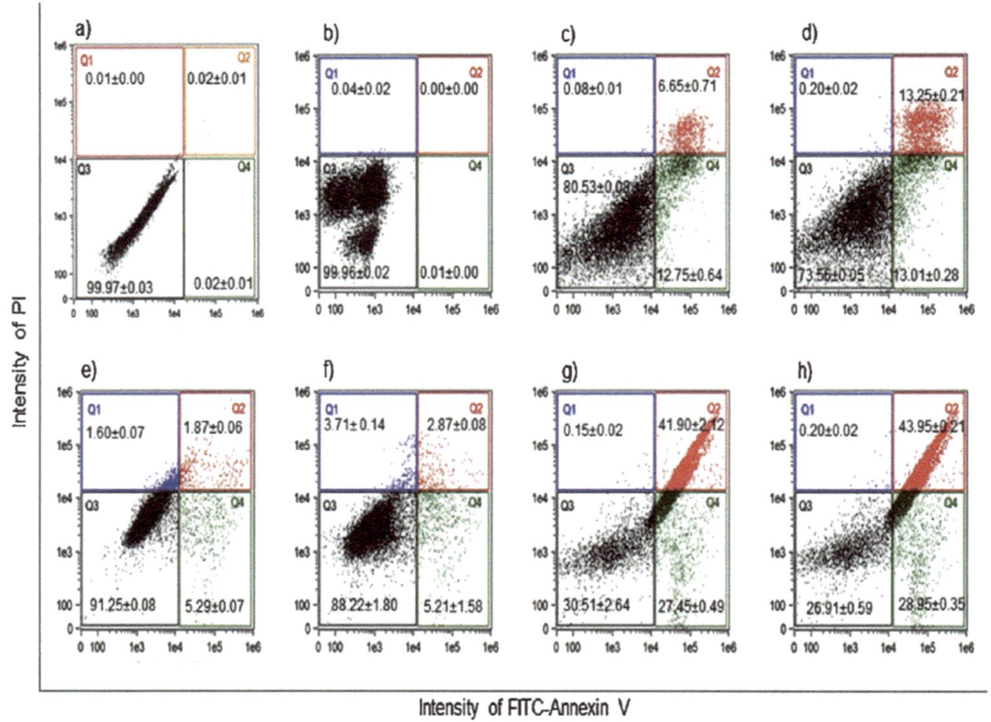

Fig. 8.4 Apoptosis events observed in B16F10 cells after treatment with formulations. (**a**) Untreated cells; (**b**) free STAT3 siRNA; (**c**, **d**) AuNP-CS/SA/CS containing 338μM and 675μM of AuNP; (**e**, **f**) AuNP-CS/scrambled-siRNA/CS at 0.25 nM and 0.5 nM; (**g**, **h**) AuNP-CS/STAT3-siRNA/CS at 0.25 nM and 0.5 nM, respectively. Dot plots are representative of three independent experiments. Reproduced with permission from Labala et al. (2016). © 2016 Elsevier BV

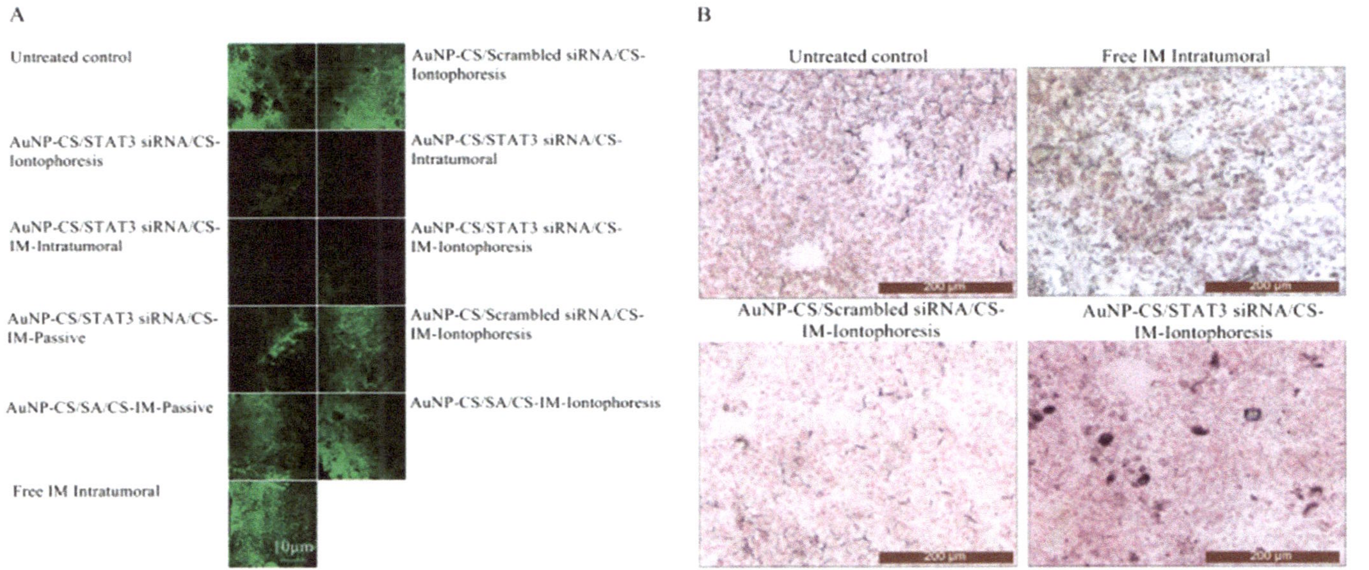

Fig. 8.5 (**a**) Immunohistochemical analysis of STAT3 protein expression in cryosections of tumors treated with different formulations. Images were showed in bright field and dark field, where emission in the 510–530 nm wavelength was because of binding of FITC labeled anti-STAT3 antibody to STAT3 protein. Bar represents 10μm. (**b**) Histological examination of tumor cryosections after treatment with different formulations. Cryosections (15μm thick) were counter stained using hematoxylin. Scale bar represents 200μm. Reproduced with permission from Labala et al. (2017). © 2017 Elsevier BV

and IL-4 isolated from the splenocytes demonstrated CD8+ T-cell mediated cellular and humoral immune response by the DC targeting Au-SGSH-MART1 that lysed the melanoma B16F10 cells in co-culture as detected by LDH leakage (Fig. 8.6). Therefore, this novel DC targeting DNA immunization using gold nanoparticles could be a potential therapy against melanoma (Gulla et al. 2019).

8.3.1.3 Biosynthesized Gold Nanoparticles

Green synthesized gold nanoparticles are mostly biocompatible and effective in treating various diseases including cancers. In this regard, our group biologically synthesized gold nanoparticles using leaf extract of *Butea monosperma* (BM). The synthesized gold nanoparticles (b-AuNP) were biocompatible towards endothelial cells. However, when these AuNPs were conjugated with doxorubicin (b-Au-DOX), showed significant melanoma B16F10 cells inhibition compared to free DOX (Patra et al. 2015). In a similar way, another leaf extract of *Peltophorum pterocarpum* (PP) was utilized by our group to synthesize gold nanoparticle for the delivery of Dox (b-Au-PP-Dox) to treat melanoma both in vitro (B16F10 cells) and in vivo (B16F10 tumor model). Altogether, biosynthesized gold nanoparticles based drug delivery system could be a potential alternative future therapy to treat melanoma (Mukherjee et al. 2016).

In another study, Wu et al. demonstrated that Siberian ginseng extract was used to biosynthesize gold nanoparticles (SG-GNPs) for inhibiting melanoma cells (B16) (Wu et al. 2019). The SG-GNPs were cytotoxic to the B16 murine melanoma cells mediated by increased ROS generation and induced apoptosis. The mechanism of the induction of apoptosis was revealed by q-PCR analysis where, the treatment increased apoptotic gene expression (Bid, Bad, Casp3, Casp9) and decreased anti-apoptotic Bcl2 gene expression. Thereby, biosynthesized SG-GNPs were explored as an effective anti-cancer therapy in vitro. However, detailed in vivo anti-cancer and toxicity studies are required for further application of these biosynthesized GNPs (Wu et al. 2019).

8.3.1.4 Imaging

Cancer therapy demands the early diagnosis of the diseased state. As a result, metal nanoparticles especially gold nanoparticles are excellent candidates for the uptake and detection of cancer cells as a fluorescent agent or accumulation in the cancer tissues due to EPR effect and quantification of the gold content. Thus, we hereby mentioned brief studies in gold particles as imaging agent for the diagnosis of melanoma.

In view of that, our group has synthesized gold nanoparticles using the leaf extract of *Zinnia elegans* (AuZE) which was revealed to have fluorescent property (Kotcherlakota et al. 2019a). The biosynthesized gold nanoparticles (AuZE) were demonstrated for their application in non-invasive imaging in NIR region. Interestingly, AuZE when injected into the mice intraperitoneally, it accumulated into the brain showing the brain targeting ability of the AuZE without any targeting agent. Apart from that, AuZE was investigated to have cell labeling property when incubated with B16F10 cells and injected into the mice for graft transplantation

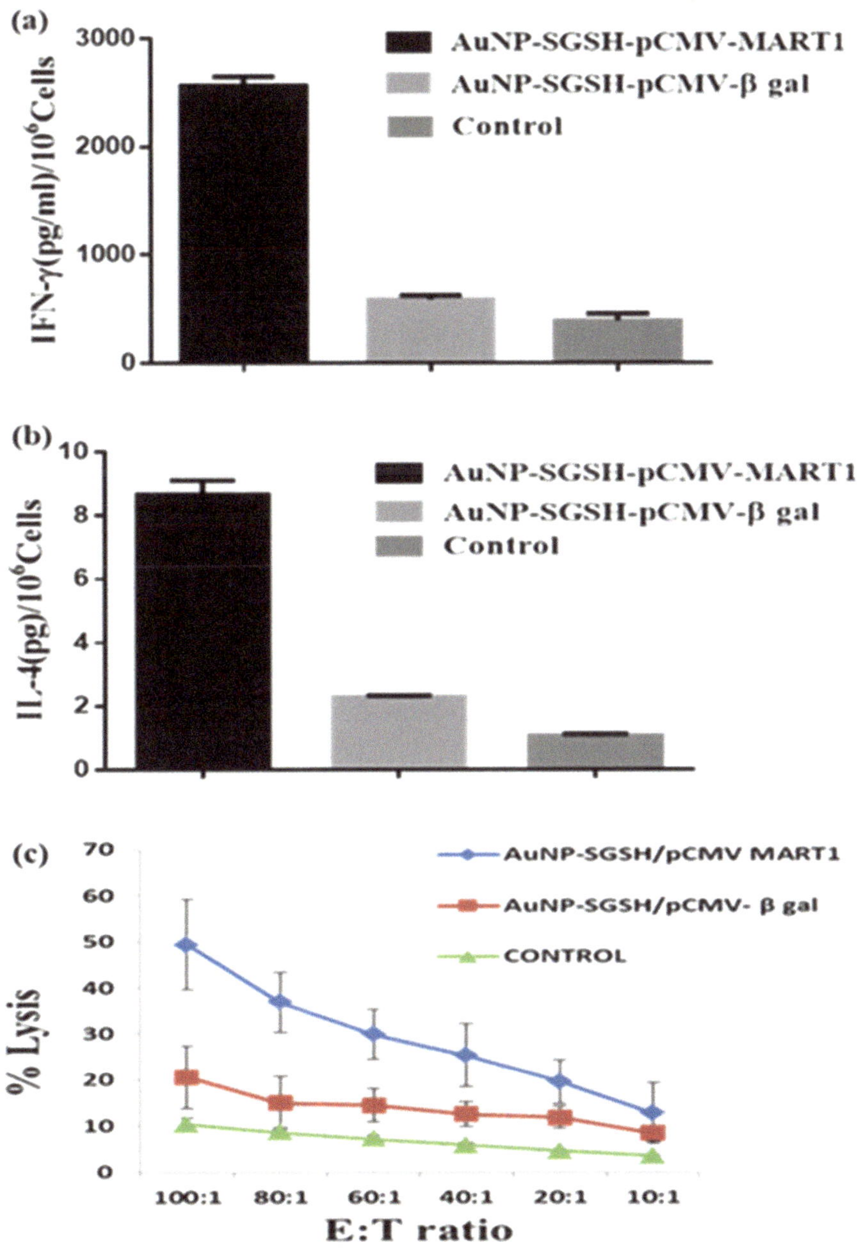

Fig. 8.6 Cellular and humoral immune responses and specific lysis of B16F10 cells by CD8+ T cells (CTLs): 6–8 weeks-old female C57BL/6J mice (each weighing 20–22 g, $n = 4$) were immunized (s.c., thrice at seven-day intervals) with nanoplexes of AuNP-SGSH and pCMV-MART1 and AuNP-SGSH and pCMV-β-gal (as negative control). (**a**, **b**) Four weeks post third immunization, splenocytes were collected, stimulated for 3 days by co-culturing with target B16F10 cells. (**a**) Amount of IFN-γ (signature cytokine for cellular immune response) and (**b**) IL-4 (signature cytokine for humoral immune response) released in the co-culture supernatants determined by ELISA ($*P < 0.005$ for

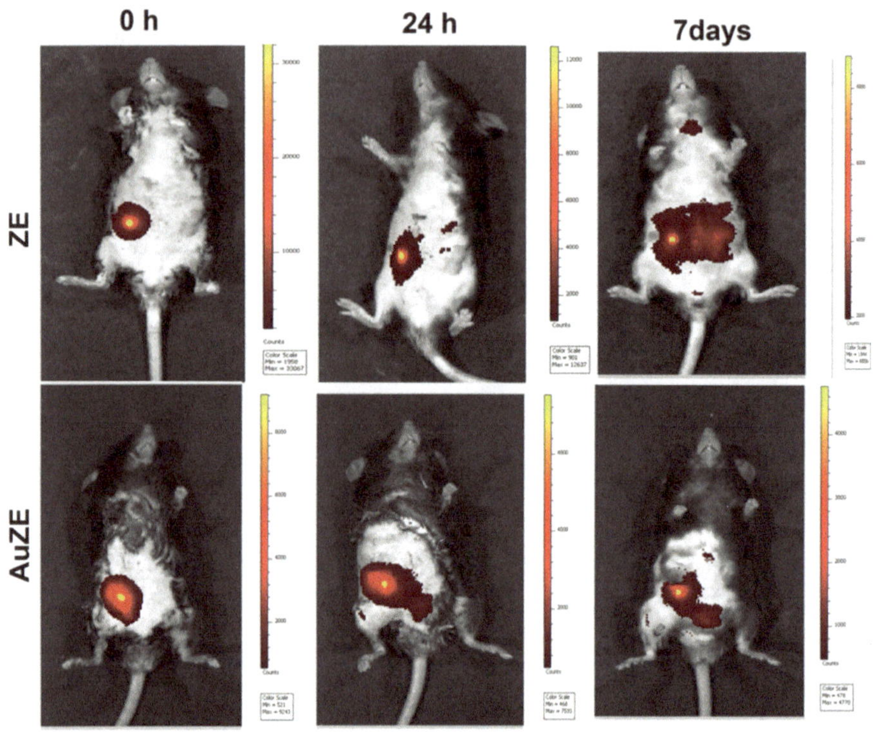

Fig. 8.7 In vivo cell transplantation applications. In vivo cell transplantation applications of ZE and AuZE-pretreated B16F10 cells. The cells treated with ZE and AuZE exhibit the fluorescence signals in the mice body. The top row indicates the ZE-pretreated B16F10 cell-injected mice with fluorescence signal up to 7 days. Similarly, the bottom row shows the AuZE-pre-incubated B16F10 cells transplanted into mice and their fluorescence signals up to 7 days. Reproduced with permission from Kotcherlakota et al. (2019a). Copyright © 2019 American Chemical Society

biology. The administered B16F10 cells pre-incubated with AuZE in C57BL6 mice showed strong fluorescence up to 7 days (Fig. 8.7). This application of AuZE, however could be beneficial for the theranostic potential to treat melanoma (Kotcherlakota et al. 2019a).

Recently, Lara et al. used gold nanoparticles for double-labeling of melanoma extracellular vesicles (EVs) with the goal of specific uptake and fluorescence imaging towards other cancer cells and metastatic tumors (Lara et al. 2020). The authors synthesized gold nanoparticles and conjugated with folic acid to augment internalization and trafficking through the endocytic or multivesicular bodies (MVB)

Fig. 8.6 (continued) AuNP-SGSHpCMV-MART1 vs. control). (**c**) Splenocytes were collected 28 days post the third immunization and the percentage of target melanoma cell lysis (CTL responses) was measured by quantifying the LDH leakage from the lysed B16F10 cells after 4 h incubation (**P* < 0.005 for AuNP-SGSHpCMV-MART1 vs control). Reproduced with permission from Gulla et al. (2019). © Royal Society of Chemistry 2020

pathway for secretion inside the extracellular vesicles (EVs) of B16F10 cells. The gold nanoparticles encapsulated EVs were further fluorescently labeled for dual application of imaging and gold quantification in metastasized tumor tissues. Therefore, this study provides a valuable tool for targeting of gold nanoparticle based distribution and interaction of EVs in metastatic nodules of mice for theranostic application in the treatment of melanoma or other cancers (Lara et al. 2020).

8.3.1.5 Photothermal and Photodynamic Therapy

Photothermal therapy is a process of in situ, minimally invasive therapeutic approach using laser irradiation especially at NIR to convert into heat energy in order to thermally ablate the cancer cells. Metal nanoparticles, particularly the noble metal nanoparticles (Au, Ag, Pt) aids as photosensitizing agents owing to their property of surface plasmon resonance (SPR), absorbs the light energy to generate heat energy into the specific region contributes to the photodynamic therapy. In line with this, recent reports on the application of gold nanoparticles in the photothermal and photodynamic therapy of melanoma are discussed herewith.

Apart from the delivery of chemotherapeutic drugs or genes, gold nanoparticles are well known for their radioactivity or photothermal therapy in various cancers including melanoma. Kim et al. used AuNP of 50 nm size for kilovoltage X-ray therapy of melanoma. With the concentration of 320μM of 50 nm AuNP showed dose-enhancement effect in human melanoma cells and improvement of radio response of 150 kVp X-ray treatment (Kim and Kim 2017). Another group used liposome gold nanoparticles for the delivery of curcumin (Au-Lipos Cur NPs) that act as an in situ adjuvant for photothermal therapy of melanoma. The photothermal transduction of the Au-Lipos Cur NPs was through the absorption of the NIR light (780 nm) due to the SPR of gold coating that generated heat using the light energy. The authors demonstrated the biocompatibility of only Au-Lipos NPs without curcumin and before laser irradiation. However, Au-Lipos Cur NPs augmented the cytotoxicity of the B16F10 melanoma cells upon laser irradiation as indicated by cell viability and propidium iodide dead cell staining (Fig. 8.8) (Singh et al. 2018).

Later this group found that the curcumin trapped inside the Au-Lipo NPs was released as nanocrystals which amalgamate to form curcumin microcrystals (CMCs) due to the NIR irradiation (Alvi et al. 2019). The in vivo photothermal treatment with the Au-Lipo Cur NPs demonstrated the localized curcumin release that increases the specific site temperature increase which serves as adjuvant that leads to reduction of tumor volume in B16 melanoma tumor model. At the end of the experiment, excised tumors show remains of melanoma cells in the reduced tumor and H&E staining revealed an accumulation of curcumin in the tumor sections (Fig. 8.9). Therefore, gold nanoparticles are successful in the induction of photothermal therapy in melanoma cells with sustained release of hydrophobic curcumin microcrystals (Alvi et al. 2019).

In a similar way, Aishwarya et al. synthesized gold nanoparticles using the bacteria *E. coli* and conjugated a photosensitizer drug 5-aminolevulinic acid (ALA) to activate protoporphyrin IX (PpIX) through irradiation in B16 F10 melanoma and A431 epidermoid carcinoma cells (Aishwarya and Sanjay 2018). When

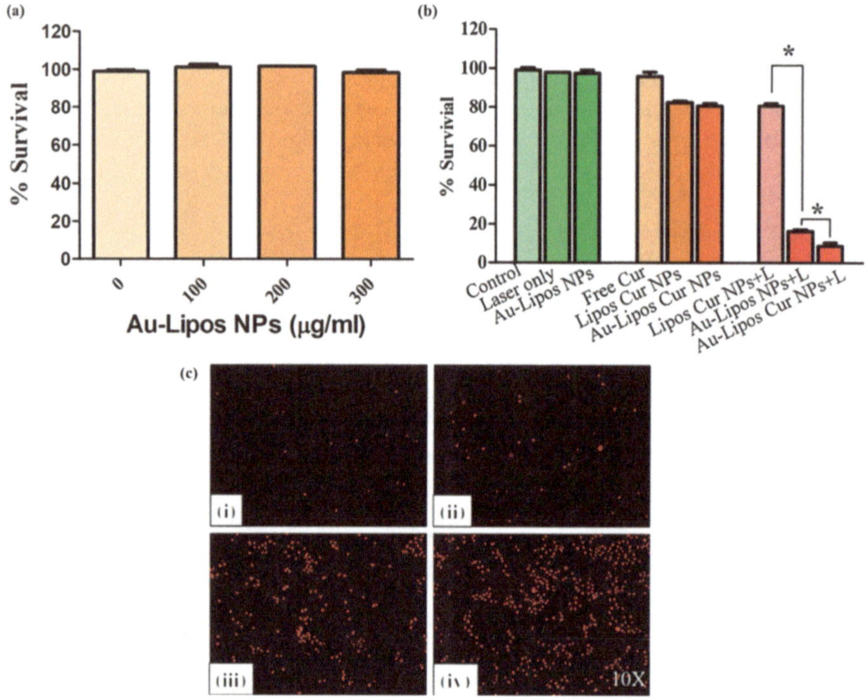

Fig. 8.8 (**a**) Viability of cells incubated with different concentration of Au-Lipos nanoparticles ranging from 100 to 300 g/ml in L929 cell lines (mouse fibroblast) for 48 h. (**b**) Evaluation of in situ photothermal adjuvant effect of curcumin in B16 F10 cells. Free Cur, Lipos Cur NPs and Au-Lipos Cur NPs were incubated with cells for 4 h before laser irradiation. Twelve hours after laser treatment MTT assay was performed to assess the cell viability. (*$P < 0.05$ compared to Lipos Cur NPs + laser (L) treated group). (**c**) Propidium iodide staining of dead cells (1) Control (2) Free Cur (3) Au-Lipos NPs (4) Au-Lipos Cur NPs after 5 min of 780 nm laser irradiation. Reproduced with permission from Singh et al. (2018). © 2017 Elsevier BV

the cells were treated with the gold-5-ALA nanoconjugate and irradiated, showed enhanced cytotoxicity along with generation of ROS compared to pure gold nanoparticles and free drug. Thus, gold nanoparticle assisted photodynamic therapy enhances the anti-melanoma activity (Aishwarya and Sanjay 2018).

8.3.2 Silver (Ag) Nanoparticles

Silver nanoparticles (AgNPs) have multifunctional biological properties mainly as antibacterial, anti-cancer, imaging, photothermal agent, drug delivery vehicle, etc. Based on these properties of AgNPs, it is broadly used in the treatment of various diseases. Here, the anti-melanoma activities of AgNPs will be elaborated from various case studies.

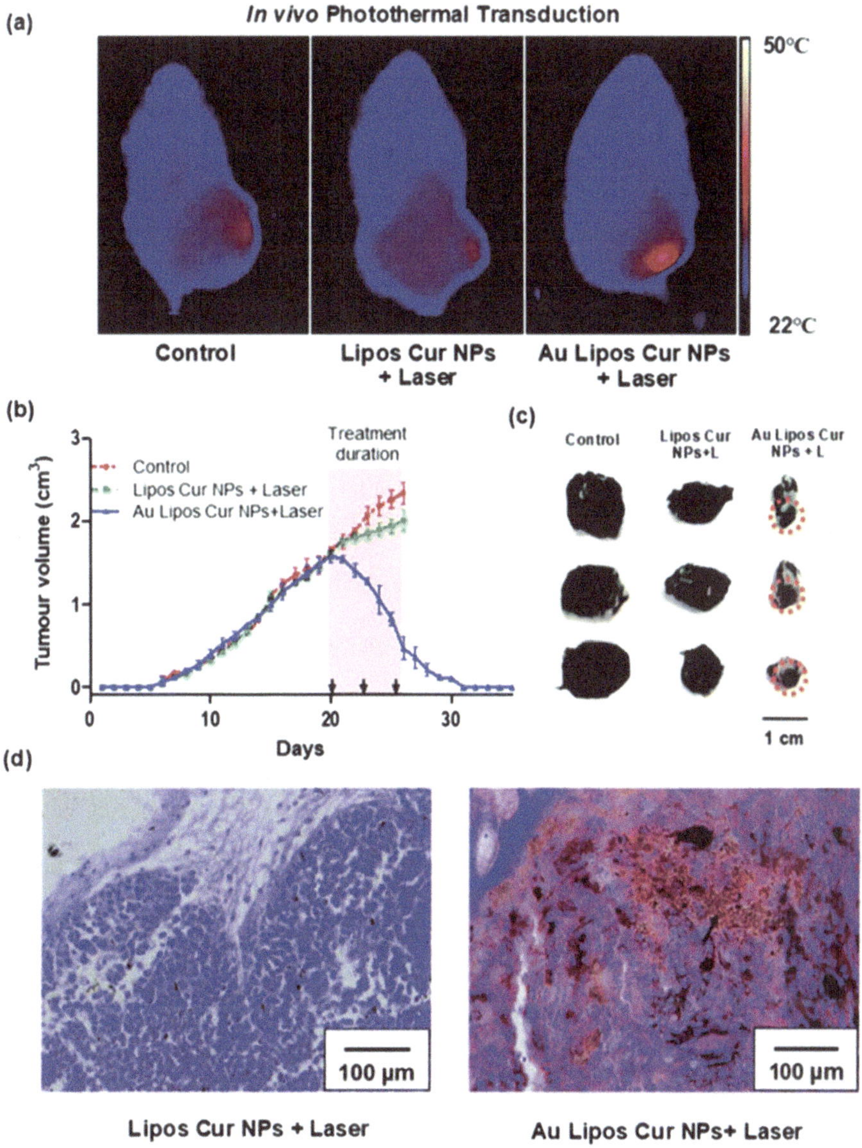

Fig. 8.9 (**a**) In vivo photothermal transduction of Au-Lipos Cur NP thermal imaging of animals after laser treatment showing a localized temperature increase. (**b**) Tumor volume from the day of cell implantation to the end of treatment. Arrows represent days of nanoparticle injection and subsequent laser irradiation. (**c**) Representative image of the isolated tumor after the end of treatment. Dashed circle shows the presence of remnant melanoma on inverted skin. (**d**) H & E staining of isolated tumor sections (black arrow represents the presence of curcumin as a depot after treatment). Reproduced with permission from Alvi et al. (2019). © Royal Society of Chemistry 2020

To begin with, our group has already demonstrated numerous studies on AgNPs to be the future therapeutics. In one of the study, AgNPs were biologically synthesized using leaf extract of *Olax scandens* that had theranostic potential (Mukherjee et al. 2014). The as-synthesized colloidal b-AgNPs exhibited multiple benefits such as antibacterial, anti-cancer, imaging capability due to the fluorescence property of the extract, and delivery of chemotherapeutic drug. The treatment of b-AgNPs to the B16 melanoma cells showed dose-dependent cytotoxicity by induction of apoptosis and ROS generation. Moreover, the b-AgNPs revealed fluorescence property that was detected in B16 cells on treatment. Thus, AgNPs serve as excellent therapeutic as well as diagnostic tool for the detection and treatment of melanoma (Mukherjee et al. 2014).

Recently, our group reported a unique nanomedicine that comprises silver and Prussian blue to form silver Prussian blue analogs nanoparticles (SPBANPs) for the treatment of both bacterial infections and cancers. This nanoformulation inhibited B16F10 cells in vitro along with in vivo melanoma growth in C57BL6/J mice. The nanocomplex significantly reduced the tumor volume and weight as well as increasing the survivability of the treated mice with melanoma. On investigating the biodistribution of the SPBANPs showed higher accumulation in the tumor tissues than other organs due to EPR effect (Fig. 8.10). Moreover, the SPBANPs were biocompatible in the in vivo system. These 2-in-1 properties of the SPBANPs are proved to have beneficial role for the treatment of melanoma and bacterial diseases (Mukherjee et al. 2019).

Apart from our group, another research team, Capanema et al. also demonstrated dual activity of AgNPs complex for the treatment of melanoma and bacterial infections (Capanema et al. 2019). The authors' synthesized AgNPs encapsulated carboxymethylcellulose (CMC) polymer hybrid hydrogel conjugated with doxorubicin (AgNP@CMC-DOX) that significantly reduced the cell viability of A375 human melanoma cells with enhanced uptake of these nanocomplex. The anti-cancer activity of the AgNP@CMC-DOX hydrogel owes to the dual toxic properties of silver and DOX. The same nanohydrogel was also successful in the inhibition of both Gram-positive and Gram-negative bacteria. To this end, the silver based nanocomplex hydrogel could be a future anti-cancer and antibacterial for topical application (Capanema et al. 2019). Valenzuela-Salas et al. synthesized silver nanoparticle (AgNP) capped with polyvinylpyrrolidone (PVP) that has anti-proliferative and anti-tumor activity against melanoma. These AgNPs inhibited the B16F10 cell proliferation, induced apoptosis, and generated ROS. In animal model, melanoma tumor was drastically reduced in the presence of AgNPs without any detectable genotoxic effect. Therefore, AgNPs could be used as a potential anti-melanoma strategy (Valenzuela-Salas et al. 2019).

In parallel to the chemically synthesized nanoparticles, biologically synthesized silver nanoparticles are also effective in photodynamic therapy for treating melanoma. To this end, bacterial strain *Bacillus licheniformis* was used to synthesize silver nanoparticles (AgNPs) that was further conjugated with 5-aminolevulinic acid (5-ALA) for photodynamic therapy (Shivashankarappa and Sanjay 2019). The cytotoxicity of the conjugated nanoparticles was higher than the free drug and

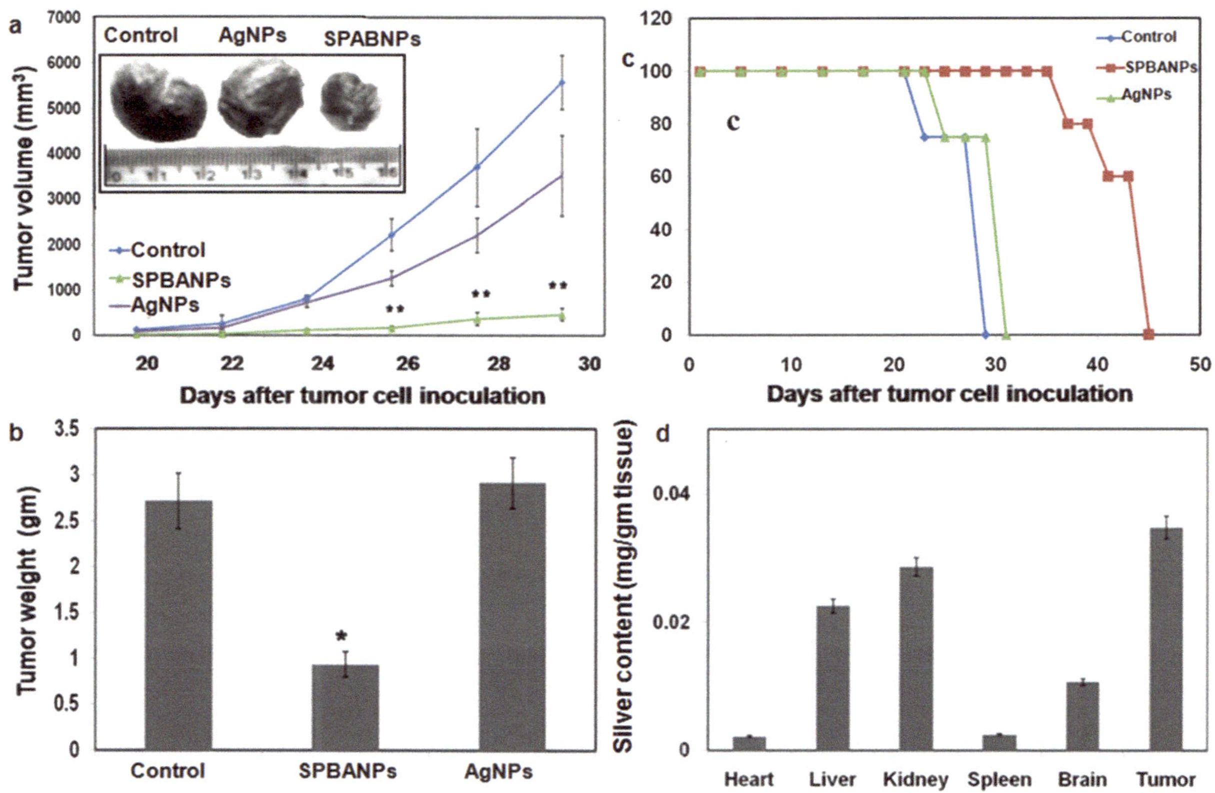

Fig. 8.10 (**a**) Tumor regression study of SPBANPs in allograft mice (C57BL6/J) melanoma tumor model (IP injection of SPBANPs and AgNP at 1 mg/kg [$n = 5$; ** represents $p < 0.005$]); doses were administered on day 20, 22, 24, 26, and 28. Inset demonstrates the representative images of the tumors from

pure silver nanoparticles in both murine melanoma (B16F10) and human melanoma (A431) cells. On the radiation exposure after conjugated AgNPs treatment to the cells showed increased ROS generation due to PpIX formation leading to the inhibition of the melanoma cells. Therefore, AgNPs could be an effective carrier for the photosensitizing drugs to be useful for anti-melanoma photodynamic therapy (Shivashankarappa and Sanjay 2019). In another approach, silver nanoparticles (AgNPs) were coated with titanium dioxide (TiO_2) to form Ag@TiO_2 NPs for inducing photothermal effect in the therapy of melanoma (Nie et al. 2020). The oxides contributed by the TiO_2 on the surface provided stability, less toxicity, and a higher photothermal conversion rate of the Ag@TiO_2 NPs in both in vitro and in vivo. The nanocomplex exhibited excellent cytotoxic effect through photothermal conversion by absorbing near-infrared (NIR) light in both B16F10 cells and melanoma tumor in C57BL/6 mice model. This work demonstrated Ag@TiO_2 NPs to be efficient photothermal agents for the reduction of melanoma by local delivery (Nie et al. 2020).

8.3.3 Platinum (Pt) Nanoparticles

Being one of the noble metals, platinum also has immense biomedical importance. Platinum-based drugs and nanoparticles (PtNPs) are well studied for the treatment of various diseases including cancers. PtNPs are studied for drug or pharmaceutical compound delivery, photothermal and photodynamic therapy, etc. The recent developments of platinum nanoparticle based melanoma therapies are briefly elaborated below.

Based on the immense biomedical importance of platinum nanoparticles, our group also designed and synthesized platinum nanoparticles for drug delivery approach. The platinum nanoparticles (PtNPs) were synthesized and surface stabilized using PEG for further conjugation of chemotherapeutic drug doxorubicin (PtNPs-DOX) for drug delivery to treat melanoma (Mukherjee et al. 2020). In vitro studies on treatment with PtNPs-DOX showed inhibition of B16F10 melanoma and A549 lung carcinoma cells proliferation by inducing apoptosis. Similarly, in vivo melanoma tumor was also reduced on the administration of PtNPs-DOX to C57BL6/J mice with maximum accumulation in the tumor and unaltered body weight of the injected mice demonstrating anti-cancer and biocompatibility of the nanoparticles. Investigation of the molecular mechanism indicated up-regulation of p53 and down-regulation of SOX2 and Ki-67 proliferation marker in melanoma tissues. Along with

Fig. 8.10 (continued) control untreated, AgNP-treated, and SPBANP-treated groups, (**b**) weight of the tumors after the sacrifice of each experiment group, (**c**) survival study of C57BL6/J mice treated with SPBANPs and AgNPs, and (**d**) biodistribution of silver content (mg per gm tissue) in different organs and tumor. Reproduced with permission from Mukherjee et al. (2019). Copyright © 2019 American Chemical Society

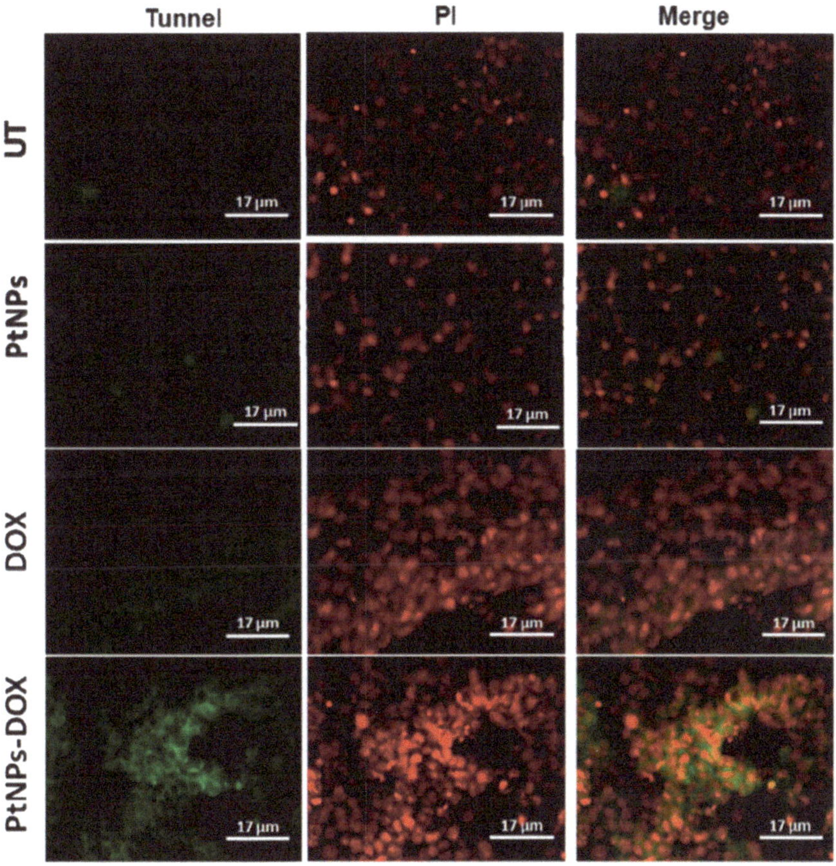

Fig. 8.11 TUNEL assay of untreated and treated (free DOX, PtNPs, and PtNPs-DOX) tumor tissue. First column represents apoptotic cells in tumor tissues (visible by green fluorescence). Second column indicates the propidium iodide staining (visible by red fluorescence), that binds to the nucleus of the apoptotic cells. Third column represents merged images of both green and red region. Images were captured at 40× magnification. Reproduced with permission from Mukherjee et al. (2020). © 2019 Elsevier BV

the increased TUNEL positive signal indicated with green fluorescence supported the induction of apoptosis in tumor tissues in PtNPs-DOX treatment (Fig. 8.11). Therefore, PtNPs could be an excellent platform for drug delivery as an alternative therapeutic strategy for the melanoma treatment (Mukherjee et al. 2020).

Another group also worked on the efficiency of PtNPs to deliver acridine mutagen ICR-191 to inhibit melanoma cells (Borowik et al. 2019). The authors developed ICR-191 attached PtNPs for enhanced mutagenic activity against cancerous cells and less toxic to the normal cells as well as survival of *Caenorhabditis elegans*. The nanoconjugate efficiently reduced the cell viability of the human melanoma cell line (MelJuSo) compared to non-cancerous HaCaT cells. Due to the fluorescence property of the acridine mutagen ICR-191, the cells up-taken the nano-conjugate fluoresce under the confocal microscope. It has been observed that the MelJuSo cells incubated with PtNP-ICR-191 showed higher and long-term fluorescence which was quenched in the HaCaT cells after certain time. The authors speculated that the quenching in the HaCaT cells happened due to the ICR-191 aggregate formation with PtNPs while maintaining the same intensity in cancer cells for long time. Thus, such platinum metal based nanoparticles should be deliberated as a prospective delivery vehicle for biologically active molecules to inhibit diseases like cancer (Borowik et al. 2019).

Likewise, a novel dendritic assembly of silver-platinum (AgPt) nanoparticles was synthesized to inhibit both bacterial infections and cancers. The as-synthesized AgPt nanoparticles showed dose-dependent cytotoxicity against melanoma A375 cells and glioblastoma U87 cells compared to human dermal fibroblast cells (HDF). The reduction of the cancer cells might be due to the selective cancer cell uptake of the nanoscale particles via enhanced permeability and retention efficiency. Therefore, this bimetallic nanoparticle could be a promising selective anti-cancer therapy in the future (Ruiz et al. 2020). Recently, PtNPs were explored for photothermal and radiotherapy against melanoma. Daneshvar et al. synthesized PtNPs for the treatment of melanoma cells by dual irradiation. B16F10 cells were treated with PtNPs and irradiated with 1.0 and 1.5 W cm^{-2} power densities of laser and 2, 4, and 6 Gy X-ray exposures. This combined radiation inhibited the melanoma cells via generation of ROS. Thus, the results encouraged for the use of PtNPs as a dual-sensitization treatment strategy of photothermal and X-ray for further clinical investigation for the treatment of melanoma tumor (Daneshvar et al. 2020).

8.4 Toxicity of Noble Metal Nanoparticles

The ubiquitous application of nanomaterials in therapeutic and diagnostic tools as well as in many consumer products exposes both humans and other living beings to these nanoscale materials. Concomitant with the activities exhibited by the nanoparticles inside biological systems, there are rising concerns about their potential toxicity due to nanoparticle–biomolecule interaction as well as cellular and immune response to these exogenous substances (Zhang et al. 2014). Studies have found that nanoparticles, by virtue of their small size can enter and be deposited in various tissues (like liver, brain, spleen, heart, lungs, gastrointestinal tract, respiratory tract, etc.) and can disrupt normal organ physiology (Nemmar et al. 2002; Takenaka et al. 2001; Garnett and Kallinteri 2006; Mostafalou et al. 2013; Radziun et al. 2011; Alshatwi et al. 2012; Pourmand and Abdollahi 2012). It is also believed that these nanoparticles may be far more toxic than their counterpart macro-particles, composed of same chemical moieties (Yang and Watts 2005). Since the current book chapter focuses on noble metal nanoparticles, it is appropriate to highlight the toxicological aspects as well as risk assessment of these noble metals.

Generally, NP toxicological profiling follows a designed set of in vitro and in vivo procedures. On cellular scale, physiological outcomes like proliferation, apoptosis, nucleic acid damage, necrosis, oxidative stress, protein degradation, etc., give a measure of the level of cytotoxicity of the nanoparticles (NPs). On the other hand, at the organismic level NPs can exert long-term systemic toxicity. As a result, in order to determine the effect of NPs in organisms, it is important to establish a representative model system and assess important systemic parameters like histopathological changes, rate of metabolism, biodistribution, regulation of homeostasis, immune response, clearance from the body, etc. Thus, based on the above physiological responses, the dose range and the time of exposure of nanoparticles to the biological system should be selected in order to make nanomedicines an integral part of clinical medicine (Yang et al. 2017).

Various factors play important role in nano–bio interaction such as NP size distribution, shape, surface charge, surface functionalization, purity, aggregation level, method of synthesis, concentration, route of administration, time of exposure, biological systems like cell line or model organism, etc. (Maurizi et al. 2018). Among all these factors, morphology is one factor that affects cytotoxic potential of NPs in contrasting ways. For instance, in case of gold nanoparticles, some studies have shown that compared to nanorods and nanospheres, other nanostructures like nanostar, nanoflower, or nanoprism are less toxic (Woźniak et al. 2017). On the contrary, another study found that nanospherical gold was more toxic than nanorods (Tarantola et al. 2011).

The first point of interaction of the nanoparticle and the cell occurs at the cell surface. Cell membrane potential plays an essential role in maintaining normal cellular homeostasis. Often it is seen that interaction of nanoparticles with cell membrane can result in anomaly in membrane potential. As for example, one study reported that PtNPs when administered in cardiomyocytes can delay depolarization–repolarization of action potentials and also depolarize resting membrane potential. This disturbance in the membrane potential coupled with disturbance in normal ion channel by PtNPs can lead to severe malfunctioning of cardiomyocytes and as such they can reduce heart rate and also block atrioventricular conduction (Lin et al. 2019). Similar results were also obtained in case of silver NPs, which can also impart cytotoxicity to cardiomyocytes by disrupting transmembrane potential and unsettle cellular ion currents. These cytotoxic effects are serious enough to induce lethal bradyarrhythmias (Lin et al. 2017).

Just like different NPs can impart cytotoxicity in a single cell line in various ways, same NP can also impart cytotoxicity to different cell lines in various ways. Additionally, the time of exposure of cells to NPs plays a crucial role in mediating cytotoxic responses. Having discussed about the role of PtNPs in inducing cardiotoxicity, the hepatotoxicity of PtNPs can result in serious lethal outcomes. Exposure of hepatocytes (HepG2 cells) to PtNPs in a sustained manner (for 24 h approximately) can result in increased ROS production, disorganization, inflammation of actin filaments, and also provoke the inflammatory cytokines like IL-1β, IL-6, IL-8, and TNF-α with resultant disruption in cell morphology and initiation of havoc inflammatory responses. PtNPs also modulate the IGF-1 dependent signal transduction pathways (Labrador-Rached et al. 2018).

Often, NPs, after entering the cells can get converted into smaller size or shapes and exert various toxic effects. TEM can be used to trace morphology and localization of NPs inside cells. Chaves et al. (Lopez-Chaves et al. 2018) showed that gold NPs after 16 h of exposure to cells (HepG2, HT-29), entered inside the cytosol from extracellular matrix. Post entry, the NPs got degraded into lower molecular weight particles and relocated inside the nucleus and also on lipid droplets. These AuNPs induced cytotoxicity by increase in ROS production, lipid peroxidation, DNA damage, and carbonyl group formation. As far as NP deposition in organs was concerned, size plays an important role. For instance, in liver and kidney, AuNPs of size 10 nm and 30 nm were found to be accumulated more while in intestine 10 nm was significantly higher. In spleen on the contrary, 60 nm particles were found abundant. In this study, AuNPs did not invoke any inflammatory response or caused any change in biochemical parameters (like glucose, urea, uric acid, triglycerides, albumin, cholesterol, γ-GT, alkaline phosphatase, GOT, and GPT) in the body of experimental animals and were found to be expelled via feces and urine (Lopez-Chaves et al. 2018).

Finally, these reports about toxic effects of NPs concomitantly raise questions about their possible effects on growth and reproduction of organisms as well as their teratogenic effects (Ema et al. 2017). Accumulation of AgNPs on testes of male mice and ovaries of female mice not only points out their effects on reproductive development of organisms but also gives a clue that these NPs can be transmitted to the next generation offsprings through germ cells. Time of exposure of NPs during gestation also plays a significant role in effect of NPs on fetuses. Exposure during early gestation led to accumulation in yolk sac, and exposure during late gestation led to accumulation in pre-natal and post-natal offspring. Pregnant mice, administered with AgNPs, possessed these NPs in breast milk and placenta. Further, delayed physical development and impaired cognitive behavior were noticeable in offsprings when pregnant mothers were exposed to AgNPs (Ema et al. 2017).

8.5 Challenges and Future Perspectives

Although the above mentioned nanomedicines have shown appreciable potential for melanoma treatment, yet health care practitioners are still apprehensive about their translation to clinical practices. This is majorly because the nanomedicines are laden with numerous challenges at various steps, starting from characterization and affectivity to safety and manufacturability. Drawbacks in the synthesis process such as difficulty to produce nanoparticles at large scale, poor stability, lack of batch-to-batch consistency, toxic chemicals, and adverse synthesis conditions impart toxicity to nanoparticles (Wang et al. 2013, 2016).

At the biological level, non-specificity, biocompatibility, evaluation of affective dose range, reactivity with biomolecules, non-uniform co-relationship between in vitro and in vivo experimental outcomes, etc., should not be ignored. These factors were serious obstacles in the path to successful patient outcomes. However, a large number of studies is being carried out, simultaneously, at both cellular and molecular level brings out convincing results about superior efficacy, safety, physicochemical properties, and pharmacodynamic profiles of nanomedicines. Further, nanomedicines have other advantages such as high transport efficacy through fine blood vessels and lymphatic endothelium. They have higher accumulation in blood and target tissues, longer circulation time, and ability to bind to targeted biomolecules, biocompatibility, reduced inflammation, longer half-life, and immune reaction in the body (Choi and Han 2018; Chowdhury et al. 2017; Howard et al. 2014; Onoue et al. 2014). All these advantages emphasize the benefits of nanotherapy over conventional treatment strategies. Taken together, the breakthrough of nanomedicine has the potential to change the course of therapeutics and drug delivery in the coming decades.

8.6 Conclusion

Failure of standard treatment strategies for melanoma to improve patient outcome has compelled doctors and scientists to turn their heads towards alternative approaches for dealing with the disease. In this regard, the unprecedented progress of nanomedicine in theranostic applications of many diseases encouraged researchers to explore their therapeutic applications in invincible diseases like cancer. To this end, this book chapter sheds light on the recent advances in adaptations of noble metal nanoparticles (Au, Ag, Pt) in therapeutics and diagnosis of melanoma. Owing to their facile methods of synthesis via chemical as well as biological routes and intrinsic functional attributes like optical, electronic, thermal, spectral, and chemical properties, they have garnered huge interest in translational scientific community, leading to exploration of their applications in biomedicine and biotechnology. Additionally, ease of modulation in terms of size, shape, and surface functionalization endowed them for clinical diagnostics and therapeutic applications in many diseases including melanoma. Hence, we have demonstrated numerous promising in vitro and in vivo reports of noble metal nanoparticles on melanoma treatment that may serve as milestones towards their clinical applications. Nevertheless, the majority of the nanodrugs are still to be approved by FDA. However, we have also emphasized the importance of gaining proper know-how about their optimization, characterization, and pharmacokinetics before their translation into clinical trials.

Acknowledgement Financial support from Nano Mission-DST (SR/NM/NS-1252/2013; GAP 570), New Delhi, to C.R.P. is duly acknowledged. A.R. is thankful to ICMR, New Delhi for supporting her Senior Research Fellowship and P.B.T. is thankful to CSIR, New Delhi for supporting her Senior Research Fellowship. We thank Director, CSIR-IICT (Ms. No. IICT/Pubs./2020/185, dated July 3, 2020) for providing all the required facilities to carry out the work.

References

Adams TG, Casagrande R (2019) Modeling the optimum Prussian blue treatment for acute radiation syndrome following 137Cs ingestion. Health Phys 116(1):88–95

Agarwal H, Nakara A, Shanmugam VK (2019) Anti-inflammatory mechanism of various metal and metal oxide nanoparticles synthesized using plant extracts: a review. Biomed Pharmacother 109:2561–2572

Ahmad MZ, Akhter S, Jain GK, Rahman M, Pathan SA, Ahmad FJ, Khar RK (2010) Metallic nanoparticles: technology overview & drug delivery applications in oncology. Expert Opin Drug Deliv 7(8):927–942

Ahmed KBA, Raman T, Anbazhagan V (2016) Platinum nanoparticles inhibit bacteria proliferation and rescue zebrafish from bacterial infection. RSC Adv 6(50):44415–44424

Aishwarya S, Sanjay K (2018) Conjugation study of 5-aminolevulinic acid with microbial synthesized gold nanoparticles to evaluate its effect on skin melanoma and epidermoid carcinoma cell lines using photodynamic cancer therapy. Gold Bull 51(1-2):11–19

Alarifi S, Ali D, Alkahtani S, Almeer RS (2017) ROS-mediated apoptosis and genotoxicity induced by palladium nanoparticles in human skin malignant melanoma cells. Oxidative Med Cell Longev 2017:8439098

Ali D, Alarifi S, Alkahtani S, AlKahtane AA, Almalik A (2015) Cerium oxide nanoparticles induce oxidative stress and genotoxicity in human skin melanoma cells. Cell Biochem Biophys 71 (3):1643–1651

Alshatwi AA, Vaiyapuri Subbarayan P, Ramesh E, Al-Hazzani AA, Alsaif MA, Alwarthan AA (2012) Al2O3 nanoparticles induce mitochondria-mediated cell death and upregulate the expression of signaling genes in human mesenchymal stem cells. J Biochem Mol Toxicol 26 (11):469–476

Alshatwi AA, Athinarayanan J, Subbarayan PV (2015) Green synthesis of platinum nanoparticles that induce cell death and G2/M-phase cell cycle arrest in human cervical cancer cells. J Mater Sci Mater Med 26(1):7

Alvi SB, Appidi T, Deepak BP, Rajalakshmi P, Minhas G, Singh SP, Khan N (2019) The "nano to micro" transition of hydrophobic curcumin crystals leading to in situ adjuvant depots for Au-liposome nanoparticle mediated enhanced photothermal therapy. Biomater Sci 7 (9):3866–3875

Amarnath K, Kumar J, Reddy T, Mahesh V, Ayyappan SR, Nellore J (2012) Synthesis and characterization of chitosan and grape polyphenols stabilized palladium nanoparticles and their antibacterial activity. Colloids Surf B Biointerfaces 92:254–261

Anantharaj S, Sakthikumar K, Elangovan A, Ravi G, Karthik T, Kundu S (2016) Ultra-small rhenium nanoparticles immobilized on DNA scaffolds: an excellent material for surface enhanced Raman scattering and catalysis studies. J Colloid Interface Sci 483:360–373

Augustine R, Dominic EA, Reju I, Kaimal B, Kalarikkal N, Thomas S (2014) Investigation of angiogenesis and its mechanism using zinc oxide nanoparticle-loaded electrospun tissue engineering scaffolds. RSC Adv 4(93):51528–51536

Balakrishnan S, Mukherjee S, Das S, Bhat FA, Raja Singh P, Patra CR, Arunakaran J (2017) Gold nanoparticles–conjugated quercetin induces apoptosis via inhibition of EGFR/PI3K/Akt–mediated pathway in breast cancer cell lines (MCF-7 and MDA-MB-231). Cell Biochem Funct 35(4):217–231

Barui AK, Jhelum P, Nethi SK, Das T, Bhattacharya D, Karri S, Patra CR (2020) Potential therapeutic application of zinc oxide nanoflowers in the cerebral ischemia rat model through neuritogenic and neuroprotective properties. Bioconjug Chem 31(3):895–906

Behnam MA, Emami F, Sobhani Z, Dehghanian AR (2018) The application of titanium dioxide (TiO2) nanoparticles in the photo-thermal therapy of melanoma cancer model. Iran J Basic Med Sci 21(11):1133

Bertrand N, Wu J, Xu X, Kamaly N, Farokhzad OC (2014) Cancer nanotechnology: the impact of passive and active targeting in the era of modern cancer biology. Adv Drug Deliv Rev 66:2–25

Bharathiraja S, Bui NQ, Manivasagan P, Moorthy MS, Mondal S, Seo H, Lee KD (2018) Multimodal tumor-homing chitosan oligosaccharide-coated biocompatible palladium nanoparticles for photo-based imaging and therapy. Sci Rep 8(1):1–16

Blanco E, Shen H, Ferrari M (2015) Principles of nanoparticle design for overcoming biological barriers to drug delivery. Nat Biotechnol 33(9):941

Bocate KP, Reis GF, de Souza PC, Junior AGO, Durán N, Nakazato G, Panagio LA (2019) Antifungal activity of silver nanoparticles and simvastatin against toxigenic species of Aspergillus. Int J Food Microbiol 291:79–86

Borowik A, Banasiuk R, Derewonko N, Rychlowski M, Krychowiak-Masnicka M, Wyrzykowski D, Piosik J (2019) Interactions of newly synthesized platinum nanoparticles with ICR-191 and their potential application. Sci Rep 9(1):1–11

Busam KG (2018) Superficial spreading melanoma pathology of melanocytic tumors, vol 1. Elsevier, Philadelphia, p 432

Buttacavoli M, Albanese NN, Di Cara G, Alduina R, Faleri C, Gallo M, Baldi F (2018) Anticancer activity of biogenerated silver nanoparticles: an integrated proteomic investigation. Oncotarget 9(11):9685

Capanema NS, Carvalho IC, Mansur AA, Carvalho SM, Lage AP, Mansur HS (2019) Hybrid hydrogel composed of carboxymethylcellulose–silver nanoparticles–doxorubicin for anticancer and antibacterial therapies against melanoma skin cancer cells. ACS Appl Nano Mater 2 (11):7393–7408

Carron S, Bloemen M, Vander Elst L, Laurent S, Verbiest T, Parac-Vogt TN (2015) Potential theranostic and multimodal iron oxide nanoparticles decorated with rhenium–bipyridine and–phenanthroline complexes. J Mater Chem B 3(21):4370–4376

Chen W, Qin M, Chen X, Wang Q, Zhang Z, Sun X (2018) Combining photothermal therapy and immunotherapy against melanoma by polydopamine-coated Al2O3 nanoparticles. Theranostics 8(8):2229

Cheng Y, Chang Y, Feng Y, Liu N, Sun X, Feng Y, Zhang H (2017) Simulated sunlight-mediated photodynamic therapy for melanoma skin cancer by titanium-dioxide-nanoparticle–gold-nanocluster–graphene heterogeneous nanocomposites. Small 13(20):1603935

Choi YH, Han H-K (2018) Nanomedicines: current status and future perspectives in aspect of drug delivery and pharmacokinetics. J Pharm Investig 48(1):43–60

Choleva TG, Gatselou VA, Tsogas GZ, Giokas DL (2018) Intrinsic peroxidase-like activity of rhodium nanoparticles, and their application to the colorimetric determination of hydrogen peroxide and glucose. Microchim Acta 185(1):22

Chowdhury A, Kunjiappan S, Panneerselvam T, Somasundaram B, Bhattacharjee C (2017) Nanotechnology and nanocarrier-based approaches on treatment of degenerative diseases. Int Nano Lett 7(2):91–122

Christopherson K, Malyapa RS, Werning JW, Morris CG, Kirwan J, Mendenhall WM (2015) Radiation therapy for mucosal melanoma of the head and neck. Am J Clin Oncol 38(1):87–89

Cozzi S, Escarpa AS, Parra DL, Jamal DN, Mitjana JMC, Edo FG, Miguelez CG (2019) Association between inflammatory bowel disease and uveal melanoma: case report of two young adults and a literature review. Rep Pract Oncol Radiother 24(1):56–59

Cui M, Zhou J, Zhao Y, Song Q (2017) Facile synthesis of iridium nanoparticles with superior peroxidase-like activity for colorimetric determination of H2O2 and xanthine. Sensors Actuators B Chem 243:203–210

D'Orazio JA, Marsch A, Veith JLWB (2011) Skin pigmentation and melanoma risk. In: Advances in malignant melanoma-clinical research perspective. IntechOpen, London, pp 39–68

Daneshvar F, Salehi F, Karimi M, Vais RD, Mosleh-Shirazi M, Sattarahmady N (2020) Combined X-ray radiotherapy and laser photothermal therapy of melanoma cancer cells using dual-sensitization of platinum nanoparticles. J Photochem Photobiol B Biol 203:111737

Das S, Roy A, Barui AK, Alabbasi MMA, Kuncha M, Sistla R, Patra CR (2020) Anti-angiogenic vanadium pentoxide nanoparticles for the treatment of melanoma and their in vivo toxicity study. Nanoscale 12(14):7604–7621

Davies H, Bignell GR, Cox C, Stephens P, Edkins S, Clegg S, Bottomley W (2002) Mutations of the BRAF gene in human cancer. Nature 417(6892):949–954

Day ES, Bickford LR, Slater JH, Riggall NS, Drezek RA, West JL (2010) Antibody-conjugated gold-gold sulfide nanoparticles as multifunctional agents for imaging and therapy of breast cancer. Int J Nanomedicine 5:445

Devi RV, Doble M, Verma RS (2015) Nanomaterials for early detection of cancer biomarker with special emphasis on gold nanoparticles in immunoassays/sensors. Biosens Bioelectron 68:688–698

Din MI, Rehan R (2017) Synthesis, characterization, and applications of copper nanoparticles. Anal Lett 50(1):50–62

Domingues B, Lopes JM, Soares P, Pópulo H (2018) Melanoma treatment in review. ImmunoTargets Ther 7:35

Duan X, Liao Y, Liu T, Yang H, Liu Y, Chen Y, Wu T (2020) Zinc oxide nanoparticles synthesized from Cardiospermum halicacabum and its anticancer activity in human melanoma cells (A375) through the modulation of apoptosis pathway. J Photochem Photobiol B Biol 202:111718

El-Kenawy AE-M, Constantin C, Hassan SM, Mostafa AM, Neves AF, de Araújo TG, Neagu M (2017) Nanomedicine in melanoma: current trends and future perspectives cutaneous melanoma: etiology and therapy. Codon Publications, Singapore

El-Readi MZ, Althubiti MA (2019) Cancer nanomedicine: a new era of successful targeted therapy. J Nanomater 2019:4927312

Ema M, Okuda H, Gamo M, Honda K (2017) A review of reproductive and developmental toxicity of silver nanoparticles in laboratory animals. Reprod Toxicol 67:149–164

Fakhar-e-Alam M, Akram MW, Iqbal S, Alimgeer K, Atif M, Sultana K, Wang ZM (2017) Empirical modeling of physiochemical immune response of multilayer zinc oxide nanomaterials under UV exposure to melanoma and foreskin fibroblasts. Sci Rep 7:46603

Fan M, Liang X, Li Z, Wang H, Yang D, Shi B (2015) Chlorambucil gemcitabine conjugate nanomedicine for cancer therapy. Eur J Pharm Sci 79:20–26

Farooq MU, Novosad V, Rozhkova EA, Wali H, Ali A, Fateh AA, Wang Z (2018) Gold nanoparticles-enabled efficient dual delivery of anticancer therapeutics to HeLa cells. Sci Rep 8(1):1–12

Freedberg DE, Rigas SH, Russak J, Gai W, Kaplow M, Osman I, Busam K (2008) Frequent p16-independent inactivation of p14ARF in human melanoma. J Natl Cancer Inst 100 (11):784–795

Garnett MC, Kallinteri P (2006) Nanomedicines and nanotoxicology: some physiological principles. Occup Med 56(5):307–311

Globocan (2019) India cancer statistics the global cancer observatory: World Health Organization

Golombek SK, May J-N, Theek B, Appold L, Drude N, Kiessling F, Lammers T (2018) Tumor targeting via EPR: strategies to enhance patient responses. Adv Drug Deliv Rev 130:17–38

Gopinath K, Karthika V, Gowri S, Senthilkumar V, Kumaresan S, Arumugam A (2014) Antibacterial activity of ruthenium nanoparticles synthesized using Gloriosa superba L. leaf extract. Chemistry 4(1):83

Gottesman MM (2002) Mechanisms of cancer drug resistance. Annu Rev Med 53(1):615–627

Gulla SK, Kotcherlakota R, Nimushakavi S, Nimmu NV, Khalid S, Patra CR, Chaudhuri A (2018) Au-CGKRK nanoconjugates for combating cancer through T-cell-driven therapeutic RNA interference. ACS Omega 3(8):8663–8676

Gulla SK, Rao BR, Moku G, Jinka S, Nimmu NV, Khalid S, Chaudhuri A (2019) In vivo targeting of DNA vaccines to dendritic cells using functionalized gold nanoparticles. Biomater Sci 7 (3):773–788

Guo J, Rahme K, He Y, Li L-L, Holmes JD, O'Driscoll CM (2017) Gold nanoparticles enlighten the future of cancer theranostics. Int J Nanomedicine 12:6131

Gupta K, Chundawat TS (2019) Bio-inspired synthesis of platinum nanoparticles from fungus Fusarium oxysporum: its characteristics, potential antimicrobial, antioxidant and photocatalytic activities. Mater Res Exp 6(10):1050–1056

Gupta B, Kumari A, Belwal S, Singh R, Fahmi N (2020) Synthesis, characterization of platinum (II) complexes of Schiff base ligands and evaluation of cytotoxic activity of platinum nanoparticles. Inorganic and Nano-Metal. Chemistry 50:1–12

GVR (2017) Melanoma therapeutics market analysis by therapy, by drugs (Opdivo, Yervoy, Mekinist+Tafinlar, Keytruda, Cotellic, Zelboraf, Imlygic, Generics), and segment forecasts, 2018–2025 Market Analysis Report, p 100

Howard M, Zern BJ, Anselmo AC, Shuvaev VV, Mitragotri S, Muzykantov V (2014) Vascular targeting of nanocarriers: perplexing aspects of the seemingly straightforward paradigm. ACS Nano 8(5):4100–4132

Ivanković S, Musić S, Gotić M, Ljubešić N (2006) Cytotoxicity of nanosize V2O5 particles to selected fibroblast and tumor cells. Toxicol In Vitro 20(3):286–294

Janetka W, Benson M (2018) Extracellular targeting of cell signaling in cancer. Wiley Online Library, Hoboken

Jiang J, Pi J, Cai J (2018) The advancing of zinc oxide nanoparticles for biomedical applications. Bioinorg Chem Appl 2018:1062562

Kalluru P, Vankayala R, Chiang C-S, Hwang KC (2016) Nano-graphene oxide-mediated In vivo fluorescence imaging and bimodal photodynamic and photothermal destruction of tumors. Biomaterials 95:1–10

Kang S, Shin W, Choi M-H, Ahn M, Kim Y-K, Kim S, Jang H (2018) Morphology-controlled synthesis of rhodium nanoparticles for cancer phototherapy. ACS Nano 12(7):6997–7008

Khazaei Z, Ghorat F, Jarrahi A, Adineh H, Sohrabivafa M, Goodarzi E (2019) Global incidence and mortality of skin cancer by histological subtype and its relationship with the human development index (HDI); an ecology study in 2018. World Cancer Res J 6:13

Kim S-R, Kim E-H (2017) Gold nanoparticles as dose-enhancement agent for kilovoltage X-ray therapy of melanoma. Int J Radiat Biol 93(5):517–526

Kim SM, Faix PH, Schnitzer JE (2017) Overcoming key biological barriers to cancer drug delivery and efficacy. J Control Release 267:15–30

Kimmel JN, Taft TH, Keefer L (2016) Inflammatory bowel disease and skin cancer: an assessment of patient risk factors, knowledge, and skin practices. J Skin Cancer 2016:4632037

Kirkwood JM, Tarhini AA, Panelli MC, Moschos SJ, Zarour HM, Butterfield LH, Gogas HJ (2008) Next generation of immunotherapy for melanoma. J Clin Oncol 26(20):3445–3455

Kora AJ, Rastogi L (2018) Peroxidase activity of biogenic platinum nanoparticles: a colorimetric probe towards selective detection of mercuric ions in water samples. Sensors Actuators B Chem 254:690–700

Kostova I (2009) Titanium and vanadium complexes as anticancer agents. Anti Cancer Agents Med Chem 9(8):827–842

Kotcherlakota R, Nimushakavi S, Roy A, Yadavalli HC, Mukherjee S, Haque S, Patra CR (2019a) Biosynthesized gold nanoparticles: in vivo study of near-infrared fluorescence (NIR)-based bio-imaging and cell labeling applications. ACS Biomater Sci Eng 5(10):5439–5452

Kotcherlakota R, Vydiam K, Jeyalakshmi Srinivasan D, Mukherjee S, Roy A, Kuncha M, Patra CR (2019b) Restoration of p53 function in ovarian cancer mediated by gold nanoparticle-based EGFR targeted gene delivery system. ACS Biomater Sci Eng 5(7):3631–3644

Labala S, Jose A, Venuganti VVK (2016) Transcutaneous iontophoretic delivery of STAT3 siRNA using layer-by-layer chitosan coated gold nanoparticles to treat melanoma. Colloids Surf B: Biointerfaces 146:188–197

Labala S, Jose A, Chawla SR, Khan MS, Bhatnagar S, Kulkarni OP, Venuganti VVK (2017) Effective melanoma cancer suppression by iontophoretic co-delivery of STAT3 siRNA and imatinib using gold nanoparticles. Int J Pharm 525(2):407–417

Labrador-Rached CJ, Browning RT, Braydich-Stolle LK, Comfort KK (2018) Toxicological implications of platinum nanoparticle exposure: stimulation of intracellular stress, inflammatory response, and akt signaling in vitro. J Toxicol 2018:1367801

Lara P, Palma-Florez S, Salas-Huenuleo E, Polakovicova I, Guerrero S, Lobos-Gonzalez L, Varas-Godoy M (2020) Gold nanoparticle based double-labeling of melanoma extracellular vesicles to

determine the specificity of uptake by cells and preferential accumulation in small metastatic lung tumors. J Nanobiotechnol 18(1):1–17
Lee AY, Jeffrey (2010) Soft tissue tumors of the hand and wrist. In: Slutsky D (ed) Principles and practice of wrist surgery. Elsevier, Berkeley, p 720
Leonardi GC, Falzone L, Salemi R, Zanghì A, Spandidos DA, Mccubrey JA, Libra M (2018) Cutaneous melanoma: from pathogenesis to therapy. Int J Oncol 52(4):1071–1080
Li J, Wang Y, Liang R, An X, Wang K, Shen G, Tao J (2015) Recent advances in targeted nanoparticles drug delivery to melanoma. Nanomedicine 11(3):769–794
Lin C-X, Yang S-Y, Gu J-L, Meng J, Xu H-Y, Cao J-M (2017) The acute toxic effects of silver nanoparticles on myocardial transmembrane potential, I Na and I K1 channels and heart rhythm in mice. Nanotoxicology 11(6):827–837
Lin C-X, Gu J-L, Cao J-M (2019) The acute toxic effects of platinum nanoparticles on ion channels, transmembrane potentials of cardiomyocytes in vitro and heart rhythm in vivo in mice. Int J Nanomedicine 14:5595
Liu Y, Sheikh MS (2014) Melanoma: molecular pathogenesis and therapeutic management. Mol Cell Pharmacol 6(3):228
Liu H, Zhang Y, Zheng S, Weng Z, Ma J, Li Y, Zheng W (2016) Detention of copper by sulfur nanoparticles inhibits the proliferation of A375 malignant melanoma and MCF-7 breast cancer cells. Biochem Biophys Res Commun 477(4):1031–1037
Liu Q, Xu N, Liu L, Li J, Zhang Y, Shen C, Tao J (2017) Dacarbazine-loaded hollow mesoporous silica nanoparticles grafted with folic acid for enhancing antimetastatic melanoma response. ACS Appl Mater Interfaces 9(26):21673–21687
Long GV, Stroyakovskiy D, Gogas H, Levchenko E, De Braud F, Larkin J, Grob J-J (2015) Dabrafenib and trametinib versus dabrafenib and placebo for Val600 BRAF-mutant melanoma: a multicentre, double-blind, phase 3 randomised controlled trial. Lancet 386(9992):444–451
Lopez-Chaves C, Soto-Alvaredo J, Montes-Bayon M, Bettmer J, Llopis J, Sanchez-Gonzalez C (2018) Gold nanoparticles: distribution, bioaccumulation and toxicity. In vitro and in vivo studies. Nanomedicine 14(1):1–12
Lu W, Huang Q, Ku G, Wen X, Zhou M, Guzatov D, Wang LV (2010) Photoacoustic imaging of living mouse brain vasculature using hollow gold nanospheres. Biomaterials 31(9):2617–2626
Mahdavi B, Shokrani P, Hejazi SH, Talebi A, Taheri A (2019) Doxorubicin-loaded PVP coated Gd2O3 NPs for effective chemoradiotherapy in melanoma. J Drug Deliv Sci Technol 53:101189
Marks JG, Miller JJ (2017) Lookingbill and Marks' principles of dermatology e-book. Elsevier Health Sciences, Amsterdam
Maurizi L, Papa A-L, Boudon J, Sudhakaran S, Pruvot B, Vandroux D, Millot N (2018) Toxicological risk assessment of emerging nanomaterials: cytotoxicity, cellular uptake, effects on biogenesis and cell organelle activity, acute toxicity and biodistribution of oxide nanoparticles. Unraveling the safety profile of nanoscale particles and materials-from biomedical to environmental applications
Miao Z, Chen S, Xu C-Y, Ma Y, Qian H, Xu Y, Lu Y (2019) PEGylated rhenium nanoclusters: a degradable metal photothermal nanoagent for cancer therapy. Chem Sci 10(21):5435–5443
Mioc M, Pavel IZ, Ghiulai R, Coricovac DE, Farcaş C, Mihali C-V, Dehelean CA (2018) The cytotoxic effects of betulin-conjugated gold nanoparticles as stable formulations in normal and melanoma cells. Front Pharmacol 9:429
Mostafalou S, Mohammadi H, Ramazani A, Abdollahi M (2013) Different biokinetics of nanomedicines linking to their toxicity; an overview. Springer, New York
Mukherjee S, Sushma V, Patra S, Barui AK, Bhadra MP, Sreedhar B, Patra CR (2012) Green chemistry approach for the synthesis and stabilization of biocompatible gold nanoparticles and their potential applications in cancer therapy. Nanotechnology 23(45):455103
Mukherjee S, Vinothkumar B, Prashanthi S, Bangal PR, Sreedhar B, Patra CR (2013) Potential therapeutic and diagnostic applications of one-step in situ biosynthesized gold nanoconjugates (2-in-1 system) in cancer treatment. RSC Adv 3(7):2318–2329

Mukherjee S, Chowdhury D, Kotcherlakota R, Patra S (2014) Potential theranostics application of bio-synthesized silver nanoparticles (4-in-1 system). Theranostics 4(3):316
Mukherjee S, Rao BR, Sreedhar B, Paik P, Patra CR (2015) Copper Prussian blue analogue: investigation into multifunctional activities for biomedical applications. Chem Commun 51 (34):7325–7328
Mukherjee S, Sau S, Madhuri D, Bollu VS, Madhusudana K, Sreedhar B, Patra CR (2016) Green synthesis and characterization of monodispersed gold nanoparticles: toxicity study, delivery of doxorubicin and its bio-distribution in mouse model. J Biomed Nanotechnol 12(1):165–181
Mukherjee S, Kotcherlakota R, Haque S, Das S, Nuthi S, Bhattacharya D, Patra CR (2019) Silver prussian blue analogue nanoparticles (SPBANPs): rationally designed advanced nanomedicine for multifunctional biomedical applications. ACS Biomater Sci Eng 6(1):690–704
Mukherjee S, Kotcherlakota R, Haque S, Bhattacharya D, Kumar JM, Chakravarty S, Patra CR (2020) Improved delivery of doxorubicin using rationally designed PEGylated platinum nanoparticles for the treatment of melanoma. Mater Sci Eng 108:110375
Mukhopadhyay R, Kazi J, Debnath MC (2018) Synthesis and characterization of copper nanoparticles stabilized with Quisqualis indica extract: evaluation of its cytotoxicity and apoptosis in B16F10 melanoma cells. Biomed Pharmacother 97:1373–1385
Nandakumar V, Vettriselvi V, Doble M (2014) Toxicity of high glycolic poly (DL-lactic-co-glycolic acid) stabilized ruthenium nanoparticles against human promyelocytic leukemia cells. RSC Adv 4(22):11438–11443
Naserzadeh P, Ansari Esfeh F, Kaviani M, Ashtari K, Kheirbakhsh R, Salimi A, Pourahmad J (2018) Single-walled carbon nanotube, multi-walled carbon nanotube and Fe2O3 nanoparticles induced mitochondria mediated apoptosis in melanoma cells. Cutan Ocul Toxicol 37 (2):157–166
Nemmar A, Hoet PM, Vanquickenborne B, Dinsdale D, Thomeer M, Hoylaerts M, Nemery B (2002) Passage of inhaled particles into the blood circulation in humans. Circulation 105 (4):411–414
Ni Q, Zhang F, Zhang Y, Zhu G, Wang Z, Teng Z, Lu G (2018) In situ shRNA synthesis on DNA–polylactide nanoparticles to treat multidrug resistant breast cancer. Adv Mater 30(10):1705737
Nie C, Du P, Zhao H, Xie H, Li Y, Yao L, Zhang M (2020) Ag@ TiO2 nanoprisms with highly efficient near-infrared photothermal conversion for melanoma therapy. Chemistry 15 (1):148–155
Niu J, Chu Y, Huang Y-F, Chong Y-S, Jiang Z-H, Mao Z-W, Gao J-Q (2017) Transdermal gene delivery by functional peptide-conjugated cationic gold nanoparticle reverses the progression and metastasis of cutaneous melanoma. ACS Appl Mater Interfaces 9(11):9388–9401
Onoue S, Yamada S, Chan H-K (2014) Nanodrugs: pharmacokinetics and safety. Int J Nanomedicine 9:1025
Oves M, Arshad M, Khan MS, Ahmed AS, Azam A, Ismail IM (2015) Anti-microbial activity of cobalt doped zinc oxide nanoparticles: targeting water borne bacteria. J Saudi Chem Soc 19 (5):581–588
Pan T, Li X, Jankovic J (2011) The association between Parkinson's disease and melanoma. Int J Cancer 128(10):2251–2260
Patra S, Mukherjee S, Barui AK, Ganguly A, Sreedhar B, Patra CR (2015) Green synthesis, characterization of gold and silver nanoparticles and their potential application for cancer therapeutics. Mater Sci Eng 53:298–309
Pourmand A, Abdollahi M (2012) Current opinion on nanotoxicology. BioMed Central, London
Radziun E, Wilczyńska JD, Książek I, Nowak K, Anuszewska E, Kunicki A, Ząbkowski T (2011) Assessment of the cytotoxicity of aluminium oxide nanoparticles on selected mammalian cells. Toxicol In Vitro 25(8):1694–1700
Rouleau L, Berti R, Ng VW, Matteau-Pelletier C, Lam T, Saboural P, Tardif JC (2013) VCAM-1-targeting gold nanoshell probe for photoacoustic imaging of atherosclerotic plaque in mice. Contrast Media Mol Imaging 8(1):27–39

Ruiz AL, Garcia CB, Gallón SN, Webster TJ (2020) Novel silver-platinum nanoparticles for anticancer and antimicrobial applications. Int J Nanomedicine 15:169
Rybka JD (2019) Radiosensitizing properties of magnetic hyperthermia mediated by superparamagnetic iron oxide nanoparticles (SPIONs) on human cutaneous melanoma cell lines. Rep Pract Oncol Radiother 24(2):152–157
Safwat MA, Soliman GM, Sayed D, Attia MA (2018) Fluorouracil-loaded gold nanoparticles for the treatment of skin cancer: development, in vitro characterization, and in vivo evaluation in a mouse skin cancer xenograft model. Mol Pharm 15(6):2194–2205
Samarasinghe RM, Kanwar RK, Kanwar JR (2012) The role of nanomedicine in cell based therapeutics in cancer and inflammation. Int J Mol Cell Med 1(3):133
Santhoshkumar J, Agarwal H, Menon S, Rajeshkumar S, Kumar SV (2019) A biological synthesis of copper nanoparticles and its potential applications green synthesis, characterization and applications of nanoparticles. Elsevier, London, pp 199–221
Saravanan M, Barik SK, MubarakAli D, Prakash P, Pugazhendhi A (2018) Synthesis of silver nanoparticles from Bacillus brevis (NCIM 2533) and their antibacterial activity against pathogenic bacteria. Microb Pathog 116:221–226
Satzger I, Mattern A, Kuettler U, Weinspach D, Voelker B, Kapp A, Gutzmer R (2010) MicroRNA-15b represents an independent prognostic parameter and is correlated with tumor cell proliferation and apoptosis in malignant melanoma. Int J Cancer 126(11):2553–2562
Sharma V, Kaushik S, Pandit P, Dhull D, Yadav JP, Kaushik S (2019) Green synthesis of silver nanoparticles from medicinal plants and evaluation of their antiviral potential against chikungunya virus. Appl Microbiol Biotechnol 103(2):881–891
Shivashankarappa A, Sanjay KR (2019) Photodynamic therapy on skin melanoma and epidermoid carcinoma cells using conjugated 5-aminolevulinic acid with microbial synthesised silver nanoparticles. J Drug Target 27(4):434–441
Siegel RL, Miller KD, Jemal A (2019) Cancer statistics, 2019. CA Cancer J Clin 69(1):7–34
Singh SP, Alvi SB, Pemmaraju DB, Singh AD, Manda SV, Srivastava R, Rengan AK (2018) NIR triggered liposome gold nanoparticles entrapping curcumin as in situ adjuvant for photothermal treatment of skin cancer. Int J Biol Macromol 110:375–382
Spain E, Gilgunn S, Sharma S, Adamson K, Carthy E, O'Kennedy R, Forster RJ (2016) Detection of prostate specific antigen based on electrocatalytic platinum nanoparticles conjugated to a recombinant scFv antibody. Biosens Bioelectron 77:759–766
Strojan P (2010) Role of radiotherapy in melanoma management. Radiol Oncol 44(1):1–12
Sturm RA (2002) Skin colour and skin cancer–MC1R, the genetic link. Melanoma Res 12 (5):405–416
Su H, Liu D-D, Zhao M, Hu W-L, Xue S-S, Cao Q, Mao Z-W (2015) Dual-enzyme characteristics of polyvinylpyrrolidone-capped iridium nanoparticles and their cellular protective effect against H2O2-induced oxidative damage. ACS Appl Mater Interfaces 7(15):8233–8242
Subramaniyan SB, Ramani A, Ganapathy V, Anbazhagan V (2018) Preparation of self-assembled platinum nanoclusters to combat Salmonella typhi infection and inhibit biofilm formation. Colloids Surf B Biointerfaces 171:75–84
Tahir K, Nazir S, Ahmad A, Li B, Shah SAA, Khan AU, Khan FU (2016) Biodirected synthesis of palladium nanoparticles using Phoenix dactylifera leaves extract and their size dependent biomedical and catalytic applications. RSC Adv 6(89):85903–85916
Takebe H, Nishigori C, Tatsumi K (1989) Melanoma and other skin cancers in xeroderma pigmentosum patients and mutation in their cells. J Investig Dermatol 92:236S–238S
Takenaka S, Karg E, Roth C, Schulz H, Ziesenis A, Heinzmann U, Heyder J (2001) Pulmonary and systemic distribution of inhaled ultrafine silver particles in rats. Environ Health Perspect 109 (suppl 4):547–551
Tang JQ, Hou XY, Yang CS, Li YX, Xin Y, Guo WW, Jiang G (2017) Recent developments in nanomedicine for melanoma treatment. Int J Cancer 141(4):646–653

Tang J, Zhou H, Hou X, Wang L, Li Y, Pang Y, Liu Y (2018) Enhanced anti-tumor efficacy of temozolomide-loaded carboxylated poly (amido-amine) combined with photothermal/photodynamic therapy for melanoma treatment. Cancer Lett 423:16–26
Tarantola M, Pietuch A, Schneider D, Rother J, Sunnick E, Rosman C, Janshoff A (2011) Toxicity of gold-nanoparticles: synergistic effects of shape and surface functionalization on micromotility of epithelial cells. Nanotoxicology 5(2):254–268
Taruttis A, Herzog E, Razansky D, Ntziachristos V (2010) Real-time imaging of cardiovascular dynamics and circulating gold nanorods with multispectral optoacoustic tomography. Opt Express 18(19):19592–19602
Tawagi E, Massmann C, Chibli H, Nadeau JL (2015) Differential toxicity of gold-doxorubicin in cancer cells vs. cardiomyocytes as measured by real-time growth assays and fluorescence lifetime imaging microscopy (FLIM). Analyst 140(16):5732–5741
Valenzuela-Salas LM, Girón-Vázquez NG, García-Ramos JC, Torres-Bugarín O, Gómez C, Pestryakov A, Bogdanchikova N (2019) Antiproliferative and antitumour effect of nongenotoxic silver nanoparticles on melanoma models. Oxidative Med Cell Longev 2019:4528241
Van Elsas A, Hurwitz AA, Allison JP (1999) Combination immunotherapy of B16 melanoma using anti–cytotoxic T lymphocyte–associated antigen 4 (CTLA-4) and granulocyte/macrophage colony-stimulating factor (GM-CSF)-producing vaccines induces rejection of subcutaneous and metastatic tumors accompanied by autoimmune depigmentation. J Exp Med 190 (3):355–366
Vankayala R, Gollavelli G, Mandal BK (2013) Highly fluorescent and biocompatible iridium nanoclusters for cellular imaging. J Mater Sci 24(8):1993–2000
Wang R, Billone PS, Mullett WM (2013) Nanomedicine in action: an overview of cancer nanomedicine on the market and in clinical trials. J Nanomater 2013:629681
Wang D, Lin Z, Wang T, Yao Z, Qin M, Zheng S, & Lu W (2016) Where does the toxicity of metal oxide nanoparticles come from: the nanoparticles, the ions, or a combination of both? Journal of Hazardous Materials 308:328-334.
Wang D, Dong H, Li M, Cao Y, Yang F, Zhang K, Zhang X (2018) Erythrocyte–cancer hybrid membrane camouflaged hollow copper sulfide nanoparticles for prolonged circulation life and homotypic-targeting photothermal/chemotherapy of melanoma. ACS Nano 12(6):5241–5252
Watson RR, Preedy VR, Zibadi S (2018) Polyphenols: prevention and treatment of human disease. Academic, New York
Wilson MA, Schuchter LM (2016) Chemotherapy for melanoma melanoma. Springer, New York, pp 209–229
Woźniak A, Malankowska A, Nowaczyk G, Grześkowiak BF, Tuśnio K, Słomski R, Jurga S (2017) Size and shape-dependent cytotoxicity profile of gold nanoparticles for biomedical applications. J Mater Sci 28(6):92
Wu F, Zhu J, Li G, Wang J, Veeraraghavan VP, Krishna Mohan S, Zhang Q (2019) Biologically synthesized green gold nanoparticles from Siberian ginseng induce growth-inhibitory effect on melanoma cells (B16). Artif Cells Nanomed Biotechnol 47(1):3297–3305
Yan S, Xia P, Xu S, Zhang K, Li G, Cui L, Yin J (2018) Nanocomposite porous microcarriers based on strontium-substituted HA-g-poly (γ-benzyl-l-glutamate) for bone tissue engineering. ACS Appl Mater Interfaces 10(19):16270–16281
Yang L, Watts DJ (2005) Particle surface characteristics may play an important role in phytotoxicity of alumina nanoparticles. Toxicol Lett 158(2):122–132
Yang Y, Qin Z, Zeng W, Yang T, Cao Y, Mei C, Kuang Y (2017) Toxicity assessment of nanoparticles in various systems and organs. Nanotechnol Rev 6(3):279–289
Yu B, Wang Y, Yu X, Zhang H, Zhu J, Wang C, Zhu H (2017) Cuprous oxide nanoparticle-inhibited melanoma progress by targeting melanoma stem cells. Int J Nanomedicine 12:2553
Zhang M, Jin J, Chang Y-N, Chang X, Xing G (2014) Toxicological properties of nanomaterials. J Nanosci Nanotechnol 14(1):717–729

Zhang X, Teodoro JG, Nadeau JL (2015) Intratumoral gold-doxorubicin is effective in treating melanoma in mice. Nanomedicine 11(6):1365–1375

Zhang B, Hu Y, Pang Z (2017) Modulating the tumor microenvironment to enhance tumor nanomedicine delivery. Front Pharmacol 8:952

Zhang Y, Bush X, Yan B, Chen JA (2019) Gemcitabine nanoparticles promote antitumor immunity against melanoma. Biomaterials 189:48–59

Zhao S, Zhu X, Cao C, Sun J, Liu J (2018) Transferrin modified ruthenium nanoparticles with good biocompatibility for photothermal tumor therapy. J Colloid Interface Sci 511:325–334

Zhou Z, Li H, Wang K, Guo Q, Li C, Jiang H, Sun M (2017) Bioreducible cross-linked hyaluronic acid/calcium phosphate hybrid nanoparticles for specific delivery of siRNA in melanoma tumor therapy. ACS Appl Mater Interfaces 9(17):14576–14589

Zhu Y, Li W, Zhao X, Zhou Z, Wang Y, Cheng Y, Zhang Q (2017) Hyaluronic acid-encapsulated platinum nanoparticles for targeted photothermal therapy of breast cancer. J Biomed Nanotechnol 13(11):1457–1467

Ethics in Nanomedicine

9

Alakesh Das, Dikshita Deka, Syed Sana Abrar, Surajit Pathak, and Antara Banerjee

Abstract

Nanomedicine contributes exceptional possibilities for novel therapeutic management. Nanomedicine moderately interlocks, exceeds, and overlaps other medical curriculum. As various approaches in Nanomedicine had progressed with enormous promise toward theranostic interventions, ethical queries also arise in conjunction. Nanomedicine is a unique niche in various facets, but it comes along with indications of dangers and uncertainties not confronted in other fields of medical practice or analysis. Some intellectuals agree that progress in the field of nanotechnology may present several ethical challenges, while others dispute that these challenges are not recent and that nanotechnology generally echoes frequent bioethical impasses. The objective of this article is to analyze some of the ethical concerns associated with Nanomedicine application and to reveal the queries and recent developments on whether Nanomedicine yields further ethical challenges keeping in view the principle of medical ethics. Such a conclusion should have significance on professional strategy and regulatory approaches and designing the policies for application in the upcoming days.

Keywords

Nanomedicine · Ethics · Nanotechnology · Challenges · Safety · Societal risks · Translational impact

---

A. Das · D. Deka · S. S. Abrar · S. Pathak · A. Banerjee (✉)
Department of Medical Biotechnology, Faculty of Allied Health Sciences, Chettinad Academy of Research and Education (CARE), Chettinad Hospital and Research Institute (CHRI), Chennai, India
e-mail: antarabanerjee@chettinadhealthcity.com

A. Malik et al. (eds.), *Nanomedicine for Cancer Diagnosis and Therapy*,
https://doi.org/10.1007/978-981-15-7564-8_9

9.1 Introduction

Currently, Nanomedicine has been considered as advancing field in scientific analyses. Nanomedicine is an expansive field that includes the development of sensors for the detection and identification of biomarkers, nanocarriers, and nanoparticles for the detection/imaging of cancers and for the delivery of therapeutic molecules. Most of the ongoing arguments surrounding the ethical problems in the field of nanomedicine are subsequent of the former technologies, as for example information technology and biotechnology (Jamison 2009). Arguments also arise over either nanomedicine has any particular ethical problem, or the ethical problems of former technologies relate to nanoscience (Sechi et al. 2014). Scientists have broadly described the possible scenarios of the ethical issues that might coincide with the advancement of Nanoscience technology. Various analyses conducted in the field of Nano-toxicology have recommended the threats comprising the ill effects of nanoparticles on the environment, humans, and fish (Patra et al. 2010; Sandler 2009). Various biotechnology and pharmaceutical associations and government firms have begun analyzing and inspecting several Nanotechnology utilization in areas of Nanomedicine. As reported, many of the Nanomedicines have been accepted for cancer therapies or are recently being tested on human trials (Resnik and Tinkle 2007). It is supposed that the intended therapeutic potential for Nanomedicine can produce capable ill effects if the accuracy becomes improperly applied or if it has higher than just the required concentration. Bottom-up synthesis from the molecular level, based either on imitating biology or on integrating components from a living structure, enhances problems about hybrid mechanisms that integrate machine and human and also reduces the preference towards Nanomedicine (Bruce 2006). Since science and technology are dealing with nanoparticles synthesis and large-scale manufacturing for drug discovery, the field of Nanomedicine is rapidly expanding. Several developing nations have assigned a considerable quantity of funding for nanotechnological analyses. In this context, the ethical and law issues involving Nanomedicine should be taken into consideration to address the effects on the environment and humans and the public reactions.

This paper, therefore, represents the ethical issues relevant to the field of Nanomedicine. Till now, however, there have been few formal analyses, arguments, or thinking regarding the ethical and social problems associated with Nanomedicine all around the globe. Therefore, it implies that we need to consider evaluation for ethical training in nanomedicine as well as initial recommendations for medical ethics and research ethics preparations for clinicians and researchers as well as for experimental analyses in nano ethics.

9.2 Nanomedicine

In recent years, the field of nanomedical research has shown promising growth. Nanomedicine may be defined as the application of Nanotechnology to the area of medicine. The area of Nanomedicine is in its budding phase, as several products are

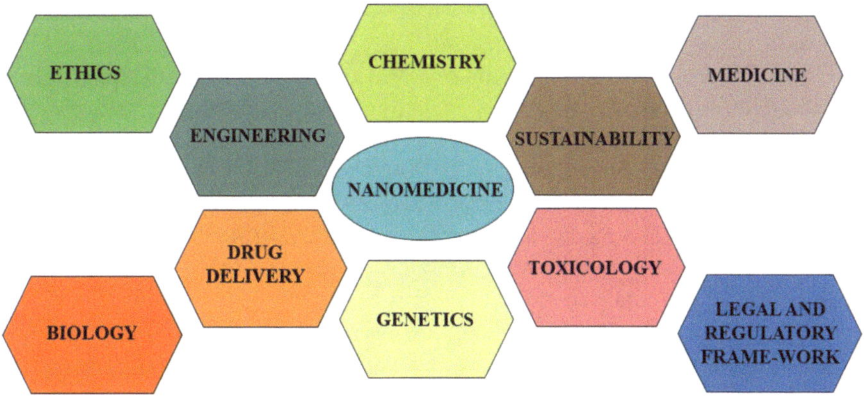

Fig. 9.1 Association of Nanomedicine with diverse fields

in the developmental stage. Development of sensors for single molecular observation, the use of nanoparticles and nanocarriers for identifying and imaging cancer, biomarkers, and ultrafast DNA sequencing are some of the many contributions of nanomedicine (Ferrari et al. 2009; Życiński 2006). Drugs like Doxil (Liposomal DOX), Lipusu (Liposomal PTX), and Abraxane (Nanoparticulate albumin/PTX) are centered out of Nanomedicine. Several such drugs have been approved by the FDA and European Medicines Agency (EMA), while the regulatory framework for these nano-enabled pharmaceutical products is being developed (Liu et al. 2016; Sharma et al. 2017). There are various kinds of organic and inorganic nanoparticles and nanomaterials like nanoshells, micelles, quantum dots, carbon nanotubes, tecto dendrimers, gold nanoparticles, etc., that are used in imaging diagnostic and several other medical applications. Nanomedicine has led to the integration of effective molecules that could not be used earlier because of being highly toxic (e.g., Mepact), exploitation of multiple mechanisms of action (e.g., Nanomag), increase in efficacy and reduction in dose and toxicity, controlled and site-specific drug targeting causing an even distribution within the body, and improvement in transport across the biological barriers. Nanomedicine thus has the potential to improve the bioavailability, dose-response, personalization, and targeting ability of conventional medicines (Ventola 2012b, 2017; Życiński 2006) and has been associated with diverse fields for application (Fig. 9.1). It can help in the advancement of detection and diagnosis of diseases, significantly improving human health.

9.3 Difference Between Nanotechnology and Nanomedicine

The convergence of various scientific fields like biology, chemistry, physics, mathematics, and engineering has led to the development of Nanotechnology. It mainly focuses on the investigation and manipulation of atoms, molecules, and submicroscopic particles that generally range within 1–100 nm. The National Nanotechnology

Initiative (NNI) of the USA describes it as a science of matter and phenomena occurring at the nanoscale level (Schottel and Karn 2016). In nanotechnology, scientists explore the natural quantum effects occurring at nanometric level, which can be effective on various properties, including biological, optical, and mechanical properties. These special characteristic properties of nanoscale materials make them different from their counterparts (Ventola 2012b).

Nanomedicine, however, is an interdisciplinary field formed by the combination of nanotechnology and medicine. It involves genomics, proteomics, molecular and cellular biology, along with bioengineering and material science. Nanomedicine deals with physiological processes at the nanoscale level and focuses on the working of biological molecules like antibodies, proteins, enzymes, and receptors. According to the European Science Foundation (ESF), Nanomedicine is the science and technology of diagnosis, treatment, and prevention of diseases, thus improving human health using molecular tools and knowledge of the human body (Resnik and Tinkle 2007; Satalkar et al. 2016).

9.4 Hype Versus Reality of Nanomedicine

Whenever a new technology is developed, a plethora of hype is created around its application. Nanomedicine has several assumptions around it, too, regarding the outcomes that this field can offer. James F Leary, in his own version of "Gartner's Hype Cycle" showed that ultimately reality takes over both hype and unfair criticism as it is based on a variety of real factors. According to him, the advancement in nanomedical technologies will create sophisticated and efficient drug delivery methods (Leary 2013). Some major hypes surrounding nanomedicine are that it will provide low cost, exceptional medical research equipment, the nanomachines will be programmed in a way to remove fatty deposits from our bloodstream and that the nanorobots which can provide protection to the human body against viruses will be a part of preventive medicine. Overall, Nanomedicine is expected to transform the existing medical diagnosis and drug delivery system. However, all this will only be turned into a reality with rational thinking and understanding of the nanoparticles, biological molecules of the human body and their interactions (Kuiken 2011; Życiński 2006). The ongoing research projects based around Nanomedicine can lead to a brighter future for medical diagnosis.

9.5 Nondiscrimination and Integrity of Nanomedicine

Ever since the concept came out, research on Nanotechnology has been experiencing a surprising advancement in several fields. The enormous advancement was accomplished by the pharmaceutical associations in the field of drug delivery, which is fabricating considerable aftermaths. At this period, due to the advancement in pharmacogenomics and pharmacogenetics: the drug delivery system (DDS) is under analysis, which brings into the spotlight the approaches of personalized medicine (PM) (Bawa and Johnson 2007; Bawa 2005; Patra et al. 2010). All these studies are being accomplished by the biggest pharmaceutical industries globally. In the year 2006, a budget of around 12.4 billion US Dollars was used, globally, by governments, associations, and investors, which is 13% higher than that spent in the year 2005 and the budgets are escalating each year. As the nanomedical commodities are very costly, the venture capitalists have to cover-up their investments; therefore, the nanomedical market is progressing only in developed nations. In developing nations however, the governments and their citizens cannot bear the nanomedical commodities. Thus, the consecutive query arises: how ethical is it to enforce extremely costly nanomedical therapies for medical systems and patients? This circumstance is generating a gap among the conditions of the health care structure in developed nations and that of the health care structure in developing nations. Moreover, an escalating count of specialists is migrating to developed nations to have access to novel nanotechnologies in the medical care structure (Graur et al. 2011). This will eventually cause a lack of researchers in developing nations. As a result, the recent medical sciences will be unapproachable for several people of lower socio-economic condition or for those in developing nations. However, in the future, there is a probable situation where only the rich will have permission to the new treatments, while the poor are declined even to have the insight of their diseases (Bawa 2005; Patra et al. 2010). On the other hand, intellectual property theft and biopiracy are also responsible for the inadequacy of necessary drugs to the poorly developed regions around the world (de SC and Nigel 2006; Sharma et al. 2017).

9.6 The Potentiality of Nanomedicine

Nanotechnology assures to benefit most industries and will have a specifically extensive effect on medicine and health care. The future effect of nanomedicine on society could be immense. Especially, Nanomedicine can enhance the quality of life of the patient, decrease socio-economic expenses correlated with healthcare, provide early recognition of pathological conditions, decrease the asperity of therapy, and lead to enhanced clinical results for the patient. Nanomedicine, in a wider sense, is the utilization of nanoscale technologies in medicinal practice, such as for detection, protection, and treatment of disease and to achieve an expanded insight of complex fundamental mechanisms of disease. Advancement in miniaturization of analytic tools, delivering nano therapies, enhanced computational and memory capacity, and enhancements in remote communications will be unified. These exertions will cross the new boundaries to the insight and practice of medicine. The fundamental aim is definitely extensive monitoring, repair, and enhancement of all biological systems of humans to improve the quality of life. Thus, Nanomedicine is not a single class of medical interference that can readily be evaluated from an ethical prospect. Nanomedicine will probably revive old questions about human improvement, justice, and dignity that have been raised several times before in the framework of pharmaceutics research, gene therapy, or cloning. Generally, Nanomedicine

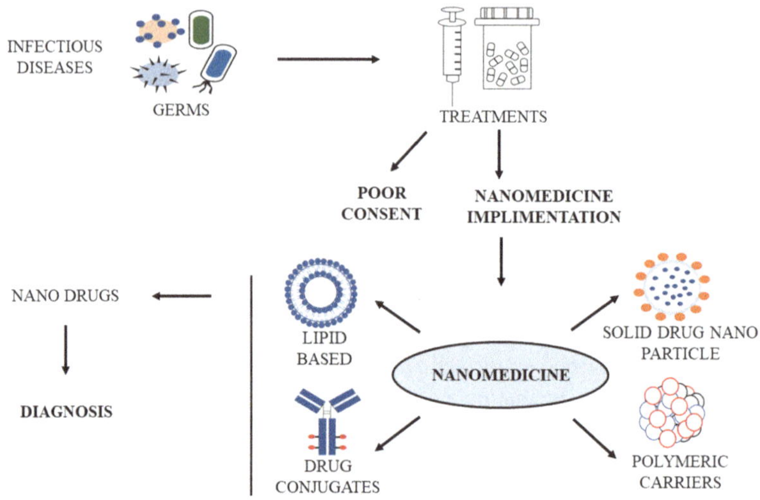

Fig. 9.2 Scope of applicability of Nanomedicine for Clinical application

interference comes under two major categories: diagnostic nanomedicine and therapeutic nanomedicine. Each of these technologies and their uses is specific, and in certain cases, novel ethical significance for their advancement, use, and approachability. The two leading types of Nanomedicine products that are presently in clinical trials are related to diagnostics and drug delivery (Bawa and Johnson 2009; Bawa et al. 2005; Sandler 2009; Sechi et al. 2014). The scope of applicability of Nanomedicine is explained in Fig. 9.2.

9.7 Biocompatibility and Toxicity of Nanostructures

The most extensively improved sector of Nanomedicine is the nano drug therapy and delivery system, which utilizes a broad range of substances to deliver effective agents to various parts of the human body. The action of nanomaterials is usually uncertain, as they may act in a different way in vivo organization when compared to in vitro system: nanoparticles can break down into smaller fragments that are lethal to the human body, or they may accumulate into larger fragments as well (Oberdörster et al. 2005a). The penetration capability and absorbance of the nano drugs at various barriers of the body are also to be considered during drug designing and testing (Fig. 9.3). Thus, it is ethically acceptable to design short- and long-term analysis to decide whether Nanomedicines actually are more efficient and secure for humans in comparison to conventional drugs. However, while running those trials, there may arise some other obstacles, such as difficulty with apprehension and insight with regard to the informed assent, given the complication of

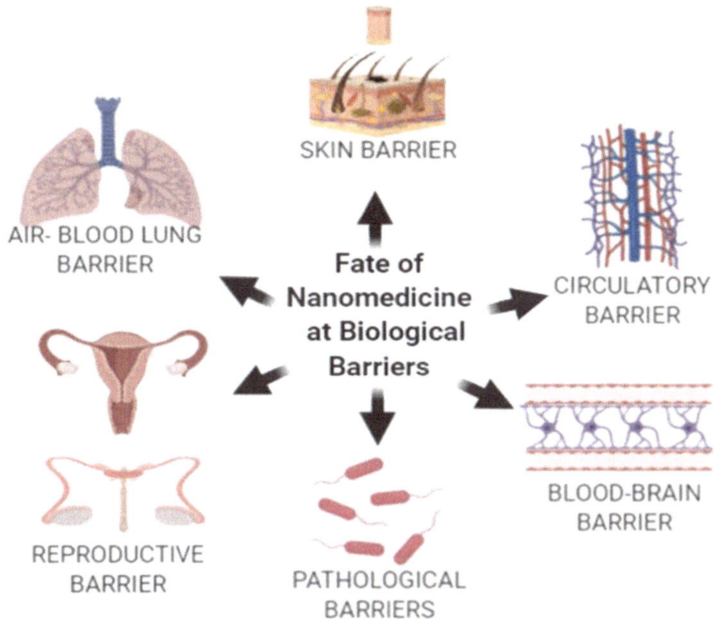

Fig. 9.3 Fate of Nano drugs to cross various barriers of the body (Created with BioRender.com)

nanotechnologies. Therefore, the long-term impacts of using Nanomedicines to date are still largely unexplained (Nel et al. 2006). To assure that the new drugs can be used securely by the people, Nanomedicine associations should be asked to conduct long-term analysis on nanomedical products followed by their initiation on the market. But this type of analysis is rarely practiced as it is not desired by current laws. Though it is clear that new approaches should be initiated, this should be done with much care and implementing safety guidelines, so as to avoid overregulating tendencies, as those would have an alarming impact on development, research, commercialization, exertion, and fair approach of the public towards Nanomedicines (Strom 2006; Ventola 2012b).

9.8 Demand of the Nanomedicine in Market

With the advancement in medical technologies, our world is moving closer to personalized and effective medical care. Nanomedicine can prove to be one of the major driving forces behind it. Recent statistics display that the global demand for Nanomedicine accounted for $111,912 million in 2016, which is expected to hit $261,063 million by 2023. The major parameters dividing the global Nanomedicine market are application, modality, indication, and region. Treatment and diagnostic are the two major divisions in terms of modality. Based on its several applications, it is categorized as drug delivery candidates, vaccines, regenerative medicine aid, and

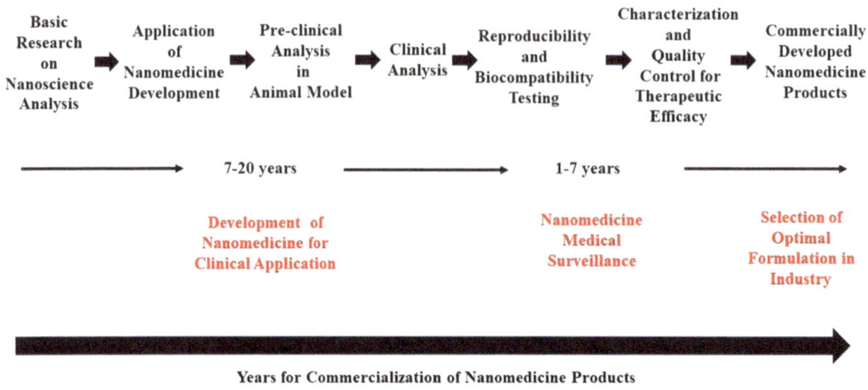

Fig. 9.4 Pipeline for the development and launching of Nanomedicine products

others. Based on further indication, their effectiveness was classified as relating to various diseases, such as immunological, oncological, neurological, urological, infectious, cardiovascular diseases, and several others. North America, Europe, and Asia-Pacific are the major regions across which the market of Nanomedicine manufacturing is based. According to the analysis conducted by Wagner et al. in 2006, there are more than 150 start-ups and small- and medium-sized enterprises based on Nanomedicine research and development projects (Siddique et al. 2019). The size of the global market for Nanomedicine was estimated to be nearly 140 billion USD in 2019. The current need for the development of early detection tools and effective diagnostic techniques can give a boost to this growth by 2025 (Chang et al. 2015; Życiński 2006). The National Science Foundation (NSF) predicts Nanomedicine being a major part of future pharmaceutical products, with the nanotechnology-based companies to be actively involved in the biomedical field (Ventola 2012b). The steps involved in the development and launching of novel nano therapeutic drugs are explained in Fig. 9.4.

9.9 Nanomedicine and Ethical Concerns

As mentioned above, the confusion surrounding the behavior of the nanoparticles and the capable impacts of exposure develops an ethical issue for those unveiled to these materials (Fig. 9.5). Evaluating the assurance of nanoparticles can be crucial due to the reason that these substances are not a united group of compounds; thus every type of substance must be evaluated separately (Oberdörster et al. 2005b; Wolf and Jones 2011). Particles less than the size of 200 nm may leave the circulatory system (CS) and are also capable of invading any human cell. Dermal penetrability is also possible, as in the central nervous system (CNS) via the olfactory mucosa. Notably, following the infiltration through the blood–brain barrier (BBB), particles could persist in the CNS, leading or inducing neurodegenerative disorders in extended usage (Obermeier et al. 2013; Yeagle 2007). The nanoparticles could

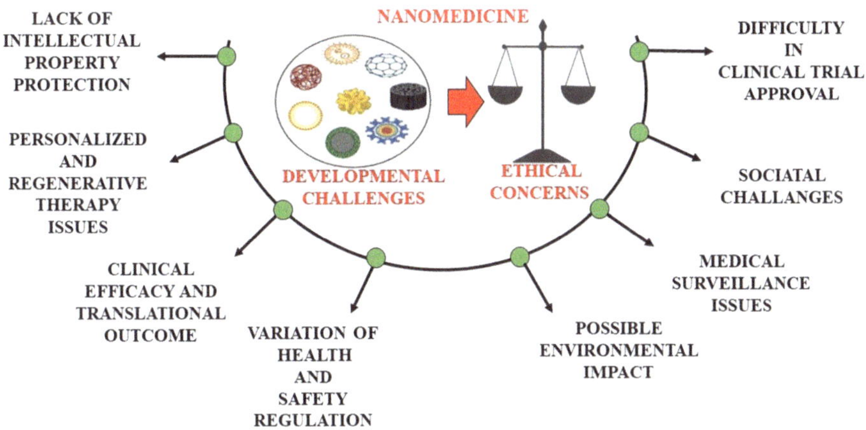

Fig. 9.5 Schematic representation of ethical aspects associated with Nanomedicine (Created with BioRender.com)

also impair via free radical impairment or can even act as teratogenic, perturbing the future generation. Some coated particles cannot be detached from the cells, and others may aggregate in the immune system. Usually, the mechanisms of interplay between the immune system and the nanoparticles are still not entirely evident. The exposure to nanomaterials can also be unintended via environmental sources like a contagion of underground water sources and soil penetration. These problems not only influence the scientists and workers initially unveiled to the nanoparticles but all the personnel along the complete chain of production, marketing, and distribution. Eventually, they can harm the consumers as well. To focus on these problems, a standardized approach for uncertainty evaluation is necessary (Allon et al. 2017; Turanlı and Everest 2016). The fine points related to ethical concerns of Nanomedicine are depicted in Fig. 9.5 and explained in the below sections.

9.9.1 Ethical Problems Associated with Translational Research Involving Nanomedicine

As recorded by Anderson and Kimmelman (2010) no broadly approved measures for analyses of threats, advantages, and significance in Phase I trials have been done with new drugs. Therefore, the challenge is initially to recognize and illustrate the deep-rooted pitfalls of translational research in an aspect that assembles with the fundamentals of transparency, liability, and decreasing the impact of harm to the participating individuals. Secondly, legal and ethical rules and protocol necessitate that researchers notify the subjects about the potential to intend of the analyses, approaches, advantages, significant uncertainties as well as forms of severe uncertainty, substitutes, privacy protections, and other necessary information that make a subject to make a decision whether to participate. Moreover, the challenge is whom to choose to go initially for human trials when it is futile to appropriately measure the uncertainties involved and when the impacts of failure are probably extensive (Allon et al. 2017; Solbakk and Zoloth 2011). Depicting on this prevailing knowledge relating to translational analyses, the recent condition of nanomedicine can be developed. Thus, the unsolvable ethical queries regarding translational analyses are common to nanomedicine and arise from: (a) Uncertainty regarding the initial unveiling of human trials to a specific type of nanomedical commodities in Phase I clinical trials. (b) Intrinsic inequity—in Phase I trials, individuals are enlisted into analysis designed not to profit them but instead to achieve safety knowledge for others. This ethical impasse may be usually acute in the context of nanomedicine, given the unawareness of the nanoparticles, including the experimental substances. (c) Frailty arising from ignorance and uncertainty. Certainly, forms of uncertainty are not limited entirely to measurable threats. This form comprises severe uncertainty, where possibilities cannot be accredited, as well as certain ignorance, where the sample space is not completely recognized, reign in translational analysis (Wynne 1992).

9.9.2 Ethical Problems in Personalized and Regenerative Therapy with Nanomedicine

Nanomedicine contributes to the emerging area of regenerative medicine and, as such, arises a number of ethical queries correlated to the idea that the human body can be created, remodeled, or regrown (Habets et al. 2016). The goal for improvement may pave the way in transforming medicine into a yet unknown entity. Nanomedicine impacts the elegant homeostasis between therapy and advancement by specifying the technological potentiality by regulating tissue elements, enabling the recovery of diseases and health conditions. Nanomedicine may be a mechanism in transforming personalized medicine to existence since nanotechnology provides targeted delivery and hence can contribute to the advancement of personalized medicine both for therapy and screening (Sharma et al. 2017). It facilitates the potentiality to personalize healthcare, conforming it to groups and individual patients. The transform of healthcare from disease-oriented to patient-oriented models comprises recent ethical challenges, chiefly regarding the data foundation required. Personalized nano diagnostics arise ethical queries concerning the scope and nature of genetic screening, for example, concerning the kind of screening and type of legal or social pressure to be practiced. Moreover, privacy issues and authority and ownership over data may be supplementary interests to be argued among regulatory bodies.

9.9.3 Ethical Concerns of Medical Surveillance

In the absence of a decisive cadenced to quantify environmental unveil or an analysis that firmly quantifies the impacts of nanosubstance exposure in humans, current medical inspection is the most reasonable substitute to analyze exposure safety

(Hartzema et al. 2013; Oberdörster et al. 2005a). Medical inspection comprises diagnosing for the pre-clinical sign of diseases for individuals showing no symptoms, allows for early detection and more potent treatment or intervention. The norm for regulating the suitability of medical investigation involves the strain of agony, the efficiency and accuracy of the analysis method, the potency of early screening, the risk of screening, and the advantages of surveillance comparative to damage (Public Health Surveillance 2008). Currently, there is no premise for aimed "nano specific" occupational medical investigations. When threat aspects are eminent and approve statistical interpretation, and when their impacts on human health are sustained by potent evidence, it is generally not challenging to make occupational or public health decisions. In these situations, ethical concerns rarely arise. However, when handling with non-measurable forms of uncertainty, as is the matter with nanotechnology, the decision-making procedure is not sustained by an adequate quantity of information and ethical impasses may arise and take root. It is though not apparent if the applicable information on nanoparticle threat is really adequate to justify medical investigation and even what minimal level of information is necessary to support decision-making is a matter of controversy (Dresser 2012; Jamison 2009).

The beneficence fundamental states that decisions should increase the profits for both the society and individuals. The approach of medical investigation of individuals unveiled to nanoparticles should maintain the advantage of appraising the employer's health situation contrary to the ethical costs. Given the limitation of the reliable analysis, challenges in illustrating the results of both physical and verification irregularity, and the lack of specific criteria for determining the ethical expenses can be extremely high.

9.9.4 Ethical Challenges Inherent to Nanomedicine Applications

The ethical impasses related to nanomedicine are not restricted to the laboratory solely. Nanomedicine increases and whets the screening and therapeutic approaches feasible for contemporary medicine. With its commitment, however, the requirement for an ethical appraisal of the purpose and significance of nanomedical novelty in screening and therapeutics arises.

Nanomedical commodities, which could determine early screening of the disorders, incite queries concerning the implication and effect of the evidences when no therapeutic option exists (Desai 2012; Ventola 2012b). Therefore, queries concerning to an individual are right to learn, but also on the right not to learn (i.e., not to unveil to excessive information that is insignificant or incidentally approved) arise.

Ethical queries also appear with respect to therapeutics. The predicted high cost of nanomedical commodities, at least in the initial phases of marketing, increase the justice fundamental arguments with socio-economic discrimination and challenged the approachability. Arguments like enabling the rich to profit, while the poor cannot access, might broaden the social difference within and among both societies and individuals (Wolf and Jones 2011).

9.9.5 Social Ethics in Public Health Systems

The progression of nanomedicine and its potent utilization increases various socio-economic queries, specifically within the situation of public health. The economic sector has hardly any reason and also inadequate funds to generate extensive information on harmful and safety issues of nanomedicine; therefore it falls on the responsibility of governments to transport public budget towards the production of what is apparently beneficial for the public and awareness of the safety and health significance of the novel technology platform, which is transforming the world. Without specific support, the potent advantages of nanomedicine will not be illustrated. However, the impact of nanomedicine on human biology is extensive; the other societal impacts of it also account to be considered. Nanotechnological advancements also impact human interplay, economics, and politics (Keiper 2007; Solbakk and Zoloth 2011; Yeagle 2007).

9.9.5.1 Impact of Nanotechnology in Developing Nations

Due to the evidence that Nanotechnology and its utilization fields are potent of being very strong and effective, the impact of this novel technology on developing nations is a matter that should not be neglected. It is obvious to assume that the impact of Nanotechnology will vary from individuals having distinct lifestyles and convenience in a different region. In the twenty-first century, developed nations having huge industries with regard to nanotechnological capability will be an essential element for the global contest (Ebbesen et al. 2006; Ebbesen 2008; Satalkar et al. 2016).

Firstly, the distinction among the definitions of developing and developed nations should be determined. The extent of progression of a nation is depended on some factors such as equality among the people, total national product, and the political balance. According to the evaluation of these factors, advancing nations have a similar scenario. Most of the people in these nations are usually devoid of some fundamental requirements such as health services and education. Secondly, the process cycle of Nanotechnology that is manufacturing, marketing, and utilization of nano-products. In this process, there are functions for different nations such as final product manufacturer, raw material manufacture, and wastes disposer. Every function for each nation can be beneficial or disadvantageous. For example, if a nation is the manufacturer of nanomaterials, it should be benefited with some financial advantage, but on the other hand, the threat of environmental deterioration, unclear employee protection, and undefined dangers arising from nano-products arise as disadvantages for that nation. However, the raw material manufacturing and marketing of these products to technological product manufacturer nations appears advantageous (Gökçay and Berna 2015; Graur et al. 2011; Leary 2013).

As a general conclusion, nanotechnology is displaying as a beneficial field for developed nations. However, the developing nations will not be able to compete contrary to the developed nations in the area of Nanotechnology. Nanotechnology, as a consequence, will limit developed nations reliability on developing nations having raw material, and if this reason causes developing nations to fall in the economy, developing nations should work on international negotiations those promise their profits.

9.9.5.2 Impact of Nanotechnology on Laborers and Managerial Issues

It is always likely to come up with certain uncertainty in every kind of Research and Development area, which is the basic characteristics of scientific research. Generally, the unpredictability of scientific analysis outcome is also unpredictable for the safety of the scientists. When discussing Nanotechnology, the unrecognized harm of the nanoparticles could be dangerous for scientists. Unknown employee protection and autonomous dangers arising from nano-products should be considered to have an impact on laborers.

Currently, there is a developing focus toward the field of Nanotechnology research. While the funds for Nanotechnology analysis in the USA was 2.1 billion USD in 2012, 16.5 billion USD has been used since 2001 (2012's budget is included). From the year 2005, nanotechnological research fund that has been used in the defense industry, environmental, and health fields was 575 billion US dollar and the fund used for the analysis for legal, ethical, and social impacts of nanotechnology was higher than 390 billion US dollars.

For the regulation of research on Nanotechnology around the world in relation to the ethical dimensionality of science and technology transformation, UNESCO initiated an "International Bioethics Committee" comprising of thirty-six experts of a distinct area from various regions in the world. The goal of this committee is to share various novel ideas and knowledge in the area of life sciences, to make suggestions in the decision taking powers and to make a platform between those public and powers. It is also crucial to increase the general awareness of individuals having distinct educational qualifications. As Nanotechnology is a promptly developing area, it is immensely necessary to consider the ethical impacts for the future (Gelfert 2012; Kearnes 2006; Wolf and Jones 2011).

9.10 Future Perspectives

In the historical advancement of medicine, there has always been an innovative dialogue and mental stress between the more idealistic scientist and the patient-oriented clinician. Similarly, in the present context, Nanomedicine is at risk of being available only to privileged societies, at least initially, but it proposes uncultivated opportunities for medical advances that might benefit underprivileged populations. When the queries rise in the framework of more traditional clinical contexts and the issues are addressed in a specific, gradual way, is called type 1 research practice. On the other hand, when there are key new fields of fundamental scientific study, the leading scientists might conceive how the medicine might be basically altered. In this case, the sense of arising science regulates, and its improvement includes a deep and basic rearrangement of medicine. In such type 2 research, the primary spotlight is often on the improvement of the basic insight and tools required for this future vision to be realized. In practice, these two aspects are in constant dialogue and the dissimilarity in the approached proposal might be unseen in certain collaborative projects. Occasionally, the mental stress is clear in the same person, who is both a scientist and a clinician. In the case of medicine, the two advances together, repetitively refining one another, till a novel, more mature kind of assimilation arises, which is referred to as type 3. It associates a basic reshaping of the logics of the resulting science and engineering so that they are reactive to the realities of advancing clinical practice settings.

The stress among the Nanomedicine impacts reflects on the ethical issues. Thus, these ethical issues have been observed as beyond the science—as the issues of integrative or human-subject preservation were one-time objections. Such an accession to ethics reflects a long-standing complication between the realms of value and facts. Yet, in Nanomedicine, this older complication is no longer justifiable. The new science calls for a fundamental reconsidering of the relationship between ethical reflection and medical research. Even though it might be too early to say what a mature type 3 nanomedicine requires, but one thing is clear: it has to include a far more nuanced, crucial consideration to the institutional, cultural, and policy circumstances that allow its own practice. Without this, the full capacity of Nanomedicine will remain suppressed.

9.11 Conclusion

Concept and misconception of risks by researchers and representatives of the public similarly play an important function in decision taking to approve or reject the technologies, and also to decide how best to reduce any specific issues. Valuable decision-making arises at each step of the process cycle. Notably, the queries may not be about how "real" the threats are, but instead, how they approach to introduce in the society, which in turn defines a favorable agreement about a society and its institutions of administrations. Some researchers and ethicists have been immensely vocal about the requirement to review the threats arising from nanotechnologies and their products, recounting multiple reasons for concern. Others recommend that present systems are adequate and insist that the present approach already identifies and deals with the threats, so adding a new committee of review will only delay the development of potentially valuable products (Jotterand 2008). Nanotechnology is also located in historical importance in which wider problems of evidence, expertise, and potentiality are being called into queries. This is when the suggestion to establish an inter-agency working committee is most significant: where crucial data may be available but is not evaluated equally or properly across managerial agencies and other significant organizations. An inter-agency working committee could reduce the gaps in awareness and types of expertise, be better potent to organize more extensive and integrative study, and more importantly, deteriorate potential issues. Novel nano-products also come in review with regard to evidence-based medicine approaches, which have a greater limit for illustrating the effectiveness and may influence the threat and advantage of study accordingly. Analysis into distinct ways of organizing pre-clinical trials, including the recommendation of introducing predictive algorithms and bioinformatics or cell-based, in vitro pre-clinical analysis in addition to the visualization approaches during and after the administration of nanomedicines may transform the complete process of analyses. Medical threat evaluation performed by quantitative risk experts, regulatory authorities, and bioethicists has not apparently considered the wider scenario of the threats, comprising the market and business threat evaluations made by the translating percepts into products. Decisions taken about the novel nano-products from this perspective from clinical trial to market introduction are core on distinct inference and priorities than those utilized by regulators and bioethicists, yet there is a specific interplay between the two decision taking approaches (Hogle 2012). One way to negotiate with threats might be to encourage trial sponsors themselves to become more deliberate about the threat and the threat practices. Triggered by financial downfall as much as natural and technological disasters, many agencies have become conscious of how immensely disasters might influence the progress of the agencies for the near and long period (Hall et al. 2012; Schottel and Karn 2016; Ventola 2012b). Regulation and communication among all entities are crucial in order to avert assumptions from being concretized into exercise and to promise an interspersed, consistent reflection on review practices as a whole. If we agree that values are ingrained in threats, threat analysis, and improvement, then adding to the supervision of Nanomedicine human trial analysis by establishing an inter-agency working committee and International ethical committee with different experts representing distinct kinds of expertise and function in society will be beneficial in acknowledging and understanding the moral, social, and scientific elements of decision taking about which is a better way to proceed. They are an essential element towards responsible novelty in Nanomedicine (Ventola 2012a). Focusing attention on the promise that certain Nanomedicine drugs behold in terms of personalized medicine and targeted drug delivery, and also the associated safety and risk factors that need to be regulated in terms of benefits to the subjects, society, and environment, the formation of global negotiations should be strengthened to illuminate the ethical and legal aspects of Nanomedicine.

Acknowledgement The authors are thankful to Chettinad Academy of Research and Education (CARE) for providing the infrastructural support and to SERB, DST, Govt. of India, for providing the financial support to complete this piece of work.

Author Contribution The idea and design of the study was conceived by Antara Banerjee. Alakesh Das, Dikshita Deka, Syed Sana Abrar, Surajit Pathak, and Antara Banerjee wrote the manuscript and designed the diagrammatic representations. All the authors read and approved the final version of the manuscript.

Funding This work was supported by the grants sanctioned to Dr. Antara Banerjee (PI) from the SERB-DST, Govt. of India with the sanction file no ECR/2017/001066 and departmental grants at CARE.

References

Allon I, Ben-Yehudah A, Dekel R, Solbakk JH, Weltring KM, Siegal G (2017) Ethical issues in nanomedicine: tempest in a teapot? Medicine. Health Care Philos 20(1):3–1

Bawa R (2005) Will the nanomedicine “patent land grab” thwart commercialization? Nanomedicine: nanotechnology. Biol Med 1(4):346–340

Bawa R, Johnson S (2007) The ethical dimensions of nanomedicine. Med Clin N Am 91 (5):881–887

Bawa R, Johnson S (2009) Emerging issues in nanomedicine and ethics. In: Nanotechnology & society. Springer, Dordrecht, pp 207–203

Bawa R, Bawa SR, Maebius SB, Flynn T, Wei C (2005) Protecting new ideas and inventions in nanomedicine with patents. Nanomedicine 1(2):150–158

Bruce D (2006) The question of ethics. Nano Today 1(1):6–7

Chang EH, Harford JB, Eaton MA, Boisseau PM, Dube A, Hayeshi R et al (2015) Nanomedicine: past, present and future–a global perspective. Biochem Biophys Res Commun 468(3):511–517

de SC, Nigel M (2006) The NELSI imperative: nano ethical, legal and social issues, and federal policy development. Nanotechnol Law Bus 3:159

Desai N (2012) Challenges in development of nanoparticle-based therapeutics. AAPS J 14 (2):282–285

Dresser R (2012) Building an ethical foundation for first-in-human nanotrials. J Law Med Ethics 40 (4):802–808

Ebbesen M (2008) The role of the humanities and social sciences in nanotechnology research and development. NanoEthics 2(1):1–3

Ebbesen M, Andersen S, Besenbacher F (2006) Ethics in nanotechnology: starting from scratch? Bull Sci Technol Soc 26(6):451–452

Ferrari M, Philibert MA, Sanhai WR (2009) Nanomedicine and society. Clin Pharmacol Ther 85 (5):466–467

Gelfert A (2012) Nanotechnology as ideology: towards a critical theory of ‘converging technologies’. Sci Technol Soc 17(1):143–144

Gökçay B, Berna AR (2015) Nanotechnology, nanomedicine; ethical aspects. Rev Romana Bioet 13(3):423–432

Graur F, Elisei R, Szasz A, Neagos HC, Muresan A, Furcea L et al (2011) Ethical issues in nanomedicine. In: International conference on advancements of medicine and health care through technology. Springer, Cham, pp 9–12

Habets MG, van Delden JJ, Bredenoord AL (2016) Studying the lay of the land: views and experiences of professionals in the translational pluripotent stem cell field. Regen Med 11 (1):63–61

Hall RM, Sun T, Ferrari M (2012) A portrait of nanomedicine and its bioethical implications. J Law Med Ethics 40(4):763–769

Hartzema AG, Reich CG, Ryan PB, Stang PE, Madigan D, Welebob E et al (2013) Managing data quality for a drug safety surveillance system. Drug Saf 36(1):49–48

Anderson JA, Kimmelman J (2010) Extending clinical equipoise to phase 1 trials involving patients: unresolved problems. Kennedy Inst Ethics J 20(1):75–98

Hogle LF (2012) Concepts of risk in nanomedicine research. J Law Med Ethics 40(4):809–802

Jamison A (2009) Can nanotechnology be just? On nanotechnology and the emerging movement for global justice. NanoEthics 3(2):129–126

Jotterand F (ed) (2008) Emerging conceptual, ethical and policy issues in bionanotechnology. Springer, Dordrecht

Kearnes M (2006) Chaos and control: nanotechnology and the politics of emergence. Paragraph 29 (2):57–50
Keiper A (2007) Nanoethics as a discipline? The New Atlantis 16:55–57
Kuiken T (2011) Nanomedicine and ethics: is there anything new or unique? Wiley Interdiscip Rev Nanomed Nanobiotechnol 3(2):111–118
Leary JF (2013) Nanomedicine–reality will trump hype! J Nanomed Biother Discov 4:125
Liu D, Yang F, Xiong F, Gu N (2016) The smart drug delivery system and its clinical potential. Theranostics 6(9):1306
Nel A, Xia T, Mädler L, Li N (2006) Toxic potential of materials at the nanolevel. Science 311 (5761):622–627
Oberdörster G, Maynard A, Donaldson K, Castranova V, Fitzpatrick J, Ausman K et al (2005a) Principles for characterizing the potential human health effects from exposure to nanomaterials: elements of a screening strategy. Part Fibre Toxicol 2(1):8
Oberdörster G, Oberdörster E, Oberdörster J (2005b) Nanotoxicology: an emerging discipline evolving from studies of ultrafine particles. Environ Health Perspect 113(7):823–829
Obermeier B, Daneman R, Ransohoff RM (2013) Development, maintenance and disruption of the blood-brain barrier. Nat Med 19(12):1584
Patra D, Haribabu E, McComas KA (2010) Perceptions of nano ethics among practitioners in a developing country: a case of India. NanoEthics 4(1):67–65
Resnik DB, Tinkle SS (2007) Ethical issues in clinical trials involving nanomedicine. Contemp Clin Trials 28(4):433–431
Sandler R (2009) Nanomedicine and nanomedical ethics. Am J Bioeth 9(10):16–17
Satalkar P, Elger BS, Shaw DM (2016) Defining nano, nanotechnology and nanomedicine: why should it matter? Sci Eng Ethics 22(5):1255–1256
Schottel BL, Karn B (2016) The national nanotechnology initiative approach to environment, health, and safety: a model for future science investments. Fed Hist 8:48
Sechi G, Bedognetti D, Sgarrella F, Eperen LV, Marincola FM, Bianco A et al (2014) The perception of nanotechnology and nanomedicine: a worldwide social media study. Nanomedicine 9(10):1475–1476
Sharma R, Mody N, Agrawal U, Vyas SP (2017) Theranostic nanomedicine; a next generation platform for cancer diagnosis and therapy. Mini Rev Med Chem 17(18):1746–1747
Siddique S, Alexander A, Yadav P, Agrawal M, Shehata AM, Shaker MA et al (2019) Nanomedicines: challenges and perspectives for future nanotechnology in the healthcare system. Sci Res Essays 14(5):32–38
Solbakk JH, Zoloth L (2011) The tragedy of translation: the case of "first use" in human embryonic stem cell research. Cell Stem Cell 8(5):479–471
Strom BL (2006) How the US drug safety system should be changed. JAMA 295(17):2072–2075
Turanlı ET, Everest E (2016) Nanomedicine. In: Low-dimensional and nanostructured materials and devices. Springer, Cham, pp 579–587
Ventola CL (2012a) The nanomedicine revolution: part 1: emerging concepts. Pharm Ther 37 (9):512
Ventola CL (2012b) The nanomedicine revolution: part 3: regulatory and safety challenges. Pharm Ther 37(11):631
Ventola CL (2017) Progress in nanomedicine: approved and investigational nanodrugs. Pharm Ther 42(12):742
Wolf SM, Jones CM (2011) Designing oversight for nanomedicine research in human subjects: systematic analysis of exceptional oversight for emerging technologies. J Nanopart Res 13 (4):1449–1445
Wynne B (1992) Uncertainty and environmental learning: reconceiving science and policy in the preventive paradigm. Glob Environ Chang 2(2):111–117
Yeagle J (2007) Nanotechnology and the FDA. VA J Law Technol 12:1
Życiński J (2006) Ethics in medical technologies: the Roman Catholic viewpoint. J Clin Neurosci 13(5):518–513

Challenges and Future Opportunities of Nanomedicine in Cancer Therapy

10

Shoba Narayan

Abstract

A review of the tumor microenvironment, its heterogeneity and challenges in infiltration into the tumor microenvironment is discussed. The relationship between tumor microenvironment and various therapeutic modalities has been evaluated and the significant advantage that tunability of therapeutic provides so as to target specific receptors and molecules in the tumor microenvironment has been discussed. In this, the advantage of nanomedicine for multifunctionality, targetability, and ability to carry therapeutic loads through active and passive modes into the tumor microenvironment has been highlighted. The review covers all forms of therapeutic strategies, including those in market space and emerging. The role of nanotech products for drug delivery and in development and extending the progress of research in the area of cancer vaccine has been described in detail. The review focuses attention more towards understanding the tumor microenvironment for the development of immunotherapy, rather than tumor killing—a perspective considered to be of high potential in the conquer of cancer.

Keywords

Tumor microenvironment · Nanoparticles · Nanomedicine · Therapeutics · Drug delivery

S. Narayan (✉)
Faculty of Allied Health Sciences, Chettinad Hospital and Research Institute, Chettinad Academy of Research and Education, Kelambakkam, Tamil Nadu, India
e-mail: shobanarayan@chettinadhealthcity.com

A. Malik et al. (eds.), *Nanomedicine for Cancer Diagnosis and Therapy*,
https://doi.org/10.1007/978-981-15-7564-8_10

Highlights

- With tumor microenvironment in focus cancer nanomedicine is emerging out of its nascent state.
- There are clear advantage for nano therapeutics in conventional, alternative, and modern therapies.
- Nanocarriers seem to be surging ahead in the development of vaccines for cancer.
- Challenges to nanomedicine are not up at the clinic but at the bottom point of nanoparticle/capsule production.

10.1 Tumor Incidences and Basis of Tumor Progression

As of 2018, 18.1 million new tumor cases were reported across the world, of which almost 50% of them died as well (Bray et al. 2018). Till a couple of decades back, the oncogene mutations were considered as the basis of tumor. Based on this consideration, tumor therapies were developed to kill the tumor cells, which led to secondary damage and treatment resistance (Vogelstein and Kinzler 1993). About a century ago, an English surgeon—S Paget, for the first time, considered tumor progression as one of interaction between tumor cells and the external environment and proposed the concept of tumor microenvironment (Cheng et al. 2020). A solid tumor differs from a hematological tumor in the expression of tumor specific antigen. While B-cell marker CD19 is universally expressed in leukemia, solid tumors have tumor associated antigens in an enriched form but are also expressed in low levels in normal cells.

10.2 Tumor Microenvironment

As cancer develops, some tumors have a pervasive growth of dense fibrous tissues around the tumor. This process is known as the desmoplastic reaction, which involves both stromal and immune cells. While immune cells are known to originate from bone marrow, the origin of stromal cells is still not clear, with a majority of researchers suggesting the origin to be normal cells in the original organ, with a few from bone marrow derived cells (Kalluri and Zeisberg 2006). Density and diversity of immune cells are related to the prognosis and prediction of efficiency of treatment. Thus, the understanding of the difference in immune cells between primary and the metastatic states in tumor microenvironment is an important step in designing immunotherapy (Duan et al. 2020).

A tumor microenvironment is one that favors the growth and expansion of the cancer cells. In the tumor microenvironment, the cells create an environment that escapes the host immune surveillance (Cheng et al. 2020) (Fig. 10.1).

Human tumors vary in composition of their microenvironment (Schumacher and Schreiber 2015). It is thus very critical that an understanding of the interactions within the tumor microenvironment is available to design new cancer therapies. Genomic analysis has provided ample information on the genetic and epigenetic

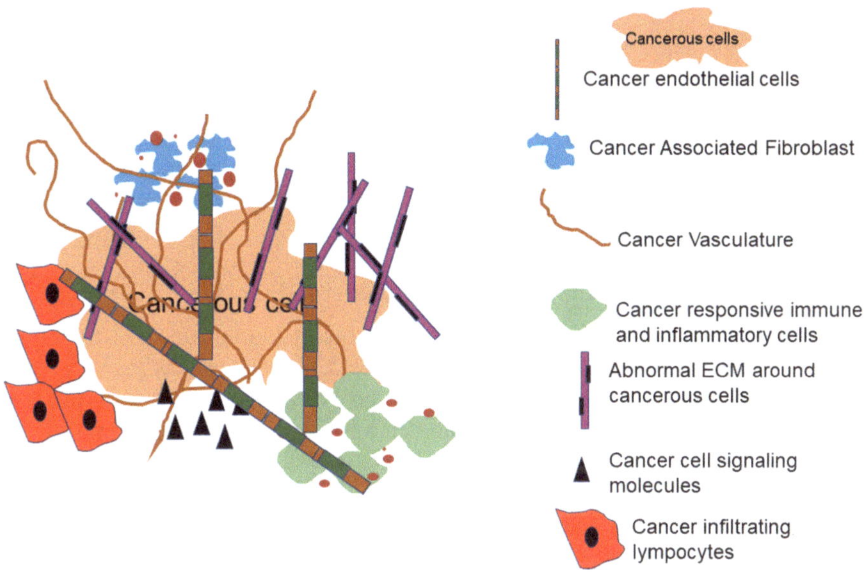

Fig. 10.1 A view of cancerous cell microenvironment

alterations in human and mouse cancer associated fibroblasts (Costea et al. 2013). Resistance to cancer cell proliferation arises from the development of alternative pathways for cell survival (Amin et al. 2015). Through tumor–stroma interactions, tumor cells and immune cells contribute to gene modifications in activated cancer associated fibroblasts. The activated cancer associated fibroblasts abundantly produce growth factors including bFGF, VEGF, PDGF, ligands of EGFR, interleukins, and TGF-β. The produced growth factors regulate tumor growth and inflammatory response either through cell-to-cell contact or cell-to-cell signaling. Some of the molecules secreted by activated cancer associated fibroblasts have inhibitory effects on tumor progression.

Thus, in short, cancer associated fibroblasts are heterogeneous and can be both tumor promoting and tumor restraining (Elyada et al. 2019; Oya et al. 2020). This, in turn, links well to the observations of oncologists who suggest that in a healthy state, the tumor microenvironment protects against tumorigenesis and in an unhealthy state becomes an accomplice. Researchers have classified tumor microenvironment non-T-cell inflamed (cold) and T-cell inflamed (hot) based on the levels of proinflammatory cytokine production and T cell infiltration. The hot cells indicate a higher level of T cell infiltration and better response to immunotherapy and accordingly, some studies have looked at the possibility of converting cold cells to hot cells (Zemek et al. 2019; Gajewski 2015).

The extracellular matrix of tumor, which comprised of collagen, fibronectin, laminin, etc., is secreted by cells in the tumor microenvironment. The cancer associated fibroblasts transform the extracellular matrix to phenotypes that promote tumor progression (Spugnini et al. 2018). While physical support to the tumor cells is provided by collagen and fibronectin, proteoglycans bind growth factors and cytokines (Wu and Dai 2017). Tumor progression also brings about changes in tumor associated collagen signatures (Malik et al. 2015). Fibrosis and extracellular matrix stiffness are part of the desmoplastic reactions and cause obstruction for effective permeation of drugs to the intratumoral area leading to the transformation of cancer cells to cancer stem cells (Najafi et al. 2020). The stiffening of the tumor tissues leads to tumor constituents displacing the surrounding normal tissues and thus tumor invading and growing in size. The mechanical force coupled with aberrant tumor vessel generates abnormal solid and fluid stress, which facilitates tumor progression and hindrance to treatment (Jain et al. 2014). The non-fluid components create solid stress. The part of solid stress that remains with the tumor after it is excised is known as growth induced stress. The solid stress has both direct and indirect effect, viz., the direct compression of cancer and stromal cells and indirect deformation of blood vessels. Compression of cells alters the gene expression, cancer cell proliferation, apoptosis, stromal cell function, extracellular matrix synthesis and organization–features typical of a tumor (Helmlinger et al. 1997a). The blood and lymphatic vessel compression reduces oxygen, nutrient, and drug delivery, leading to a hypoxic and acidic microenvironment (Helmlinger et al. 1997b).

Tumor angiogenesis which is the formation of abnormal vascular tissues and having an immature structure and high permeability, contributes to tumor microenvironment hypoxia and hypoperfusion. It is reported that the hypoxic tumor microenvironment carries cells that have high proliferation activity (Mennerich et al. 2019). Bidirectional crosslinking between hypoxia and angiogenesis results in increasing the power of each other's effect on tumor growth (Viallard and Larrivee 2017). The VEGF is an important factor for angiogenesis and progresses with activation and tube formation of endothelial cells. Cells in the tumor microenvironment activate the vascular endothelial cells by secreting VEGF (Ribeiro et al. 2013).

Besides the angiogenic effect, factors such as recruit peripheral nerves and leukocytes are also involved in tumor growth and dissemination. A neurogenic switch that gets activated by neurotrophins and extracellular vesicles attracts peripheral fibers, thus attracted fibers guiding the cancer cell dissemination. One of the ways forward for cancer therapy is to prevent cancer cell communication and tumor induced neurogenesis (Cervantes-Villagrana et al. 2020).

Small vesicles that are enriched with proteins, lipids, and nucleic acids with high levels of selectivity and molecular heterogeneity are known as exosomes. Release of exosomes transforms the matrix microenvironment. Transmission of signals and molecules to recipient cells also brings in pathophysiological functions. The tumor mediated exosomes mediate the interactions between microenvironment and tumor cells and also stimulate tumor growth through specific signaling pathways. Because of their effective material transport characteristics, exosomes can be tuned to be active therapeutic agents as well (Tang et al. 2020).

10.3 Tumor Infiltration

Even after the identification of a tumor antigen, unlike hematological cancers, where a chimeric antigen receptor (CAR-T) cell (CAR-T cells are genetically engineered cells which express antigen-specific receptor) reaches the destination through the blood stream, they encounter multiple barriers in the case of solid tumors (Martinez and Moon 2019).The major challenges include (1) the heterogeneity of the solid tumor antigen, (2) toxicity control, (3) inadequate infiltration, (4) poor proliferation and persistence, and (5) immunosuppressive tumor microenvironment (Hanahan and Coussens 2012; Lim and June 2017; Tian et al. 2020). Thus targeting a single antigen could result in tumor recurrence owing to excess growth of antigen negative cells. The receptor needs to be accompanied by co-stimulatory molecules and cytokines to overcome the toxicity.

Targeting and breaking the tumor microenvironment barrier, leading to disruption of its protective effect, are considered as an effective strategy for therapy (Villanueva and Bazhenova 2018). In this, the relevance of natural killer (NK) cells has been highlighted. NK cells are innate lymphoid cells that mediate immune responses and are able to rapidly and spontaneously recognize and kill tumor cells. NK cells for the killing of tumor cells require activation through receptors such as NKG_2D. NK cells release cytotoxic granules carrying cytolytic enzymes such as perforin and granzymes that can perform lysis and killing of tumor cells (Wang and Matosevic 2020). The significant drawback of NK cells is their poor capacity for the elimination of large solid tumors as the antitumor activity gets compromised in the presence of large number of cancer cells.

There are now approaches for engineering CAR-NK cells with enriched safety, amenability, and ease of production. Some CAR-NK cells have reached pre-clinical studies for breast cancer, neuroblastoma, etc. (Hu et al. 2019).

Macrophages are another class of mediators that are capable of lysing the tumor cells. Macrophages release excessive amounts of lysosomal enzymes and reactive oxygen metabolites post-activation (Alvaro et al. 2010). They play dual role of tumor inhibition and promotion as there are two different phenotypes. Macrophages in the tumor microenvironment are also referred to as tumor associated macrophages (Zhang et al. 2020c). In the initial stages of tumor, macrophages either directly promote antitumor response or indirectly recruit and activate immune cells. With genetic changes, the tumor associated macrophages start exhibiting immunosuppressive phenotypes and promote tumor progression (Lopez-Yrigoyen et al. 2020). A combination of high expression of CD47 and signal regulatory protein-α on the surface of the tumor associated macrophages deceives the immune system and thus makes them an accomplice for tumor progression (Hayes et al. 2020).

Dendritic cells have the ability to imbibe, process, and present tumor associated antigens. They express essential co-stimulatory ligands on cells surfaces and thus play a major role in the initiation, programming, and regulation of tumor specific immune response (Koido et al. 2010). In their lifecycle, dendritic cells, after exiting bone marrow, enter and seed all organs and tissues. On activation, the dendritic cells migrate to lymphoid tissues and initiate adaptive immunity. Based on their ability to detect tumor antigens produced by the cancer cells, dendritic cells are able to identify cancer cells easily (de Winde et al. 2020).

10.4 Tumor Microenvironment and Cancer Therapeutics

Tumor microenvironment has been described as an acidic, hypoxic, acidic, and inflammatory cell-enriched milieu. For solid tumors, it has now been recognized that the targeting of tumor microenvironment would be an effective strategy (Zhong et al. 2020).

Chemo- and radiotherapy coupled with surgical resection continues to be the common therapeutic methods for various types of cancers. Poor solubility of the drug, short half-life, faster clearance, non-specific binding or distribution, narrow therapeutic index, extensive systemic toxicity, etc. are observed in chemotherapy. The radiotherapy is limited by therapeutic efficacy, the improvement of which requires multiple doses of radiation and the ability of normal cells to withstand such radiation doses (Norouzi et al. 2020).Multidrug resistance (MDR) is a result of involvement of multiple factors and thus is classified as innate and acquired phenotypes. In general, it is accepted that the multidrug resistance is owing to the resistance developed through overexpression of ATP-binding cassette (ABC) membrane transporters. ABC membrane transporters are a family of 48 genes. The MDR associated proteins reduce the effective intracellular concentration of the drug. One of the proteins—P-gp detects and binds to a broad range of chemotherapeutics, including hydrophobic molecules. The presence of transferases such as Glutathione-S-transferases in the tumor microenvironment can metabolize the drugs and increase the expression of malignant cells. The standard methodologies to overcome MDR are (a) developing ABC transporter inhibitors, (b) modified dosage of chemotherapeutics to gain higher dosage, (c) rendering MDR genes ineffective through post-transcriptional modifications, (d) developing non-P-gp substrates as chemotherapeutics (Majidinia et al. 2020). Biomaterials in combination with radiation and chemotherapy have also shown promise to lead their way to pre-clinical trials, thus opening up the opportunity for theranostics, combination therapy, and tissue protection (Shi et al. 2020).

10.4.1 Radiotherapy

In radiotherapy, the use of α particles is gaining importance for the treatment of solid tumors. Radium is one of the elements that emit α particles. The choice of α particles for targeted therapy has gained prominence as gamma rays are massless, photons that travel through most materials and beta rays are mostly electrons that travel through tissues in a manner similar to gamma rays. α particles are the least ionizing type of particles with high potency and local specificity. The poor penetration of α particles can be overcome through the use of antibodies specific to cancer. The therapeutic model that uses antibody tagged α particles is referred to as immunoradiotherapy, still needs to evolve for solid tumors (Sharkey and Goldenberg 2011). The advantages of α particles are summarized as (a) α particles do not need oxygen for increasing their biological effectiveness, (b) α particles have much higher relative biological effect, (c) α particles can kill both dividing and non-dividing tumor cells (Kaim et al. 2009; Issa et al. 2011; Ali et al. 2020).

10.4.2 Boron Neutron Capture Therapy

Boron neutron capture therapy is attracting attention as a treatment methodology for cutaneous melanomas. An appropriate number of 10B atoms are introduced to the neoplastic cells along with 3–7 α particles to destroy tumor tissues. Boron compounds that meet the requirements of low systemic toxicity, high tumor uptake, and low normal tissue uptake are preferred. Examples of such boron compounds are mercaptoundecahydrodecaborane and boronophenylalanine (Barth et al. 2018; Sköld et al. 2010). Boron neutron capture therapy is a promising approach, which however, requires improvement in selectivity.

10.4.3 Radionucleotide Therapy

Another methodology for improving radiotherapy is the peptide receptor radionuclide therapy, where a peptide is used to target the tumor, and includes a pharmacokinetic modifier and bifunctional chelating agents and radionuclide (Bodei et al. 2009).

10.4.4 Genomic Guided Therapy

Genomic guided therapy is considered as a long-term disease control when the response rate and duration of chemotherapy is poor. Genomic therapy is employable after resistance to chemotherapy has developed or in cases such as chemotherapy-refractory sarcoma (Chen and Chen 2020).

10.4.5 New Generation Therapeutics

Inflammation plays a crucial role in the tumorigenesis and progression of cancer. The cancer metabolic program is mirrored in the metabolic milieu of the tumor microenvironment. Inflammatory molecules exert both pro- and antitumor effects. Interleukin is one such inflammatory molecule produced by CD3+ and CD4+ T lymphocytes. Interleukin is responsible for intercellular communication (Xi et al. 2020). The manner in which the T cells metabolism and function occur depends on the microenvironment conditions such as nutrient deprivation, hypoxia, and presence of toxic metabolites. In a very recent review article, Leone and Powell have tabulated the immune contexture of the tumor microenvironment. The effector cells in the microenvironment are dedicated to cell killing. They arise from innate or adaptive arms of the immune system. The antitumor effective cells are from the adaptive arm and their role is to carry out antigen specific killing of cancer cells through induction of apoptosis and cytokine secretion, viz., the $CD8^+$ T_{eff} cells. The primary role of conventional $CD4^+$ cells is one of antitumor immunity, however, a subset of $CD4^+$ cells, viz., T_H1, can also provide antitumor activity (Leone and Powell 2020). Newer versions of conventional cancer therapeutics as well as new generation therapeutics are indented for targeting specific components of the tumor microenvironment to realize antitumor activity.

In recent years, small molecules have been designed to promote T-cell response against certain cancers. They have cell penetrative ability and thus can target intracellular proteins. They also have short half-lifes and thus reduce the risk of systemic toxicity arising from limited accumulation in the circulation. These small molecules can also be combined with other molecules for targeted immunotherapy (van der Zanden et al. 2020). Immunotherapeutic approaches have included dendritic cell vaccines, immune checkpoint inhibitors, monoclonal antibodies, cytokines, and adoptive cell therapies and the mode of therapy can be passive or active. Dendritic cell vaccines are an example of active mode (Zhang and Chen 2018).

10.4.5.1 Small Molecule Inhibitors

Small molecule inhibitors are characterized by good penetration and accessibility and can overcome issues such as penetration and accessibility to cancer cells. The penetration and accessibility offered by the tumor microenvironment are an advantage for the small molecule inhibitors as they can specifically target microenvironment components (Zhong et al. 2020).

10.4.6 Micro and Small Interfering RNA

MicroRNAs (miRNAs) are 20–24 nucleotide long molecules. Their role in tumorigenesis, such as cell cycle regulation, metastasis, angiogenesis, metabolism, and apoptosis has been analyzed by various researchers. While a significant number of publications indicate regulation of gene expression through post-transcriptional regulation, some studies suggest activation of gene expression. From the data available currently, the role of miRNA in tumor suppression and as a biomarker is forthcoming. An added advantage is their ability to regulate immune checkpoints such as PD-1 and its ligand PD-L1, which are known to facilitate the creation of a tumor microenvironment that favors tumor growth and progression. Development of anticancer strategies based on miRNA mimics, and miRNA sponges are on the anvil (Iqbal et al. 2019; Vautrot et al. 2019).

Small interfering RNA (siRNA) has the ability to target any protein. Recommended as an attractive therapeutic for many diseases with overexpression of proteins, the use of siRNA for cancer therapeutics is a major attraction for researchers. Clinical translation of siRNA therapeutics is challenged by effective delivery at the site of action, with nanodelivery vehicles being the most promising. There are reports that siRNA can target even such proteins that are traditionally considered as non-targetable and their superiority over small molecule inhibitors and antibodies has been forthcoming. Targeting components of tumor microenvironment, particularly immune cells, through nanodelivery of siRNA has been under extensive investigation (Ngamcherdtrakul and Yantasee 2019). *Prodrugs:* Prodrugs, viz., molecules with low / no biological activity can be metabolized into biologically active parent drugs in the body through chemical or enzymatic reactions. In this, two or more functional motifs are combined through cleavable linkers. Through the appropriate mechanisms, the links can be cleaved, and the parent drug released. Disulfide based prodrugs can be self-assembled nanomedicines, prepared from drug–drug conjugates. The choice of the linker is based on its stability during circulation so as to avoid premature drug release and high self-immolation rate in the tumor cells. The number of disulfide prodrugs under in vivo test is very low currently (Wang et al. 2020a).

10.4.7 Tumor Associated Macrophages

In the tumor associated macrophages, there are two types of cells, M1 and M2, which are classified according to the secretion of cytokines, growth factors, and proteases. M1 type promotes inflammation and participates in immune response, has antitumor activity and ability to distinguish between healthy and non-healthy cells. M2, on the other, inhibits the inflammatory reaction, clears debris, and promotes angiogenesis and tumor progression (Jeannin et al. 2018). At this stage, the tumor associated macrophages also secrete IL-6 that activates STAT3 in cancer cells and produce resistance to drugs such as cisplatin and doxorubicin. Based on this knowledge, therapeutics that block recruitment of monocytes (Carlumab and Bindarit as classic examples) inhibit the activity of tumor associated macrophages (Chlorophosphonate and zoledronic acid as examples), regulate their phenotypes that are being developed (Hu5F9-G4, CP-870,893 as class examples) (Zhang et al. 2020c).

10.4.8 FAKs

Focal adhesion kinase (FAK) is a non-receptor protein tyrosine kinase regulated by integrin signaling. FAK expression is upregulated in different types of cancers and therapeutics have aimed at reducing or inhibiting the activity of FAK. FAK also contributes to tumor progression by regulating multiple factors in the tumor microenvironment. One of the first efforts to block FAK signaling was through the expression of antisense oligos, which in recent years have moved to the generation of small molecule inhibitors that block FAK activity. Over a period of time, tumors have developed remarkable resistance to chemotherapeutics. The addition of FAK inhibitors has had an effect on tumor remission. In addition to this, the addition of immunomodulating agents in combination with FAK inhibitors has also led to better treatment strategies (Murphy et al. 2020).

10.4.9 Hyperthermia and PTT

When the temperature of the tumor cell is increased preferentially over the normal cells through microwaves, ultrasound, laser, or other waves, cell death occurs. This process is known as hyperthermia. When near infrared light is used to activate a photosensitizer, it converts a light photon to heat and the process is known as photothermal therapy. One of the well research photothermal therapeutic agents is gold nanoparticles. The surface plasmon effect in gold nanoparticles increases the radiative properties. Cellular internalization of gold nanoparticles is a challenge and here, the ability of gold nanorods with a favorable surface plasmon resonance in the near infrared region comes as an advantage (Norouzi et al. 2018).

10.5 Nanomaterials in Cancer Therapy

Pharmaceutical history of nanoparticles in therapeutics started with liposomes. Over the years, the therapeutic index of nanoparticles has improved, with efficacy increasing and toxicity decreasing. It is now recognized that the adverse effect of chemotherapeutics can be overcome by nanoparticulate systems. However, a cause of concern is the reticuloendothelial system—a defense system of the bloodstream, which can rapidly remove nanoparticles from blood. Ou et al., have traced the historical timeline of developments in nanomedicine, starting with liposome structure being published in 1964, to targeted liposomes in 1980, Doxil in 1995, polymeric micelle paclitaxel in 2007, iron oxide nanoparticles in 2010, and BIND-014 in 2011.

One of the significant advantages of nanomedicine is in its ability to design therapeutics with multiple functional elements. A survey of the literature indicates some common functions such as drug solubilization, protection of drug against degradation, drug carrier with immune-evasive properties and targeting, carrier having properties such as triggered release of drug, ability to enhance permeation of cell structure, the carrier being able to carry other functional molecules such as imaging, and finally ability to perform combination therapy.

10.5.1 Solubilization

With a large number for chemotherapeutics being poorly water soluble, use of surfactants and other solubilizers along with the therapeutic was introduced. This required the administration of corticosteroids and antihistamines to avoid side effects (Yardley 2013). Nanomedicine thus offers a safer alternative. In the first generation nanotherapeutics, albumin was considered as carrier. Newer variants with PEG, polysaccharides, etc. as carriers have emerged over time. While it is a known fact that nanomedicines can be administered at higher dosages, studies relating to optimal dosing, infusion rates, etc. are still not conclusive enough. Nanotherapeutics also has advantage of delivery of higher drug concentration owing to higher drug loading capacity of the nanoparticles.

10.5.2 Degradation

One of the common problems in drug delivery is the enzymatic and mechanical degradation of drugs. Drugs such as siRNA, microRNA, antisense oligonucleotides, etc. are very sensitive to degradation. In addition to this, the negative charge on the drug, such as in the case of oligonucleotides prevents efficient internalization. The use of nanodelivery vehicles is towards (a) protecting the drug from enzymes that are in circulation and in extracellular space, and (b) aid cellular uptake and lysosomal escape (Shen et al. 2012). Based on this concept, a few chemically modified oligonucleotides such as fomivirsen are already in the market. One of the major concerns for such chemically modified oligonucleotides is the safety during clinical use, with some studies indicating side effects and even deaths.

10.5.3 Immunoevasion

Surface modification with anti-fouling polymers, self-peptides, and cell coatings is considered a way forward to avoid immunological recognition. One of the clinically approved strategies is to use PEG—a stealth polymer. Such conjugation through a steric barrier created reduces the binding of plasma opsonins and prevents the interaction with cells (Pasut and Veronese 2012). The pegylated version of doxorubicin– doxil is a classic example of a drug under this category where a decrease in cardiotoxicity risk is observable. Through 40 years of research in this area, researchers have now established that pegylation prolongs the circulation time of the drug but does not improve substantially the tumor accumulation. Similarly, pegylation delays the immunological clearance and does not prevent the same. A source of concern however on pegylated drugs is that the prolonged usage results in the generation of PEG antibodies which are responsible for accelerated blood clearance (Ishida et al. 2003). Popularly known as the ABC phenomenon, the pegylated liposomes on generation of PEG antibodies are rapidly cleared by the immune system leading to shorter circulation time as against their indented role of longer circulation times.

10.5.4 Combination Therapy

A major advantage seen in many nanotherapeutic development studies is in the combination of various components for same end effect. Combining various types of chemotherapeutic or chemotherapeutics with photodynamic or photothermal therapeutics has been observed in several research publications. Co-encapsulation within a nanocapsule is one such methodology. Further expansion of this concept includes those of combining therapeutics with imaging for development of a new class of products called as theranostics (Ryu et al. 2014).

10.5.5 Targeting

Surface conjugation of nanoparticles with molecular targeting ligands helps the drug carrier recognize biomolecular targets to bind so that the drug directly reaches the overexpressed molecules on the surface of the tumor. Literature is upbeat about several target ligands and their use for functionalization of nanoparticles. Some of them that have reached pre-clinical or clinical trials are MM310, an ephrin type A receptor 2-targeted docetaxel containing liposome, BIND-014, a docetaxel containing polymeric nanoparticle targeted to prostate-specific membrane antigen, and a whole host of functionalities that target $\alpha V\beta 3$ integrin receptor or folate receptor (Garcia-Bennett et al. 2011; Daniels et al. 2012).The manipulation of gold nanoparticle chemistry is one of the well-researched areas leading to combination therapy. Designing gold nanorods that are functionalized with peptides that bind to the KDR domain of cancer cells is said to provide for blocking of angiogenesis and also phototherapy (Narayan et al. 2013).

Nanoparticles can be designed for active and passive targeting of anticancer drugs, leading to their elevated levels in intracellular regions. In the case of active targeting, the nanoparticles can be engineered to be based on the tumor microenvironment and a ligand directed targeting can be achieved (El-Readi and Althubiti 2019). A further advantage is based on the multifunctionality of the nanoparticles (Fig.10.2).

The accumulation of nanoparticles in the tumor is considered as one of interaction of the nanoparticle with cells in the tumor microenvironment. Some of the well-researched nanoparticle-tumor microenvironment cell interactions include those with tumor associated macrophages, which promotes intratumoral uptake of nanoparticles (Miller et al. 2015). Many of the reported multifunctional nanoparticles have very good imaging and therapeutic effects. The drawback, however, is the tumor intrinsic barrier and tumor heterogeneity lead in vivo low therapeutic efficacy. A new way to overcome this is the image guided delivery of nanoparticles where techniques like

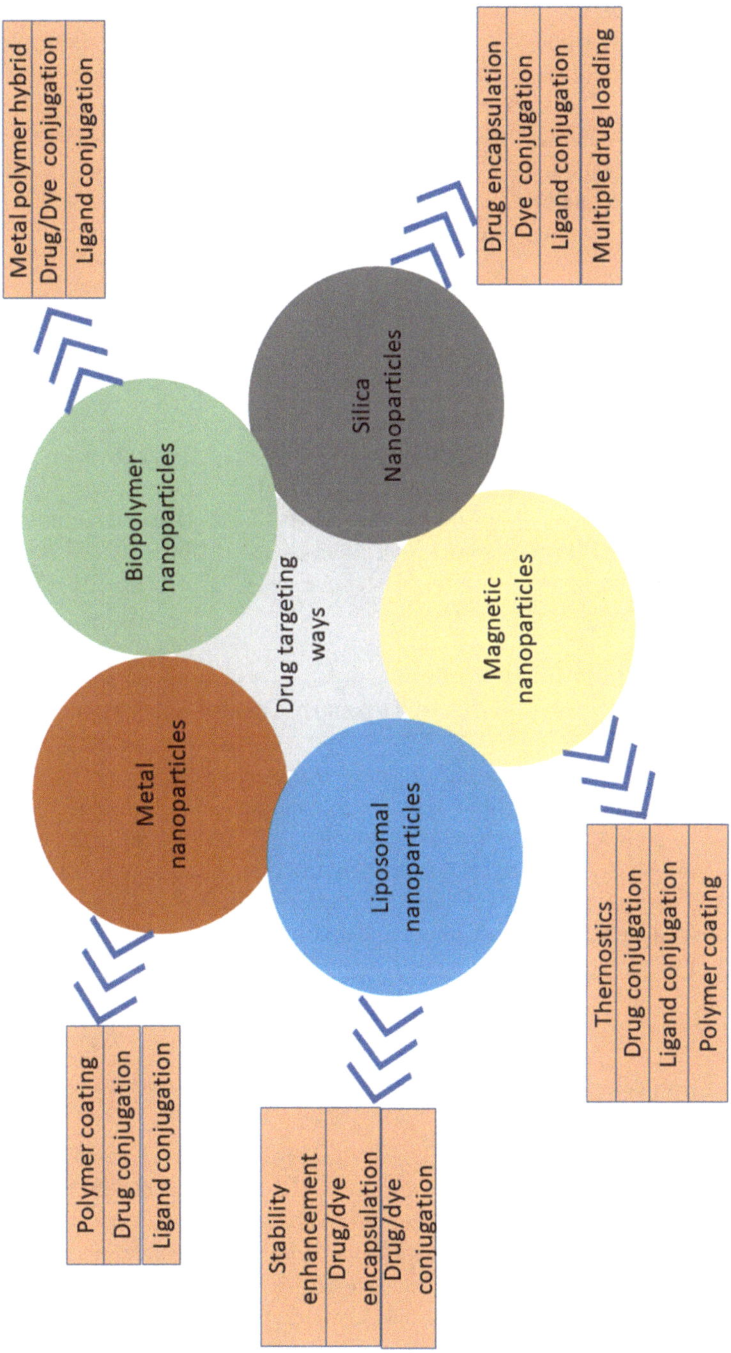

Fig. 10.2 Drug targeting methods for nanoparticles

CT, MRI, PET, and x-ray provide interactive feedback for enabling the localization of nanomedicine (Rai 2014).

Many of these targeting therapeutics have had undesired failure. Some of the observed areas of concerns are (a) increased immunological recognition and clearance due to presence of surface ligands, (b) increased size leading to decreased extravasation and intratumor penetration, and (c) binding site barrier, where the high affinity binding of ligand to target molecule prevents further drug diffusion throughout tumor. Owing to one or more of the above, drugs such as BIND-014 had to be withdrawn after the pre-clinical trials (Wolfram and Ferrari 2019).

10.5.6 Triggered Activation

Stimuli such as pH, glutathione levels, elevated levels of enzymes, etc. that occur in the tumor microenvironment have been identified as triggers for the activation of release of therapeutics from the nanoparticle carriers. Other common strategies also include stimuli such as heat, ultrasound, magnetic field, etc. One such drug that has reached Phase III trials is ThermoDox, a thermosensitive liposomal formulation which releases doxorubicin at temperatures above 39 °C (Dou et al. 2017).

10.6 Promising Nanoparticle Types in Cancer Therapeutics

Nanoparticles, amongst several other features are considered the ideal choice for immunotherapy. Properties such as size, shape, charge, elasticity, carrier function, ability to be engineered to carry multifunctionality, targeting ligands, etc., are some features commonly sought. The tumor microenvironment has a number of immunocompetent cells that can be modulated by cancer cells. Nanoparticles can carry immunomodulatory agents to both tumor and immunocompetent cells, leading to the regulation of phenotypes and functions (Comparetti et al. 2018).

10.6.1 Liposomes

A phospholipid based colloidal drug delivery system based on a bilayer of aqueous media and lipid layers are termed as liposomes and their sizes can be as small as 20 nm. The significant promise that liposomes offered for therapeutics is in its ability to incorporate both hydrophilic and hydrophobic drug molecules, thus increasing the span of active molecules for therapeutics. Liposomal variants of conventional drugs such as doxorubicin are already in the market space.

10.6.2 Polymers, Nanocapsules, and Nanoparticles

Composed of a hydrophilic–lipophilic combination, the polymeric nanocapsules can carry hydrophobic drugs in their lipid core. High drug loading and sustained release are the important features of these class of nanoproducts. Lipid nanocapsules or particles have been found to be suitable to overcome the P-gp mediated drug resistance. In this subsection, the growing relevance of polysaccharides can also not be undermined.

10.6.3 Micelles

Facile synthesis, biodegradability, non-toxicity make micelles a good candidate to carry drug payloads. Features such as pH responsive drug release can be obtained when micelles are composed of lipids such as dilauroyl phosphatidylcholine and deoxycholic acid. Micelles can also be coupled with photothermal therapy (Zhang and Chen 2018).

10.6.4 Polysaccharides

The use of polysaccharide nanoparticles and nanoformulations as carriers for small molecules for tissue regeneration has been reviewed in detail (Narayan 2019). Extensive investigations on the role of particle size in the self-assembly processes of collagen for tissue engineering applications have been reported (Vedhanayagam et al. 2015, 2017, 2019, 2020). Predominantly used in tissue regeneration such as cardiomyocyte differentiation through delivery of drugs such as 5-Azacytidine (Rachel et al. 2020), the use of polysaccharides in cancer therapeutics is increasing. There are reports that chitosan based nanoformulations can enhance the anticancer efficacy of natural product drugs such as hesperetin (Mary Lazer et al. 2018).

10.6.5 Gold Nanoparticles

The use of gold nanorods for photothermal therapy is established. Amine functionalized silica coated gold nanostructures have electrostatic and covalent binding to model proteins such as BSA, with nanoparticle curvature and crosslinking agent influencing the biosafety and cellular response (Narayan et al. 2014). There are a number of studies that indicate the potential for coupling photothermal therapy and immunotherapy. The high biocompatibility of gold nanoparticles comes handy for delivery them intravenously and thus accumulating them in the target cell, taking due to advantage of the EPR effect. Gold nanostructures are also one of the most studied, in terms of the influence of shape on the desired functionality, in this case photothermal therapy. In immunotherapy gold nanoparticles can be used for carrying cancer antigen and immune adjuvants. While the debate on the ideal shape of gold nanoparticles for cancer therapy continues, the gold nanostars have been reported to have an edge on account of its ability to enhance light absorption and high photon-to-heat conversion efficiency arising from plasmonic effect. It is suggested that the combination of photothermal therapy and immunotherapy can give a vaccine like effect (Liu et al. 2018).

10.6.6 Iron Oxide Nanoparticles

Iron oxide nanoparticles have been reported as potent carriers for vaccines. Superparamagnetic iron oxide (SPION) has been reported to be a delivery vehicle for ovalbumin and as an immune potentiator. Iron oxide can also polarize immune cells such as dendritic cells to get increased immune response against tumors (Surendran et al. 2018). Cancer theranostics has benefited tremendously from magnetic nanoparticles. The unique physico-chemical properties have led to magnetic resonance imaging contrasts, easy functionalizations, low toxicity, and good biodegradability. The T1/T2 relaxation ability comes hand in imaging, biosensors, magnetic hyperthermia, photothermal ablation, etc. Several magnetic nanoparticles are today approved by the US FDA for iron deficiency, iron replacement therapy, lymph node metastases, imaging, and MRI (Mukherjee et al. 2020).

SPIONs can be conjugated with drugs to obtain drug delivery systems with unique features such as magnetic targetability, in vivo imaging, magnetic therapy, and combined delivery with anticancer drugs. Researchers have pointed out that targeting moieties for SPIONs can vary from transferrin to antibodies, folates, and targeting peptides, which can be recognized by the overexpressed integrin in the tumor microenvironment (Zhi et al. 2020).

10.6.7 Dendrimers

One of the significant expectations for treatment of solid tumors is in nanodelivery of drugs. A well-designed nano vehicle is required as the tumor microenvironment presents several barriers to the diffusion of nanoparticles into the tumor. This includes poor blood perfusion, high elevated interstitial blood pressure, and a dense tumor matrix where in vivo drug enrichment is a major obstacle.

Common aspects of nanoparticle-based drug delivery vehicles that determine the antitumor activity are particle size, surface charge, and particle shape. With the knowledge gained in the last decade on nanoparticles with a size-shrinkable effect, the initial large size could enable longer blood circulation time, which then can reduce itself to gain deeper penetration into the tumor (Jia et al. 2020).

With CAF being an important barrier to penetration of nanoparticles, transformable drug carriers based on cleavable peptides that are responsive to fibroblast activation protein-α overexpressed on CAF surfaces have been looked at by researchers. In this direction, PAMAM dendrimers crosslinked with peptide (Asp-Ala-Thr-Gly-Pro-Ala) and having a controllable release of doxorubicin through disulfide bonds and targeted release through hyaluronic acid have been reported. On docking to CAFs, the dendrimer structure disintegrates to smaller nanoparticles and expose the CAFs (Hou et al. 2019).

Intelligent nanoparticles can be engineered to shrink in size through enzyme triggered events (Hu et al. 2018). In addition to size variations, the surface charge also needs to be modulated to alter the in vivo behavior. Thus, engineered nanoparticles with size and charge variability have been recently considered as a well doctored strategy for solid tumor treatability.

Surface charge of nanoparticles determines its roles and actions in the tumor microenvironment. A tunable surface charge enhances the therapeutic and diagnostic efficacy of nanoparticles. One of the requirements in this area is a charge reversal, i.e. from anionic to cationic or the reverse depending on the tumor microenvironment and the target site (Zhang et al. 2020a).

In a very recent effort Jia et al., reported the synthesis of poly(2-ethyl-2-oxazoline)-poly(methacryloyl sulfadimethoxine) and coupled it to polyamidoamine-doxorubicin at physiological environment. The resultant compound PEPSD/PAM/DOX was obtained through electrospinning and had an intact ~80 nm structure with prolonged circulation time. PEPSD, in tumor environment, protonates and demonstrated a charge reversal and a size of ~20 nm (Jia et al. 2020).

10.6.8 Carbon Nanotubes

Formed from graphene sheets, carbon nanotubes can single walled, or multi-walled. Diameter and length of single walled carbon nanotubes can be in the range of 0.5–3.0 nm and 20–1000 nm, which for multiwalled can be 1.5–100 nm and 1–50 μm, respectively. Carbon nanotubes owing to their excellent surface properties have gained the attention of medical researchers. On the support of their aspect ratio, cell penetration, and anisotropic conductivity along the axis, researchers have identified carbon nanotubes as ideal for molecular talks (Comparetti et al. 2018; Sanginario et al. 2017; Sheikhpour et al. 2017). The empty spaces in the tube are ideal for drug cargo as well. The reactive surfaces of carbon nanotubes are ideal for functionalization and targeting (Mahajan et al. 2018).

There are some adverse effects such as pneumoconiosis induced by carbon nanotubes through a range of pathways and cellular process, with potential to lead to cancer through inhaled nanomaterials (Dong and Ma 2019).

10.7 Cancer Vaccines

The purpose of cancer vaccines has been described as one of stimulator of tumor specific immune response. It needs to provide defensive protection by activating the adaptive immune system, which can in turn kill the cancer cells. A proposed mechanism of action consists of the following steps:

- Tumor antigen is taken up and processed by antigen presenting cells like dendritic cells.
- The antigen presenting cells migrate to vaccine draining lymph node and present relevant antigens to CD8+ T cells.
- The CD8+ T cells recognize the tumor cells and kill them.
- The mechanism of cancer cell killing includes perforin/granzyme pathway and/or cell–cell interaction.

Initiating a response from T cells requires several activation signals. The first one is that the naïve T cells recognize the antigen bound to dendritic cells (Signal 1). Signal 1 alone leads to induction of Treg cells and thus for full activation a Signal 2, i.e. co-stimulatory signal on T cells is required, which in turn is coupled to Signal 3, viz., the cytokine signals. Adjuvants for Signal 1 improve antigen stability, delivery, processing, and presentation to T cells (Bowen et al. 2018). Adjuvants such as gold nanoparticles, alum, oil/water emulsions, lipid vesicles, etc. have been reported. Heat Shock Proteins are also known to facilitate Signal 1 response. Adjuvants for Signal 2 include saponins and agonistic antibodies, which are predominantly activating ligands for immune receptors. Chitosan has been reported as adjuvant for Signal 3 and Signal 1.

Some of the potential cancer vaccines are presented below:

10.7.1 Neoantigen

It has been recognized that the ideal target for cancer therapy is one that is taken out of cancer mutation rate or unique signature. The targets for the therapeutics are thus called neoantigens. Specific T cells are responsible for clinical response to recognize neoantigens. The efficiency of drugs that control the immune evasive tactics of cancers is referred to as cancer mutation load. Through exome sequencing, a patient's mutanome is identifiable. Neoantigen therapy thus refers to the extent of a patient's immune system to perform the task of cancer killing. The activities in killing include (a) securing a mutational heterogeneity, (b) cancer neoantigen release, (c) cancer neoantigen presentation, (d) priming and activation, (e) T cell trafficking, and (f) cancer cell killing. The neoantigen therapies are administered in combination with immunomodulatory drugs. Some studies suggest that immunogenic neoantigen candidates are not the drivers of cancer development. A poor HLA binding affinity of neoantigens could result in immune responses (Hodge et al. 2020).

Mutant KRAS: Mutan KRAS is a genetic driver for multiple cancers. Neoantigens encoded by KRAS mutations can be tumor specific, with high immunogenicity to deliver precision cancer vaccines and to promote anti-tumor immune response (Zhang et al. 2020b).

10.7.2 Nucleic Acid Vaccines

DNA and mRNA vaccines deliver genetic information encoding tumor antigens to the host cell. The host cell then produces immune responses against the cancer cells that express the tumor antigens. The methodology is restricted by choice of tumor antigen, insufficient immunogenicity, and immunosuppressive character of cancer (Jahanafrooz et al. 2020).Gene encoding mRNA, found in the cytoplasm of eukaryotic cells, based on its dual mode of action, safety profile, and ease of manufacture have been considered as a good source for enabling vaccine antigen expression. It also has an adjuvant activity. Similarly, synthetic DNA vaccines induce robust antitumor immunity.

10.7.3 Human Papillomavirus Vaccine

Prophylactic vaccines, viz. quadrivalent HPV vaccine, bivalent HPV vaccine, and nonavalent HPV vaccine, are today commercially available with a track record of 90% protection against human papillomavirus. Therapeutic vaccines aim to stimulate cell mediated immunity and kill the infected cells as against neutralizing antibodies (Wang et al. 2020b).

In a recent article, Roy et al., have reviewed the literature on various different cancer vaccines in the clinical space, their limitations and advantages, and the progress of work relating to overcoming the challenges (Roy et al. 2020).

Carriers for cancer vaccines are from literature recognized as smart materials and nanocarriers can be utilized to deliver antigen components for inducing immunization. Known examples of nanocarriers for vaccines are a blend of lipidic and polymeric materials. Peptide functionalized nanocarriers have also been reported to have an activity to cytotoxic T cells. Beg et al., have summarized some of the most important cancer vaccines delivered through nano vehicles (Beg et al. 2020).

Nanocarriers for vaccines have replaced viral vector-based delivery of genetic vaccines, thus providing much-desired stability, life, and biodegradability. Nanocarriers are safe and biocompatible and can contain genes and antigens. Similar to all other nano products for industrial application, further extensive trials on safety and efficacy are to be checked. Choice of nanocarrier from among a host of possibilities would depend on antigen loading efficiency, zeta potential, and controlled release profile. A major advantage of nanocarriers for the vaccine is in its ability to carry both the antigens and adjuvants together (Kroll et al. 2019). The ease with which both can be bound to the same nanoparticle through electrostatic interactions, incorporation, or encapsulation, chemical conjugation is determined by choice of nanoparticles or combinations. The nanoparticle choices vary from liposomes to antigen proteins. Polysaccharide gels and polymeric nanoparticles can also act as depots and release antigens and adjuvants slowly over a period of time.

At this point, the opportunity that encapsulation strategies provide is worth discussing with a typical example of arsenic trioxide, which has good therapeutic efficacy against leukemia. However, the single/combined use of arsenic trioxide has not found use in solid tumors owing to severe systemic toxicity and renal elimination. Encapsulation of arsenic trioxide in nanovehicles can still give a chance for arsenic trioxide and similar molecules for the treatment of cancer (Fu et al. 2020).

Nanodelivery of peptides and proteins vaccines which otherwise have failed to elicit immune response has been reported to improve vaccine efficacy. Protein nanoparticles are highly organized structures having advantageous features such as organized structure and biodegradability. It can be functionalized both inside and outside the protein cage and between subunits of the macromolecule (Neek et al. 2019).

10.8 Market Opportunities and Challenges

The extensive range of intrinsic and acquired multidrug resistance is one of the major causes of cancer based deaths today. The ability of nanomedicine approach to overcome such multidrug resistance is one of the significant advantages. Engineering the nanocarriers for active drug targeting, leading to selective drug accumulation in the cancer cells and also being able to work as per the tumor microenvironment are other significant advantages. Strategies for targeting cancer drugs and vaccines and development of multifunctional personalized treatment profiles are other advantages of nanomedicine (Montane et al. 2020). A nano drug delivery system today is expected to deliver chemo (or alternative to chemo) therapeutics or even a combination of them in a passive or active targeted manner through pathways that overcome multidrug resistance (Bar-Zeev et al. 2017).The strengths and opportunities of nanocarriers based on the information available in the literature are presented in Table 10.1.

While immunotherapy has tremendous potential, its limits start with the similarities between normal and cancer cells. The surface antigens in both types of cells are more or less similar. The limits of immunotherapy arise from major similarities between normal cells and cancer cells, where the surface antigens are more or less same. This leads to a situation where the cancer stem cells would repopulate the tumor in a fast manner as soon as the therapeutic is withdrawn. New range of therapeutics that would enable the body's natural defense to fight cancer is needed. Non-toxic therapeutics are the distant goal (Johnson et al. 2014).

Norouzi et al., have tabulated the clinically approved cancer nanomedicines in a recent article (Norouzi et al. 2020). Interestingly, a large number of them such as Doxil and Myocet (Doxorubicin), Mepact (Mifamurtide), Marqibo (Vincristine sulfate), Onivyde (Irinotecan), and Vyxeos (Cytarabine and Daunorubicin) are liposomal formulations. It is reported that of the 2400 clinical studies on liposomal nanocarriers, 1800 are for cancer treatment. In all of the examples of products in clinical trials, the use of liposomal formulations while possibly reducing toxicity does not eliminate the toxicity of the drug itself. For instance, Doxil use has reported side effects such as hand-foot syndrome, blisters on hand and soles of feet, etc. This has been attributed to the long-circulation leading to accumulation in healthy and susceptible tissues (Liu et al. 2018). There are also reports that spherical forms of

Table 10.1 Strengths and Opportunities for Nanostructures as Cancer Therapeutic Carriers

Nanostructure	Strengths	Opportunities
Metal and metal oxide	• Easy to synthesize and functionalize • Good stability and versatility • Modifiable optical and electronic properties	• Improvement in biodegradability • Reduction in toxicity, especially from metal ions if present • Overcoming functionalization needs for solubility
Polymers	• Good for hydrophilic drugs • Biodegradable and biocompatibl • Low toxicity • Can be functionalized for targeting	• Increase in circulation time • Reduction in cytotoxicity
Liposomes	• Biocompatible • Tunable structures	• Shelf life increase • Reduced drug leakage • Increase in circulation time
Dendrimers	• Stability • Shelf life • Surface area and loading capacity • Biodegradability and biocompatibility	• Facile synthesi • Toxicity of G2 and above
Proteins	• Low toxicity • High biocompatibility and biodegradability	• Improving drug loading capacity
Carbon nanotubes	• Penetration into tumor cells • Good drug loading	• Solubility • Biodegradability • Toxicity reduction
Quantum dots	• Solubility • Sensors and imaging	• Biodegradability improvemen • Reduction in cytotoxicity
Biopolymers	• Natural resources • Biocompatible and biodegradable • Conjugation chemistry	• Encapsulation efficiency • Enzymatic degradation

liposomes undergo change to non-spherical forms leading to adverse effects (Szebeni et al. 2002, 2011, 2012). This indicates that the safety profile of liposomal and other nanocarriers are structure dependent and thus very sensitive to manufacture process (Wibroe et al. 2016).

Nanoformulation itself can be considered as a barrier to the progress of use of nanomedicine in clinical practice. It has been suggested that payload transfer is at best 1% (Wilhelm et al. 2016). A blueprint for safety assessment of nanomedicines indicates five levels of assessment or more. This includes (a) the characterization of the nanomaterial in terms of its physical and chemical properties, viz., size, shape, charge, release profile, dissolution, band gap, porosity, crystallinity, and so on, (b) toxicity mechanisms such as oxidative stress, cationic toxicity, ion shedding, fibrosis, lysis, etc., (c) abiotic and mechanistic in vitro assays, (d) in vivo studies, and (e) patient adverse event report and management.

Tumor specific improvements in the accumulation of drugs are improved when nanoparticles have targeting ligands attached. Barriers to production of nanoparticles in large scales and absence of transparent regulatory norms are other challenges. Quality assurance parameters such as consistency, composition, loading capacity, self-assembly, ligand binding density, biodegradability, etc. require standard methods of evaluation. A balance between complexity and simplicity is the way forward for nanomedicine.

It is documented that 23% of all publications in nanoparticles during 2018 is related to cancer treatment and diagnosis. Of this, only 17% were published in medical research areas, indicating a more synthesis-characterization driven approach than disease-cure driven approach (Salvioni et al. 2019). A significant number of publications have overexpressed optimism based on pre-clinical studies reported. On a pessimistic note the number of nanovehicles approved for marketing may not even touch two digit mark. Administration methodology and its influence on therapeutic or targeting efficiency are still in nascent research. However, from studies focused on EPR effect, the current focus has moved to that of tumor microenvironment triggering major ambitions in developing marketable products.

Understanding the relationship between treatment efficacy and immune system response is another area of research. The challenge in this area has been the low efficacy of animal models. Avoiding phagocytosis and enabling molecular targeting through engineering of nanoparticle surface still continues to enthuse chemists than medical scientists. This however has the advantage that nanoformulations can deliver a host active drug candidates which otherwise cannot be used or tried in clinical practice.

Nanotheranostics has the potential to harness the advantages of nanoscience for combining therapy with diagnosis. In cancer therapy, nanotheranostics can take advantage of well-defined characteristics of the tumor microenvironment (Wong et al. 2020). Personalization of nano systems through a plug and play approach to achieve desired penetration, circulation, target, release modality coupled with imaging makes nanotheranostics the future of cancer treatment.

Based on the positive notes on the creativity of nanochemists to play around with functionalization, structure, and shape of nanoparticles there is still hope for a host of nanoformulations to be used as therapeutic and vaccine for cancer. As described in *Nature Nanotechnology in 2019, nanomedicine for cancer has only two directions to go—the first one is to debate whether clinical translation of nanomaterials should be accelerated or whether long standing drug delivery paradigms are to be challenged* (Nature 2019).

There is an urgent need to move from short term cancer management strategies such as delaying tumor growth to long-term permanent disease management. Pairing of nanomaterial research with dosing conditions and optimization of efficacy and safety needs to go parallell. An assessment of phenotype response is suggested as a guide to rational drug design.

Acknowledgement SN thanks Chettinad Academy of Research and Education for support.

References

Ali F, Hosmane NS, Zhu YH (2020) Boron chemistry for medical applications. Molecules 25(4). https://doi.org/10.3390/molecules25040828

Alvaro T, de la Cruz-Merino L, Henao-Carrasco F, Rodriguez JLV, Baz DV, de Villena MCM, Provencio M (2010) Tumor microenvironment and immune effects of antineoplastic therapy in lymphoproliferative syndromes. J Biomed Biotechnol doi:https://doi.org/10.1155/2010/846872

Amin ARMR, Karpowicz PA, Carey TE, Arbiser J, Nahta R, Chen ZG, Dong J-T, Kucuk O, Khan GN, Huang GS, Mi S, Lee H-Y, Reichrath J, Honoki K, Georgakilas AG, Amedei A, Amin A, Helferich B, Boosani CS, Ciriolo MR, Chen S, Mohammed SI, Azmi AS, Keith WN, Bhakta D, Halicka D, Niccolai E, Fujii H, Aquilano K, Ashraf SS, Nowsheen S, Yang X, Bilsland A, Shin DM (2015) Evasion of anti-growth signaling: a key step in tumorigenesis and potential target for treatment and prophylaxis by natural compounds. Semin Cancer Biol 35:S55–S77. https://doi.org/10.1016/j.semcancer.2015.02.005

Barth RF, Zhang Z, Liu T (2018) A realistic appraisal of boron neutron capture therapy as a cancer treatment modality. Cancer Commun 38(1):36. https://doi.org/10.1186/s40880-018-0280-5

Bar-Zeev M, Livney YD, Assaraf YG (2017) Targeted nanomedicine for cancer therapeutics: towards precision medicine overcoming drug resistance. Drug Resist Update 31:15–30. https://doi.org/10.1016/j.drup.2017.05.002

Beg S, Alharbi KS, Alruwaili NK, Alotaibi NH, Almalki WH, Alenezi SK, Altowayan WM, Alshammari MS, Rahman M (2020) Nanotherapeutic systems for delivering cancer vaccines: recent advances. Nanomedicine (Lond) 15(15):1527–1537. https://doi.org/10.2217/nnm-2020-0046

Bodei L, Ferone D, Grana CM, Cremonesi M, Signore A, Dierckx RA, Paganelli G (2009) Peptide receptor therapies in neuroendocrine tumors. J Endocrinol Investig 32(4):360–369. https://doi.org/10.1007/bf03345728

Bowen WS, Svrivastava AK, Batra L, Barsoumian H, Shirwan H (2018) Current challenges for cancer vaccine adjuvant development. Expert Rev Vaccines 17(3):207–215. https://doi.org/10.1080/14760584.2018.1434000

Bray F, Ferlay J, Soerjomataram I, Siegel RL, Torre LA, Jemal A (2018) Global cancer statistics 2018: GLOBOCAN estimates of incidence and mortality worldwide for 36 cancers in 185 countries. CA Cancer J Clin 68(6):394–424. https://doi.org/10.3322/caac.21492

Cervantes-Villagrana RD, Albores-Garcia D, Cervantes-Villagrana AR, Garcia-Acevez SJ (2020) Tumor-induced neurogenesis and immune evasion as targets of innovative anti-cancer therapies. Signal Transduct Target Ther 5(1):23. https://doi.org/10.1038/s41392-020-0205-z

Chen HW, Chen TWW (2020) Genomic-guided precision therapy for soft tissue sarcoma. Esmo Open 5(2). https://doi.org/10.1136/esmoopen-2019-000626

Cheng YQ, Wang SB, Liu JH, Jin L, Liu Y, Li CY, Su YR, Liu YR, Sang X, Wan Q, Liu C, Yang L, Wang ZC (2020) Modifying the tumour microenvironment and reverting tumour cells: new strategies for treating malignant tumours. Cell Prolif 53(8):e12865. https://doi.org/10.1111/cpr.12865

Comparetti EJ, Pedrosa VD, Kaneno R (2018) Carbon nanotube as a tool for fighting cancer. Bioconjug Chem 29(3):709–718. https://doi.org/10.1021/acs.bioconjchem.7b00563

Costea DE, Hills A, Osman AH, Thurlow J, Kalna G, Huang X, Murillo CP, Parajuli H, Suliman S, Kulasekara KK, Johannessen AC, Partridge M (2013) Identification of two distinct carcinoma-associated fibroblast subtypes with differential tumor-promoting abilities in oral squamous cell carcinoma. Cancer Res 73(13):3888–3901. https://doi.org/10.1158/0008-5472.Can-12-4150

Daniels TR, Bernabeu E, Rodríguez JA, Patel S, Kozman M, Chiappetta DA, Holler E, Ljubimova JY, Helguera G, Penichet ML (2012) The transferrin receptor and the targeted delivery of therapeutic agents against cancer. Biochim Biophys Acta 1820(3):291–317. https://doi.org/10.1016/j.bbagen.2011.07.016

de Winde CM, Munday C, Acton SE (2020) Molecular mechanisms of dendritic cell migration in immunity and cancer. Med Microbiol Immunol 209(4):515–529. https://doi.org/10.1007/s00430-020-00680-4

Dong J, Ma Q (2019) Integration of inflammation, fibrosis, and cancer induced by carbon nanotubes. Nanotoxicology 13(9):1244–1274. https://doi.org/10.1080/17435390.2019.1651920

Dou Y, Hynynen K, Allen C (2017) To heat or not to heat: challenges with clinical translation of thermosensitive liposomes. J Control Release 249:63–73. https://doi.org/10.1016/j.jconrel.2017.01.025

Duan QQ, Zhang HL, Zheng JN, Zhang LJ (2020) Turning cold into hot: firing up the tumor microenvironment. Trends Cancer 6(7):605–618. https://doi.org/10.1016/j.trecan.2020.02.022

El-Readi MZ, Althubiti MA (2019) Cancer nanomedicine: a new era of successful targeted therapy. J Nanomater 2019:13. https://doi.org/10.1155/2019/4927312

Elyada E, Bolisetty M, Laise P, Flynn WF, Courtois ET, Burkhart RA, Teinor JA, Belleau P, Biffi G, Lucito MS, Sivajothi S, Armstrong TD, Engle DD, Yu KH, Hao Y, Wolfgang CL, Park Y, Preall J, Jaffee EM, Califano A, Robson P, Tuveson DA (2019) Cross-species single-cell analysis of pancreatic ductal adenocarcinoma reveals antigen-presenting cancer-associated fibroblasts. Cancer Discov 9(8):1102–1123. https://doi.org/10.1158/2159-8290.Cd-19-0094

Fu X, Li YS, Zhao J, Yu LL, Luo RG, Liang QR, Tang Q (2020) Will arsenic trioxide benefit treatment of solid tumor by nano-encapsulation? Mini-Rev Med Chem 20(3):239–251. https://doi.org/10.2174/1389557519666191018155426

Gajewski TF (2015) The next hurdle in cancer immunotherapy: overcoming the non–T-cell–inflamed tumor microenvironment. Semin Oncol 42(4):663–671. https://doi.org/10.1053/j.seminoncol.2015.05.011

Garcia-Bennett A, Nees M, Fadeel B (2011) In search of the holy grail: folate-targeted nanoparticles for cancer therapy. Biochem Pharmacol 81(8):976–984. https://doi.org/10.1016/j.bcp.2011.01.023

Hanahan D, Coussens LM (2012) Accessories to the crime: functions of cells recruited to the tumor microenvironment. Cancer Cell 21(3):309–322. https://doi.org/10.1016/j.ccr.2012.02.022

Hayes BH, Tsai RK, Dooling LJ, Kadu S, Lee JY, Pantano D, Rodriguez PL, Subramanian S, Shin J-W, Discher DE (2020) Macrophages show higher levels of engulfment after disruption of cis interactions between CD47 and the checkpoint receptor SIRP alpha. J Cell Sci 133(5). https://doi.org/10.1242/jcs.237800

Helmlinger G, Netti PA, Lichtenbeld HC, Melder RJ, Jain RK (1997a) Solid stress inhibits the growth of multicellular tumor spheroids. Nat Biotechnol 15(8):778–783. https://doi.org/10.1038/nbt0897-778

Helmlinger G, Yuan F, Dellian M, Jain RK (1997b) Interstitial pH and pO(2) gradients in solid tumors in vivo: high-resolution measurements reveal a lack of correlation. Nat Med 3(2):177–182. https://doi.org/10.1038/nm0297-177

Hodge K, Supabphol S, Kumar P, Poomipak W, Pisitkun T (2020) Recent developments in neoantigen-based cancer vaccines. Asian Pac J Allergy Immunol 38(2):91–101

Hou L, Chen DD, Hao LS, Tian CY, Yan YS, Zhu L, Zhang HJ, Zhang Y, Zhang ZZ (2019) Transformable nanoparticles triggered by cancer-associated fibroblasts for improving drug permeability and efficacy in desmoplastic tumors. Nanoscale 11(42):20030–20044. https://doi.org/10.1039/c9nr06438a

Hu C, Cun XL, Ruan SB, Liu R, Xiao W, Yang XT, Yang YY, Yang CY, Gao HL (2018) Enzyme-triggered size shrink and laser-enhanced NO release nanoparticles for deep tumor penetration and combination therapy. Biomaterials 168:64–75. https://doi.org/10.1016/j.biomaterials.2018.03.046

Hu WL, Wang GS, Huang DS, Sui MH, Xu YB (2019) Cancer immunotherapy based on natural killer cells: current progress and new opportunities. Front Immunol 10:1205. https://doi.org/10.3389/fimmu.2019.01205

Iqbal MA, Arora S, Prakasam G, Calin GA, Syed MA (2019) MicroRNA in lung cancer: role, mechanisms, pathways and therapeutic relevance. Mol Asp Med 70:3–20. https://doi.org/10.1016/j.mam.2018.07.003

Ishida T, Maeda R, Ichihara M, Irimura K, Kiwada H (2003) Accelerated clearance of PEGylated liposomes in rats after repeated injections. J Control Release 88(1):35–42. https://doi.org/10.1016/S0168-3659(02)00462-5

Issa F, Kassiou M, Rendina LM (2011) Boron in drug discovery: Carboranes as unique pharmacophores in biologically active compounds. Chem Rev 111(9):5701–5722. https://doi.org/10.1021/cr2000866

Jahanafrooz Z, Baradaran B, Mosafer J, Hashemzaei M, Rezaei T, Mokhtarzadeh A, Hamblin MR (2020) Comparison of DND and mRNA vaccines against cancer. Drug Discov Today 25 (3):552–560. https://doi.org/10.1016/j.drudis.2019.12.003

Jain RK, Martin JD, Stylianopoulos T (2014) The role of mechanical forces in tumor growth and therapy. Annu Rev Biomed Eng 16:321–346. https://doi.org/10.1146/annurev-bioeng-071813-105259

Jeannin P, Paolini L, Adam C, Delneste Y (2018) The roles of CSFs on the functional polarization of tumor-associated macrophages. FEBS J 285(4):680–699. https://doi.org/10.1111/febs.14343

Jia N, Li WP, Liu D, Wu SY, Song BH, Ma JZ, Chen DW, Hu HY (2020) Tumor microenvironment stimuli-responsive nanoparticles for programmed anticancer drug delivery. Mol Pharm 17 (5):1516–1526. https://doi.org/10.1021/acs.molpharmaceut.9b01189

Johnson BE, Mazor T, Hong C, Barnes M, Aihara K, McLean CY, Fouse SD, Yamamoto S, Ueda H, Tatsuno K, Asthana S, Jalbert LE, Nelson SJ, Bollen AW, Gustafson WC, Charron E, Weiss WA, Smirnov IV, Song JS, Olshen AB, Cha S, Zhao Y, Moore RA, Mungall AJ, Jones SJM, Hirst M, Marra MA, Saito N, Aburatani H, Mukasa A, Berger MS, Chang SM, Taylor BS, Costello JF (2014) Mutational analysis reveals the origin and therapy-driven evolution of recurrent glioma. Science 343(6167):189. https://doi.org/10.1126/science.1239947

Kaim W, Hosmane NS, Záliš S, Maguire JA, Lipscomb WN (2009) Boron atoms as spin carriers in two- and three-dimensional systems. Angew Chem Int Ed 48(28):5082–5091. https://doi.org/10.1002/anie.200803493

Kalluri R, Zeisberg M (2006) Fibroblasts in cancer. Nat Rev Cancer 6(5):392–401. https://doi.org/10.1038/nrc1877

Koido S, Homma S, Hara E, Namiki Y, Takahara A, Komita H, Nagasaki E, Ito M, Ohkusa T, Gong JL, Tajiri H (2010) Regulation of tumor immunity by tumor/dendritic cell fusions. Clin Dev Immunol. https://doi.org/10.1155/2010/516768

Kroll AV, Jiang Y, Zhou J, Holay M, Fang RH, Zhang L (2019) Biomimetic nanoparticle vaccines for cancer therapy. Adv Biosyst 3(1):1800219. https://doi.org/10.1002/adbi.201800219

Leone RD, Powell JD (2020) Metabolism of immune cells in cancer. Nat Rev Cancer 20 (9):516–531. https://doi.org/10.1038/s41568-020-0273-y

Lim WA, June CH (2017) The principles of engineering immune cells to treat cancer. Cell 168 (4):724–740. https://doi.org/10.1016/j.cell.2017.01.016

Liu Y, Crawford BM, Vo-Dinh T (2018) Gold nanoparticles-mediated photothermal therapy and immunotherapy. Immunotherapy 10(13):1175–1188. https://doi.org/10.2217/imt-2018-0029

Lopez-Yrigoyen M, Cassetta L, Pollard JW (2020) Macrophage targeting in cancer. Ann N Y Acad Sci. https://doi.org/10.1111/nyas.14377

Mahajan S, Patharkar A, Kuche K, Maheshwari R, Deb PK, Kalia K, Tekade RK (2018) Functionalized carbon nanotubes as emerging delivery system for the treatment of cancer. Int J Pharm 548(1):540–558. https://doi.org/10.1016/j.ijpharm.2018.07.027

Majidinia M, Mirza-Aghazadeh-Attari M, Rahimi M, Mihanfar A, Karimian A, Safa A, Yousefi B (2020) Overcoming multidrug resistance in cancer: recent progress in nanotechnology and new horizons. IUBMB Life 72(5):855–871. https://doi.org/10.1002/iub.2215

Malik R, Lelkes PI, Cukierman E (2015) Biomechanical and biochemical remodeling of stromal extracellular matrix in cancer. Trends Biotechnol 33(4):230–236. https://doi.org/10.1016/j.tibtech.2015.01.004

Martinez M, Moon EK (2019) CAR T cells for solid tumors: new strategies for finding, infiltrating, and surviving in the tumor microenvironment. Front Immunol 10:21. https://doi.org/10.3389/fimmu.2019.00128

Mary Lazer L, Sadhasivam B, Palaniyandi K, Muthuswamy T, Ramachandran I, Balakrishnan A, Pathak S, Narayan S, Ramalingam S (2018) Chitosan-based nano-formulation enhances the anticancer efficacy of hesperetin. Int J Biol Macromol 107(Pt B):1988–1998. https://doi.org/10.1016/j.ijbiomac.2017.10.064

Mennerich D, Kubaichuk K, Kietzmann T (2019) DUBs, hypoxia, and cancer. Trends Cancer 5 (10):632–653. https://doi.org/10.1016/j.trecan.2019.08.005

Miller MA, Zheng Y-R, Gadde S, Pfirschke C, Zope H, Engblom C, Kohler RH, Iwamoto Y, Yang KS, Askevold B, Kolishetti N, Pittet M, Lippard SJ, Farokhzad OC, Weissleder R (2015) Tumour-associated macrophages act as a slow-release reservoir of nano-therapeutic Pt (IV) pro-drug. Nat Commun 6(1):8692. https://doi.org/10.1038/ncomms9692

Montane X, Bajek A, Roszkowski K, Montornes JM, Giamberini M, Roszkowski S, Kowalczyk O, Garcia-Valls R, Tylkowski B (2020) Encapsulation for cancer therapy. Molecules 25(7). https://doi.org/10.3390/molecules25071605

Mukherjee S, Liang L, Veiseh O (2020) Recent advancements of magnetic nanomaterials in cancer therapy. Pharmaceutics 12(2). https://doi.org/10.3390/pharmaceutics12020147

Murphy JM, Rodriguez YAR, Jeong K, Ahn EYE, Lim STS (2020) Targeting focal adhesion kinase in cancer cells and the tumor microenvironment. Exp Mol Med 52(6):877–886. https://doi.org/10.1038/s12276-020-0447-4

Najafi M, Farhood B, Mortezaee K, Kharazinejad E, Majidpoor J, Ahadi R (2020) Hypoxia in solid tumors: a key promoter of cancer stem cell (CSC) resistance. J Cancer Res Clin Oncol 146 (1):19–31. https://doi.org/10.1007/s00432-019-03080-1

Narayan S (2019) Chitosan-based nanoformulation as carriers of small molecules for tissue regeneration. In: Jana S, Jana S (eds) Functional chitosan: drug delivery and biomedical applications. Springer, Singapore, pp 321–342. https://doi.org/10.1007/978-981-15-0263-7_11

Narayan S, Krishnan S, Chadha A (2013) Double edged sword-designing gold nanorods functionalized with KDR-binding peptides for effective blocking of angiogenesis and photothermal therapy. Third international conference on multifunctional hybrid and nanomaterials

Narayan S, Rajagopalan A, Reddy JS, Chadha A (2014) BSA binding to silica capped gold nanostructures: effect of surface cap and conjugation design on nanostructure–BSA interface. RSC Adv 4(3):1412–1420. https://doi.org/10.1039/C3RA45887C

Nature (2019) The two directions of cancer nanomedicine. Nat Nanotechnol 14(12):1083–1083. https://doi.org/10.1038/s41565-019-0597-5

Neek M, Kim TI, Wang SW (2019) Protein-based nanoparticles in cancer vaccine development. Nanomed Nanotechnol Biol Med 15(1):164–174. https://doi.org/10.1016/j.nano.2018.09.004

Ngamcherdtrakul W, Yantasee W (2019) siRNA therapeutics for breast cancer: recent efforts in targeting metastasis, drug resistance, and immune evasion. Transl Res 214:105–120. https://doi.org/10.1016/j.trsl.2019.08.005

Norouzi H, Khoshgard K, Akbarzadeh F (2018) In vitro outlook of gold nanoparticles in photothermal therapy: a literature review. Lasers Med Sci 33(4):917–926. https://doi.org/10.1007/s10103-018-2467-z

Norouzi M, Amerian M, Amerian M, Atyabi F (2020) Clinical applications of nanomedicine in cancer therapy. Drug Discov Today 25(1):107–125. https://doi.org/10.1016/j.drudis.2019.09.017

Oya Y, Hayakawa Y, Koike K (2020) Tumor microenvironment in gastric cancers. Cancer Sci 111:2696–2707. https://doi.org/10.1111/cas.14521

Pasut G, Veronese FM (2012) State of the art in PEGylation: the great versatility achieved after forty years of research. J Control Release 161(2):461–472. https://doi.org/10.1016/j.jconrel.2011.10.037

Rachel K, Pathak S, Moorthi A, Narasimhan S, Murugesan R, Narayan S (2020) 5-Azacytidine incorporated polycaprolactone-gelatin nanoscaffold as a potential material for cardiomyocyte differentiation. J Biomater Sci Polym Ed 31(1):123–140. https://doi.org/10.1080/09205063.2019.1678796

Rai P (2014) Theranostic nanomedicine for imaging-guided treatment of cancer. Abstracts of papers of the American Chemical Society, p 247

Ribeiro MF, Zhu H, Millard RW, Fan G-C (2013) Exosomes function in pro- and anti-angiogenesis. Curr Angiogenes 2(1):54–59

Roy S, Sethi TK, Taylor D, Kim YJ, Johnson DB (2020) Breakthrough concepts in immune-oncology: cancer vaccines at the bedside. J Leukoc Biol 108(4):1455–1489. https://doi.org/10.1002/jlb.5bt0420-585rr

Ryu JH, Lee S, Son S, Kim SH, Leary JF, Choi K, Kwon IC (2014) Theranostic nanoparticles for future personalized medicine. J Control Release 190:477–484. https://doi.org/10.1016/j.jconrel.2014.04.027

Salvioni L, Rizzuto MA, Bertolini JA, Pandolfi L, Colombo M, Prosperi D (2019) Thirty years of cancer nanomedicine: success, frustration, and hope. Cancers (Basel) 11(12):1855. https://doi.org/10.3390/cancers11121855

Sanginario A, Miccoli B, Demarchi D (2017) Carbon nanotubes as an effective opportunity for cancer diagnosis and treatment. Biosensors (Basel) 7(1). https://doi.org/10.3390/bios7010009

Schumacher TN, Schreiber RD (2015) Neoantigens in cancer immunotherapy. Science 348 (6230):69–74. https://doi.org/10.1126/science.aaa4971

Sharkey RM, Goldenberg DM (2011) Cancer radioimmunotherapy. Immunotherapy 3(3):349–370. https://doi.org/10.2217/imt.10.114

Sheikhpour M, Golbabaie A, Kasaeian A (2017) Carbon nanotubes: a review of novel strategies for cancer diagnosis and treatment. Mater Sci Eng C 76:1289–1304. https://doi.org/10.1016/j.msec.2017.02.132

Shen H, Sun T, Ferrari M (2012) Nanovector delivery of siRNA for cancer therapy. Cancer Gene Ther 19(6):367–373. https://doi.org/10.1038/cgt.2012.22

Shi S, Vissapragada R, Abi Jaoude J, Huang C, Mittal A, Liu E, Zhong J, Kumar V (2020) Evolving role of biomaterials in diagnostic and therapeutic radiation oncology. Bioact Mater 5 (2):233–240. https://doi.org/10.1016/j.bioactmat.2020.01.011

Sköld K, H-Stenstam B, Diaz AZ, Giusti V, Pellettieri L, Hopewell JW (2010) Boron neutron capture therapy for glioblastoma multiforme: advantage of prolonged infusion of BPA-f. Acta Neurol Scand 122(1):58–62. https://doi.org/10.1111/j.1600-0404.2009.01267.x

Spugnini EP, Logozzi M, Di Raimo R, Mizzoni D, Fais S (2018) A role of tumor-released exosomes in paracrine dissemination and metastasis. Int J Mol Sci 19(12):E3968. https://doi.org/10.3390/ijms19123968

Surendran SP, Moon MJ, Park R, Jeong YY (2018) Bioactive nanoparticles for cancer immunotherapy. Int J Mol Sci 19(12). https://doi.org/10.3390/ijms19123877

Szebeni J, Baranyi L, Savay S, Milosevits J, Bunger R, Laverman P, Metselaar JM, Storm G, Chanan-Khan A, Liebes L, Muggia FM, Cohen R, Barenholz Y, Alving CR (2002) Role of complement activation in hypersensitivity reactions to doxil and HYNICPEG liposomes: experimental and clinical studies. J Liposome Res 12(1–2):165–172. https://doi.org/10.1081/lpr-120004790

Szebeni J, Muggia F, Gabizon A, Barenholz Y (2011) Activation of complement by therapeutic liposomes and other lipid excipient-based therapeutic products: prediction and prevention. Adv Drug Deliv Rev 63(12):1020–1030. https://doi.org/10.1016/j.addr.2011.06.017

Szebeni J, Bedocs P, Rozsnyay Z, Weiszhar Z, Urbanics R, Rosivall L, Cohen R, Garbuzenko O, Bathori G, Toth M, Buenger R, Barenholz Y (2012) Liposome-induced complement activation and related cardiopulmonary distress in pigs: factors promoting reactogenicity of Doxil and AmBisome. Nanomed Nanotechnol Biol Med 8(2):176–184. https://doi.org/10.1016/j.nano.2011.06.003

Tang ZY, Li DP, Hou SP, Zhu X (2020) The cancer exosomes: clinical implications, applications and challenges. Int J Cancer 146(11):2946–2959. https://doi.org/10.1002/ijc.32762

Tian YG, Li YL, Shao YP, Zhang Y (2020) Gene modification strategies for next-generation CAR T cells against solid cancers. J Hematol Oncol 13(1):16. https://doi.org/10.1186/s13045-020-00890-6

van der Zanden SY, Luimstra JJ, Neefjes J, Borst J, Ovaa H (2020) Opportunities for small molecules in cancer immunotherapy. Trends Immunol 41(6):493–511. https://doi.org/10.1016/j.it.2020.04.004

Vautrot V, Chanteloup G, Elmallah M, Cordonnier M, Aubin F, Garrido C, Gobbo J (2019) Exosomal miRNA: small molecules, big impact in colorectal cancer. J Oncol. https://doi.org/10.1155/2019/8585276

Vedhanayagam M, Mohan R, Nair BU, Sreeram KJ (2015) Nanorod mediated collagen scaffolds as extra cellular matrix mimics. Biomed Mater 10(6). https://doi.org/10.1088/1748-6041/10/6/065010

Vedhanayagam M, Nidhin M, Duraipandy N, Naresh ND, Jaganathan G, Ranganathan M, Kiran MS, Narayan S, Nair BU, Sreeram KJ (2017) Role of nanoparticle size in self-assemble processes of collagen for tissue engineering application. Int J Biol Macromol 99:655–664. https://doi.org/10.1016/j.ijbiomac.2017.02.102

Vedhanayagam M, Nair BU, Sreeram KJ (2019) Effect of functionalized gold nanoparticle on collagen stabilization for tissue engineering application. Int J Biol Macromol 123:1211–1220. https://doi.org/10.1016/j.ijbiomac.2018.11.179

Vedhanayagam M, Anandasadagopan S, Nair BU, Sreeram KJ (2020) Polymethyl methacrylate (PMMA) grafted collagen scaffold reinforced by PdO-TiO2 nanocomposites. Mater Sci Eng C 108. https://doi.org/10.1016/j.msec.2019.110378

Viallard C, Larrivee B (2017) Tumor angiogenesis and vascular normalization: alternative therapeutic targets. Angiogenesis 20(4):409–426. https://doi.org/10.1007/s10456-017-9562-9

Villanueva N, Bazhenova L (2018) New strategies in immunotherapy for lung cancer: beyond PD-1/PD-L1. Ther Adv Respir Dis 12:1753466618794133. https://doi.org/10.1177/1753466618794133

Vogelstein B, Kinzler KW (1993) The multistep nature of cancer. Trends Genet 9(4):138–141. https://doi.org/10.1016/0168-9525(93)90209-z

Wang J, Matosevic S (2020) Functional and metabolic targeting of natural killer cells to solid tumors. Cell Oncol 43(4):577–600. https://doi.org/10.1007/s13402-020-00523-7

Wang Q, Guan JK, Wan JL, Li ZF (2020a) Disulfide based prodrugs for cancer therapy. RSC Adv 10(41):24397–24409. https://doi.org/10.1039/d0ra04155f

Wang RJ, Pan W, Jin L, Huang WM, Li YH, Wu D, Gao C, Ma D, Liao SJ (2020b) Human papillomavirus vaccine against cervical cancer: opportunity and challenge. Cancer Lett 471:88–102. https://doi.org/10.1016/j.canlet.2019.11.039

Wibroe PP, Ahmadvand D, Oghabian MA, Yaghmur A, Moghimi SM (2016) An integrated assessment of morphology, size, and complement activation of the PEGylated liposomal doxorubicin products Doxil (R), Caelyx (R), DOXOrubicin, and SinaDoxosome. J Control Release 221:1–8. https://doi.org/10.1016/j.jconrel.2015.11.021

Wilhelm S, Tavares AJ, Dai Q, Ohta S, Audet J, Dvorak HF, Chan WCW (2016) Analysis of nanoparticle delivery to tumours. Nat Rev Mater 1(5). https://doi.org/10.1038/natrevmats.2016.14

Wolfram J, Ferrari M (2019) Clinical cancer nanomedicine. Nano Today 25:85–98. https://doi.org/10.1016/j.nantod.2019.02.005

Wong XY, Sena-Torralba A, Alvarez-Diduk R, Muthoosamy K, Merkoci A (2020) Nanomaterials for nanotheranostics: tuning their properties according to disease needs. ACS Nano 14(3):2585–2627. https://doi.org/10.1021/acsnano.9b08133

Wu T, Dai Y (2017) Tumor microenvironment and therapeutic response. Cancer Lett 387:61–68. https://doi.org/10.1016/j.canlet.2016.01.043

Xi C, Zhang GQ, Sun ZK, Song HJ, Shen CT, Chen XY, Sun JW, Qiu ZL, Luo QY (2020) Interleukins in thyroid cancer: from basic researches to applications in clinical practice. Front Immunol 11:14. https://doi.org/10.3389/fimmu.2020.01124

Yardley DA (2013) Nab-paclitaxel mechanisms of action and delivery. J Control Release 170 (3):365–372. https://doi.org/10.1016/j.jconrel.2013.05.041

Zemek RM, De Jong E, Chin WL, Schuster IS, Fear VS, Casey TH, Forbes C, Dart SJ, Leslie C, Zaitouny A, Small M, Boon L, Forrest ARR, Muiri DO, Degli-Esposti MA, Millward MJ, Nowak AK, Lassmann T, Bosco A, Lake RA, Lesterhuis WJ (2019) Sensitization to immune checkpoint blockade through activation of a STAT1/NK axis in the tumor microenvironment. Sci Transl Med 11(501):eaav7816. https://doi.org/10.1126/scitranslmed.aav7816

Zhang H, Chen J (2018) Current status and future directions of cancer immunotherapy. J Cancer 9 (10):1773–1781. https://doi.org/10.7150/jca.24577

Zhang MZ, Chen XX, Li C, Shen X (2020a) Charge-reversal nanocarriers: an emerging paradigm for smart cancer nanomedicine. J Control Release 319:46–62. https://doi.org/10.1016/j.jconrel.2019.12.024

Zhang Y, Ma JA, Zhang HX, Jiang YN, Luo WH (2020b) Cancer vaccines: targeting KRAS-driven cancers. Expert Rev Vaccines 19(2):163–173. https://doi.org/10.1080/14760584.2020.1733420

Zhang XY, Li WN, Sun JL, Yang ZX, Guan QX, Wang R, Li XY, Li YJ, Feng YF, Wang YH (2020c) How to use macrophages to realise the treatment of tumour. J Drug Target. https://doi.org/10.1080/1061186x.2020.1775236

Zhi DF, Yang T, Yang J, Fu S, Zhang SB (2020) Targeting strategies for superparamagnetic iron oxide nanoparticles in cancer therapy. Acta Biomater 102:13–34. https://doi.org/10.1016/j.actbio.2019.11.027

Zhong SW, Jeong JH, Chen ZK, Chen ZH, Luo JL (2020) Targeting tumor microenvironment by small-molecule inhibitors. Transl Oncol 13(1):57–69. https://doi.org/10.1016/j.tranon.2019.10.001